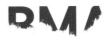

D1583621

A Companion to Specialist Surgical Practice

Series Editors
O. James Garden
Simon Paterson-Brown

CORE TOPICS IN GENERAL AND EMERGENCY SURGERY

SIXTH EDITION

Edited by

Simon Paterson-Brown

MBBS MPhil MS FRCS(Ed) FRCS(Engl) FCS(HK) FFST(RCSEd)

Honorary Clinical Senior Lecturer, Clinical Surgery,
The University of Edinburgh; Consultant General and
Upper Gastrointestinal Surgeon, Royal Infirmary of Edinburgh,
Edinburgh, UK

Hugh M. Paterson

BMedSci MBChB MD FRCS(Ed)

Clinical Senior Lecturer Coloproctology,
The University of Edinburgh; Honorary Consultant
Colorectal Surgeon, Western General Hospital, Edinburgh, UK

For additional online content visit ExpertConsult.com

ELSEVIER Edinburgh   London   New York   Oxford   Philadelphia   St Louis   Sydney   2019

ELSEVIER

First edition 1997
Second edition 2001
Third edition 2005
Fourth edition 2009
Fifth edition 2014
Sixth edition 2019

Notice

Practitioners and researchers must always rely on their own experience and knowledge in evaluating and using any information, methods, compounds or experiments described herein. Because of rapid advances in the medical sciences, in particular, independent verification of diagnoses and drug dosages should be made. To the fullest extent of the law, no responsibility is assumed by Elsevier, authors, editors or contributors for any injury and/or damage to persons or property as a matter of products liability, negligence or otherwise, or from any use or operation of any methods, products, instructions, or ideas contained in the material herein.

ISBN: 978-0-7020-7247-5

Printed in Great Britain
Last digit is the print number: 9 8 7 6 5 4 3 2

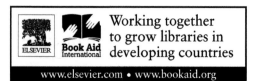

Working together
to grow libraries in
developing countries

www.elsevier.com • www.bookaid.org

Content Strategist: Laurence Hunter
Content Development Specialist: Lynn Watt
Project Manager: Umarani Natarajan
Design: Miles Hitchen
Illustration Manager: Nichole Beard
Illustrator: MPS North America LLC

Contents

Contents

Series Editors' preface

The *Companion to Specialist Surgical Practice* series has now come of age. This Sixth Edition takes the series to a different level since it was first published in 1997. The intention from the outset was to ensure that we could support the educational needs of those in the later years of specialist surgical training and of consultant surgeons in independent practice who wished for contemporary, evidence-based information on the subspecialist areas relevant to their general surgical practice. Although there still seems to be a role for larger reference surgical textbooks, and having contributed to many of these, we appreciate that it is difficult for them to keep pace with changing surgical practice.

This Sixth Edition continues to keep abreast of the increasing specialisation in general surgery. The rise of minimal access surgery and therapy, and the desire of some subspecialities, such as breast and vascular surgery, to separate away from 'general surgery' may have proved challenging in some countries. However, they also underline the importance for all surgeons of being aware of current developments in their surgical field. This series as a consequence continues to place emphasis on the need for surgeons to deliver a high-quality emergency surgical practice. The importance of evidence-based practice remains throughout, and authors have provided recommendations and highlighted key resources within each chapter. The ebook version of the textbook has also enabled improved access to the reference abstracts and links to video content relevant to many of the chapters.

We have recognised in this Sixth Edition that new blood is required to maintain the vitality of content. We are indebted to the volume editors, and contributors, who have stood down since the last edition and welcome the new leadership on several volumes. The contents have been comprehensively updated by our contributors and editorial team. We remain grateful for the support and encouragement of Laurence Hunter and Lynn Watt at Elsevier. We trust that our original vision of delivering an up-to-date affordable text has been met and that readers, whether in training or independent practice, will find this Sixth Edition an invaluable resource.

O. James Garden, CBE, BSc, MBChB, MD, FRCS (Glas), FRCS(Ed), FRCP(Ed), FRACS(Hon), FRCSC (Hon), FACS(Hon), FCSHK(Hon), FRCSI(Hon), FRCS(Engl)(Hon), FRSE
Regius Professor of Clinical Surgery, Clinical Surgery, The University of Edinburgh and Honorary Consultant Surgeon, Royal Infirmary of Edinburgh, Edinburgh, UK

Simon Paterson-Brown, MBBS, MPhil, MS, FRCS(Ed), FRCS(Engl), FCSHK, FFST(RCSEd)
Honorary Clinical Senior Lecturer, Clinical Surgery, The University of Edinburgh and Consultant General and Upper Gastrointestinal Surgeon, Royal Infirmary of Edinburgh, Edinburgh, UK

Editors' preface

While surgical subspecialisation within the speciality of 'General Surgery' remains central to the delivery of overall general surgical care, there is an increasing realisation that the core topics of general surgery, including emergency surgery, are a fundamental part of this practice. This requires the general surgeon to see and treat undifferentiated referrals and conditions outwith their normal everyday elective and emergency 'specialist' practice.

This volume of the Sixth Edition of the *Companion to Specialist Surgical Practice* series provides the background information on these key areas of general surgery for all practising general surgeons in both the elective and emergency situation. It has been divided into two main sections: the first includes the core topics relevant to all general surgeons and the second, those related to the care of emergency patients. As with previous editions of the Companion series, this volume should be considered as complementary to the other more specialist volumes, while still encompassing all those emergency areas that remain within the remit of the general surgeon.

In everyday practice there remains a group of emergency patients who, having been resuscitated and a diagnosis reached, might be better served by referral to a colleague or unit with the relevant subspecialist interest. This volume discusses those conditions that the general surgeon might be expected to deal with and, where appropriate, identifies those that might be better managed by a 'specialist'. In such cases the reader will be referred to the relevant specialist volume of this series.

Acknowledgements

We are both grateful to our long-suffering wives and families for their ongoing support and understanding in the time taken for us to complete the Sixth Edition of this volume of *Core Topics in General and Emergency Surgery* for the *Companion to Specialist Surgical Practice* series. The success of this volume, as for previous editions, very much lies in the quality of the chapters written by our co-authors and we are extremely grateful to all of them for the hard work that has gone into writing, or re-writing, each chapter. The additional workload required in the timely delivery of concise, well-referenced and up-to-date chapters for a book such as this, by busy practising surgeons, should never be underestimated. We would also like to recognise the help and support of Elsevier, and particularly Lynn Watt, in the production of this volume.

We would also would like to acknowledge and offer grateful thanks for the input of all previous editions' contributors, without whom this new edition would not have been possible.

Simon Paterson-Brown
Hugh M. Paterson
Edinburgh

Evidence-based practice in surgery

Critical appraisal for developing evidence-based practice can be obtained from a number of sources, the most reliable being randomised controlled clinical trials, systematic literature reviews, meta-analyses and observational studies. For practical purposes three grades of evidence can be used, analogous to the levels of 'proof' required in a court of law:

1. **Beyond all reasonable doubt.** Such evidence is likely to have arisen from high-quality randomised controlled trials, systematic reviews or high-quality synthesised evidence such as decision analysis, cost-effectiveness analysis or large observational datasets. The studies need to be directly applicable to the population of concern and have clear results. The grade is analogous to burden of proof within a criminal court and may be thought of as corresponding to the usual standard of 'proof' within the medical literature (i.e. $P < 0.05$).

2. **On the balance of probabilities.** In many cases a high-quality review of literature may fail to reach firm conclusions due to conflicting or inconclusive results, trials of poor methodological quality or the lack of evidence in the population to which the guidelines apply. In such cases it may still be possible to make a statement as to the best treatment on the 'balance of probabilities'. This is analogous to the decision in a civil court where all the available evidence will be weighed up and the verdict will depend upon the balance of probabilities.

3. **Not proven.** Insufficient evidence upon which to base a decision, or contradictory evidence.

Depending on the information available, three grades of recommendation can be used:

a. Strong recommendation, which should be followed unless there are compelling reasons to act otherwise.

b. A recommendation based on evidence of effectiveness, but where there may be other factors to take into account in decision-making, for example the user of the guidelines may be expected to take into account patient preferences, local facilities, local audit results or available resources.

c. A recommendation made where there is no adequate evidence as to the most effective practice, although there may be reasons for making a recommendation in order to minimise cost or reduce the chance of error through a locally agreed protocol.

✔✔ Evidence where a conclusion can be reached **'beyond all reasonable doubt'** and therefore where a **strong recommendation** can be given. This will normally be based on evidence levels:
- Ia. Meta-analysis of randomised controlled trials
- Ib. Evidence from at least one randomised controlled trial
- IIa. Evidence from at least one controlled study without randomisation
- IIb. Evidence from at least one other type of quasi-experimental study.

✔ Evidence where a conclusion might be reached **'on the balance of probabilities'** and where there may be other factors involved which influence the recommendation given. This will normally be based on less conclusive evidence than that represented by the double tick icons:
- III. Evidence from non-experimental descriptive studies, such as comparative studies and case–control studies
- IV. Evidence from expert committee reports or opinions or clinical experience of respected authorities, or both.

Evidence that is associated with either a **strong recommendation** or **expert opinion** is highlighted in the text in panels such as those shown above, and is distinguished by either a double or single tick icon, respectively. The references associated with double-tick evidence are listed as Key References at the end of each chapter, along with a short summary of the paper's conclusions where applicable. The full reference list for each chapter is available in the ebook.

The reader is referred to Chapter 1, 'Evaluation of surgical evidence' in the volume *Core Topics in General and Emergency Surgery* of this series, for a more detailed description of this topic.

Contributors

Iain D. Anderson, MBE, MD, FRCS(Eng, Edin, Glas), FRACS(Hon)
Consultant Surgeon, Intestinal Failure Unit, Salford Royal NHS Foundation Trust, Salford, UK

Robert Baigrie, BSc, MBChB, FRCS, MD
Adjunct Professor, Surgery, The University of Cape Town and Groote Schuur Hospital, Cape Town, Republic of South Africa

Ian Bailey, MBChB, MS, FRCS(GS)
Consultant Surgeon, Acute General Surgery, University Hospital Southampton, Southampton, UK

Andrew C. de Beaux, FRCSEd, MD, MBChB
Consultant General and Upper GI Surgeon, Department of General Surgery, Royal Infirmary of Edinburgh; Honorary Senior Lecturer, The University of Edinburgh, Edinburgh, UK

Maurizio Cecconi, MD, FRCA
Reader, Intensive Care Medicine, General Intensive Care Unit, St George's University Hopsitals NHS Foundation Trust, London, UK

Saxon Connor, MBChB, FRACS
Consultant HPB Surgeon, Department of Surgery, Christchurch Hospital, Christchurch, New Zealand

Dafydd A. Davies, MD, MPhil, FRCSC
Division Head, Division of Paediatric General and Thoracic Surgery, Trauma Program Medical Director, IWK Health Centre; Paediatric Trauma Director, Nova Scotia Trauma Program; Assistant Professor, Dalhousie University, Nova Scotia, Canada

Chris Deans, MBChB(Hons), FRCS, MD
Part-time Senior Lecturer, Clinical Surgery School of Clinical Sciences, The University of Edinburgh; Consultant General and Upper Gastrointestinal Surgeon, Royal Infirmary of Edinburgh, Edinburgh, UK

Thomas M. Drake, MBChB, BMedSci
Department of Clinical Surgery, The University of Edinburgh, Edinburgh, UK

Jonathan C. Epstein, MA, MD, FRCS
Consultant Surgeon, Intestinal Failure Unit, Salford Royal NHS Foundation Trust, Salford, UK

Timothy Forgan, BSc(Hons), MBBCh, MMed(Surg), FCS(SA), Cert Gastroenterology(SA)Surg
Consultant Colorectal Surgeon, Tygerberg Academic Hospital; Senior Lecturer, Surgery, Stellenbosch University, Cape Town, Republic of South Africa

Sarah A. Goodbrand, MBChB, BMSc, MD, FRCS
Colorectal Department, Western General Hospital, Edinburgh, UK

Ewen M. Harrison, MBChB, PhD, FRCS
Consultant HPB Surgeon, Clinical Surgery, Royal Infirmary of Edinburgh; Senior Lecturer, Clinical Surgery, The University of Edinburgh, Edinburgh, UK

Steven D. Heys, BMedBiol, MBChB, MD, PhD, FRCS(Eng), FRCS(Ed), FRCS(Glas), FHEA
Dean of the School of Medicine, Medical Sciences and Nutrition, University of Aberdeen; Honorary Consultant Surgeon, NHS Grampian, Aberdeen, UK

Scott R. Kelley, MD, FACS, FASCRS
Assistant Professor of Surgery, Colon and Rectal Surgery, Mayo Clinic, Rochester, MN, USA

Jacob C. Langer, MD
Professor of Surgery, University of Toronto, Attending Surgeon, Paediatric General and Thoracic Surgery, The Hospital for Sick Children, Toronto, Ontario, Canada

David W. Larson, MD, MBA
Chair, Colon and Rectal Surgery; Professor of Surgery; Mayo Clinic, Rochester, MN, USA

Kristoffer Lassen, MD, PhD
Consultant Surgeon/Professor, Department of Gastrointestinal Surgery/HPB-Section, Oslo University Hospital at Rikshospitalet, Oslo Faculty of Medicine, University of Tromsø, Norway

James Lau, MD
Professor of Surgery, The Chinese University of Hong Kong; Director, Endoscopy Centre, Prince of Wales Hospital, Hong Kong, PR China

Contributors

B. James Mander, MBBS, BSc, FRCS, MS, FRCS(Gen)
Consultant Colorectal Surgeon and Honorary Senior Lecturer, Colorectal Unit, Western General Hospital, Edinburgh, UK

Katherine McAndrew, MBChB
General Intensive Care Unit, St George's University Hospitals NHS Foundation Trust, London, UK

Craig McIlhenny, MBChB, FRCS(Urol), PGC, Med, FFST(Ed)
Consultant Urological Surgeon, NHS Forth Valley, Larbert, UK

Pradeep H. Navsaria, MBChB, MMed, FCS(SA), FACS, Trauma Surgery
General Trauma Surgeon, Groote Schuur Hospital; Professor, University of Cape Town, Cape Town, Republic of South Africa

Valentin Neuhaus, MD, PD
Trauma Centre, Groote Schuur Hospital, Cape Town, Republic of South Africa; Department of Trauma Surgery, University Hospital Zurich, Zurich, Switzerland

Andrew John Nicol, MBChB, FCS(SA), PhD
Director of the Trauma Centre, Surgery, Groote Schuur Hospital; Professor Surgery, University of Cape Town, Cape Town, Republic of South Africa

Iain J. Nixon, MBChB, FRCS(ORL-HNS), PhD
ENT Consultant Surgeon, NHS Lothian; Honorary Clinical Senior Lecturer, The University of Edinburgh, Edinburgh, UK

Gabriel C. Oniscu, MD, FRCS
Consultant Transplant Surgeon, Transplant Unit, Royal Infirmary of Edinburgh; Honorary Clinical Senior Lecturer, Clinical Surgery, The University of Edinburgh, Edinburgh, UK

Hugh M. Paterson, BMedSci, MBChB, MD, FRCS(Ed)
Clinical Senior Lecturer Coloproctology, The University of Edinburgh; Honorary Consultant Colorectal Surgeon, Western General Hospital, Edinburgh, UK

Simon Paterson-Brown, MBBS, MPhil, MS, FRCS(Ed), FRCS(Engl), FCS(HK), FFST(RCSEd)
Honorary Clinical Senior Lecturer, Clinical Surgery, The University of Edinburgh; Consultant General and Upper Gastrointestinal Surgeon, Royal Infirmary of Edinburgh, Edinburgh, UK

Andrew Rhodes, FCRP, FFICM, FRCA, MD(res)
Medical Director, Consultant in Anaesthesia and Intensive Care Medicine, St George's University Hospitals NHS Foundation Trust, London, UK

William G. Simpson, MBChB, FRCS
Consultant Chemical Pathologist, Clinical Biochemistry, Aberdeen Royal Infirmary; Honorary Senior Lecturer, School of Medicine, Aberdeen University, Aberdeen, UK

Bruce R. Tulloh, MB, MS, FRACS, FRCS
Consultant General and Upper Gastrointestinal Surgeon, Royal Infirmary of Edinburgh and Honorary Clinical Senior Lecturer, University of Edinburgh, UK

Diana A. Wu, MBChB
Clinical Research Fellow, Transplant Unit, Royal Infirmary of Edinburgh, Clinical Surgery, The University of Edinburgh, Edinburgh, UK

Hon Chi Yip, MBChB
Resident Specialist, Department of Surgery, The Chinese University of Hong Kong, Hong Kong, PR China

1

Evaluation of surgical evidence

Thomas M. Drake
Ewen M. Harrison

Introduction to surgical evidence

Evidence-based medicine is a recent innovation. It has only been over the past two centuries that scientific methods have become the accepted means of establishing the most effective treatments and tests. Nowhere in medicine has this transformation been more vibrant than in surgical disciplines, where numerous innovations have paved the way for the treatments of today. This transformation, however, has not been plain sailing.

The first person to coin the phrase 'evidence-based medicine' was Dr David Eddy, who argued that medical decision-making and policy should be supported by quantitative data.[1] One of the forefathers of evidence-based medicine in the UK, Archie Cochrane, strongly advocated the use of controlled experiments and randomisation methods to reduce bias in research in order to arrive at the most reliable answer. The eponymous Cochrane Collaboration began in 1993, in response to Cochrane's call for better evidence to underpin medical decision-making.

The generation of high-quality evidence in surgery can be particularly difficult. The reasons underpinning this are fourfold. Firstly, performing surgery is a complex intervention. There are many variables to consider when designing research studies, including postoperative care, variation in surgical techniques and factoring in the natural learning curves required for surgeons to learn new approaches or operative procedures.

Secondly, there is evidence that surgeons themselves are divided in their attitudes to research. A survey of

Australian surgeons found many believed their own clinical practice was superior to clinical guidelines; that evidence-based surgery had an adverse effect on clinical decision-making; and that not using evidence did not adversely affect patient care. Such attitudes present a major barrier to the uptake of evidence in surgery and require addressing if outcomes and patient care are to be the best they can be.[2]

Thirdly, many operations have ancient origins, are performed for a given indication and lead to a resolution of the disease process, i.e. they are held to be effective. As such, there may be limited scientific evidence for these procedures as it would be seen as unethical to deny patients an effective and established treatment in the context of a research study.

Finally, a lack of funding and interest in surgical research has led to research studies becoming the exception rather than the norm. Currently it is unusual for a patient undergoing surgery to be enrolled in a research study. When these different factors are considered in context, it is unsurprising that in 1998 surgical research was compared to a 'comic opera' by the editor of *The Lancet*.[3]

Over the past decade, considerable improvements have been made. In a short space of time, several large initiatives have been launched by Royal Colleges and collaborations have led to new surgery-specific research frameworks (e.g. the IDEAL framework, see below) being introduced. This is proving to be successful, with surgical research increasingly being published in the world's largest medical journals.

Changing the world with evidence

In order for surgical research to change practice and influence patient care, it must address a new question or an area of genuine clinical uncertainty. The uncertainty as to which treatment is best is described as 'clinical equipoise'. One of the key assumptions for the ethical conduct of any interventional research is that equipoise exists, that is, there must be genuine uncertainty as to which treatment is best for a given patient group. If clinical equipoise does not exist and it is definitively known that one treatment is better, it is unethical to knowingly expose patients to the inferior treatment.

Any research study being evaluated should be read in full, considering the following:

- Who is the patient population or target condition?
- What was the intervention (for interventional research, i.e. clinical trials) or exposure (for observational research)?
- What was the comparison (or control group)?
- How was the effect of the intervention measured, and was it measured accurately?
- Are there any sources of bias or confounding present?
- What was the result?
- Is this study relevant to my clinical practice?

In this chapter we will discuss each point in further detail.

Formulating a clinical question

The first step in the design of a clinical research study is to formulate a study hypothesis or question. Understanding the constituent parts of a clinical hypothesis is key to evaluating the relevance and quality of surgical research studies.

A simple, structured approach can be used to formulate clinical questions. This approach takes into account several important aspects of a clinical research study:

- 'P' – Population (those patients with the target condition)
- 'I' – Intervention or exposure (the intervention or exposure being studied)
- 'C' – Comparison (the control group that the intervention is being compared to)
- 'O'– Outcomes (what was the outcome of interest and how was it measured)
- 'S' – Study design (how the study was conducted).

For example, we may study antibiotics in the treatment of adults with acute appendicitis. In this situation, antibiotics are used to reduce complications of appendicitis and reduce the necessity for surgical intervention. Using the PICOS approach:

- P – The population is adults with non-perforated acute appendicitis
- I – The intervention is antibiotics
- C – The comparison group is that of usual clinical care (appendicectomy)
- O – The primary outcome is complication rate, defined using a validated grading system
- S – The study design is a randomised controlled trial.

Study population or target condition

A study population is a group of participants selected from a general population on the basis of specific characteristics. Having a clearly defined study population is key to ensuring research is clinically relevant and can answer a specific question. If a target condition is used as the basis for selecting a study population, validated diagnostic criteria should be applied.

The basis for the inclusion of particular patients in a study should be systematic, to avoid bias. The best way of ensuring a sample is both representative and free from selection bias is to approach every eligible patient in a consecutive manner. This is often referred to as a consecutive sample.

Specific study populations may have special considerations that must be taken into account in the study design. An example of this may be an older age group, where visual or hearing impairment may present difficulties with particular data collection methods, e.g. telephone interviews.

Intervention or exposure

The intervention is the main variable changed in the treatment group. In observational research, patients and clinicians decide which treatment will be received. As no direct experimental intervention occurs, the variable is termed the 'exposure'.

When considering an intervention for surgical research, particular care must be given to delivering interventions in a standardised manner. Variation in how a treatment may be delivered should be considered during the design process. For example, in a study of a new surgical technique or approach, ensuring all patients receive a similar treatment usually requires training in the delivery of the new intervention. Standardising the surgical intervention may include an assessment within the research study to determine whether an acceptable level of competence has been achieved. A good study protocol will help to address this (more about study protocols can be found in the Bias section below).

The acceptability of the intervention must also be given due thought. If an intervention is not acceptable to patients, it will be very difficult to convince patients (and research ethics committees) to participate. One means of ensuring interventions are acceptable is to involve patient representatives when designing research studies. These patient representatives are part of the study design team and provide feedback to investigators on the best means of ensuring studies are conducted in a feasible and acceptable manner.

Comparison

The comparison describes the control group the intervention or exposure of interest is being evaluated against. This group should be sufficiently similar to the intervention group to ensure valid conclusions may be drawn as to the true effects of the intervention.

In controlled trials, the comparison group may receive a *placebo* in order to reduce bias and maintain blinding. However, a study is usually more meaningful clinically if the comparison group receives the current gold standard of clinical care, so as to create a group where the new treatment can be compared directly with the current best therapy.

If the control group differs from the intervention group, bias may be introduced leading to invalid conclusions. This is of particular concern in observational research, such as case-control studies, where the comparison group is selected directly by investigators.

Outcome

A study outcome is the variable by which the effect of the intervention or exposure of interest is measured. In order for an outcome to be useful, several properties of the chosen measure should be considered:

- Incidence – the outcome of interest should be sufficiently common. The more common the outcome of interest, the smaller the sample size required to demonstrate a difference between treatment groups.

- Directness – the outcome of interest should directly measure what the intervention is ultimately intended to achieve. For example, intraoperative warming devices are designed to keep the patient warm, thereby reducing postoperative complications. Therefore, any study investigating the efficacy of intraoperative warming devices should use postoperative complications as a primary outcome, rather than looking at differences in temperature (a *surrogate* outcome in this example).

- Definition – outcomes should be measured using clearly defined criteria. Preferably these criteria should be used widely across the field so all studies are measuring the same outcome in the same way, for example the Response Evaluation Criteria In Solid Tumours (RECIST) for the assessment of tumour progression.[4]

- Relevance – outcomes should be relevant to the research question and to patient care. What may be relevant to clinicians may not be equally relevant to patients. To this end, patient representatives should be consulted when selecting study outcomes. Often quality of life and functional outcomes are of primary concern to patients.

- Timing – outcomes must be measured at appropriate time intervals, which are relevant to the timeframe where the outcome of interest would be expected to occur. For example, measuring an outcome at 48 hours following a procedure may be relevant for postoperative bleeding, but not for surgical site infection.

- Reliability – the chosen outcome measure should reliably detect an event and should be standardised for all patients. This is particularly important for multicentre research, or large-scale trials where multiple observers are judging outcomes. Here, having a standardised means of assessing an outcome is essential to ensure that all patients are being assessed in the same way, otherwise the results of the study may be inaccurate.

Patient reported outcome measures (PROMS) are outcomes reported by patients themselves. Examples of PROMS include validated generic quality of life questionnaires (e.g. EQ-5D, HR-QoL). Alternatively, PROMS may focus on specific areas of interest, such as sexual function or continence, which are of particular importance in pelvic surgery.[5,6]

Cost-effectiveness is sometimes used as an outcome measure. This is often used by clinical governance bodies to decide whether a treatment represents value for money and should be recommended for use.[7]

Occasionally, different outcomes may be combined to form a single measure. This is known as a composite measure. The use of composite outcome measures can enable researchers to measure two or more outcomes simultaneously, or can allow for better statistical efficiency for the number of patients in a study. An example may be unplanned critical care admission or death, where both represent a major complication, but are pooled to generate a greater number of events in order to reduce the sample size required for demonstrating the effectiveness of a treatment.

Study designs

There are many study designs available to answer clinical questions. Study design methodology is constantly evolving; however, all types of study can be broadly divided and subdivided into the following categories:

- **Primary research** (research at the individual patient level)
  - Randomised trial
  - Prospective cohort study
  - Retrospective cohort study
  - Cross-sectional study
  - Case-control study
  - Case series
  - Case report
- **Secondary research** (research that considers multiple sources of primary research)
  - Systematic review
  - Systematic review with meta-analysis.

Figure 1.1 provides a useful means of identifying the type of study where the article may not be explicit as to its design.[8]

Evidence may be classified according to the Oxford Centre of Evidence-based Medicine (CEBM), which divides evidence according to the risk of bias. These classifications are commonly referred to as the 'level of evidence' (Table 1.1).[9]

Another way of classifying studies is using the 'pyramid of evidence' (**Fig. 1.2**). The pyramid provides a simplified means to consider the advantages of one study design over another, taking into account the inherent properties of each and classifying them according to the likelihood of giving a reliable answer as close to the 'true value' as possible.

This pyramid of evidence is accompanied by several caveats. First of all, not all questions can be answered by a randomised controlled trial,

either due to lack of equipoise (where it would be unethical to conduct a trial) or for logistical reasons (where a trial would be too expensive or simply unfeasible). Secondly, a poorly conducted study may give an inaccurate, or unreliable answer compared to a well-conducted study of a different design. For example, a small poorly conducted randomised trial may not provide a better answer to a question than a large, well-conducted prospective cohort study. Here is where the Oxford CEBM classification and GRADE assessments (Grading of Recommendations Assessment, Development and Evaluation, discussed below) are useful to help determine whether there can be certainty in the body of evidence for a given research question.[9,10]

Systematic reviews and meta-analyses

At the top of the pyramid are systematic reviews and meta-analyses, which evaluate multiple sources of evidence for a given clinical question. These sources may take the form of randomised trials, cohort studies or even case-control studies. Systematic searching methods are used to attempt to find every possible study relevant to the clinical question of interest. These methods often include searching multiple databases, searching the references of key articles in the field and contacting experts to ask if they have suggestions for potential studies to include.[11] Once all studies that may be eligible are screened, each study is critically appraised (see Critical appraisal section). This approach of systematically identifying each and every possible study, followed by close scrutiny of the study methods, is then synthesised into the final review. The arising systematic review then should present an overarching and balanced view of the evidence for a given clinical question.

Meta-analysis describes the use of statistical methods to combine the numeric results of similar studies in order to derive a more precise point estimate of the true treatment effect than is possible from any individual study. This is often combined with a systematic review, where the results of studies are combined after being screened for inclusion. Combining studies in this manner is referred to as 'pooling'.

An important part of meta-analysis is an assessment of the similarity between different studies of the same clinical question. Variation between studies is termed heterogeneity and takes two forms, clinical and statistical. Clinical heterogeneity concerns how clinically similar a population in one study is to another. It is unlikely to make sense to combine the results of two trials examining the same treatment in two distinct populations, for instance, adults and children.

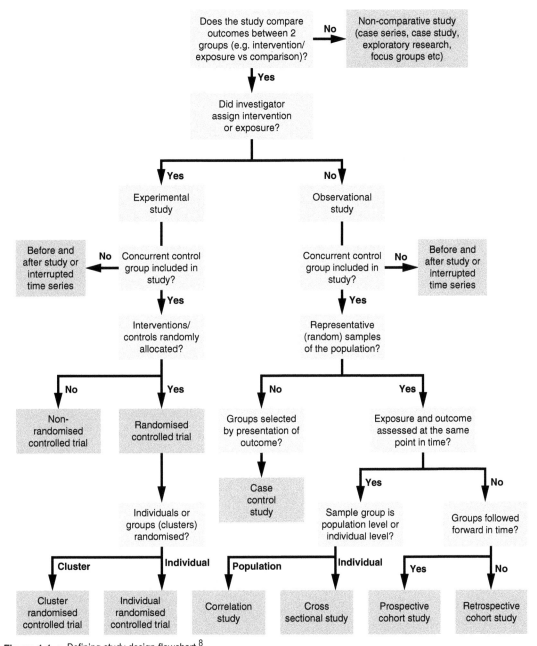

Figure 1.1 • Defining study design flowchart.[8]
Reproduced with permission from National Institute for Health and Care Excellence. https://www.nice.org.uk/process/pmg4/chapter/introduction.

Statistical heterogeneity refers to the differences in the actual results of included studies and whether these are likely to be due to chance (sampling error) or true differences in outcome. The I-squared statistic is useful here and is 0% when all included trials provide a similar result. If studies show completely contradicting results, the I-squared statistic is 100%, meaning the combined result likely lacks any real meaning.[11] A rule-of-thumb for the interpretation of the I-squared statistic is as follows:

- 0% to 30% – Low level of statistical heterogeneity
- 30% to 50% – Moderate level of statistical heterogeneity
- 50% to 100% – Substantial level of statistical heterogeneity.

Table 1.1 • Oxford CEBM levels of evidence

Level of evidence	Interventional study	Diagnostic accuracy
1a	Systematic review of randomised controlled trials (RCT)	Systematic review of level 1 diagnostic studies
1b	Individual RCT with narrow confidence interval	Validated cohort study with good reference standards
1c	Where all patients with condition have previously died without fail, but with the intervention tested some survive	Studies with a diagnostic sensitivity or specificity so high the result can rule in or out a diagnosis with very high accuracy
2a	Systematic review of cohort studies	Systematic review of level 2 or higher diagnostic studies
2b	Individual cohort study or low-quality RCT	Exploratory cohort study with good reference standards, or only validated on split-sample databases
2c	Ecological studies	
3a	Systematic review of case-control studies	Systematic review of level 3b or higher studies
3b	Individual case-control study	Non-consecutive study, or study without consistently applied reference standard
4	Case series and poor quality cohort and case-control studies	Case series and poor quality cohort and case-control studies
5	Expert opinion without explicit critical appraisal	Expert opinion without explicit critical appraisal

Source: Oxford Centre for Evidence-based Medicine – Levels of Evidence (March 2009) – CEBM. http://www.cebm.net/oxford-centre-evidence-based-medicine-levels-evidence-march-2009/.

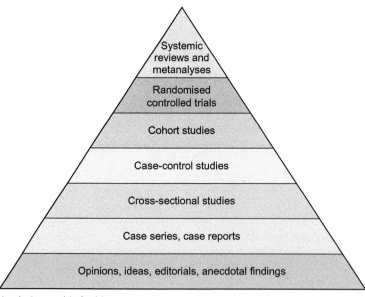

Figure 1.2 • The classical pyramid of evidence.

Randomised controlled trials

Randomised controlled trials are primary research studies that test the effect of an intervention using experimental methods. After participants are recruited they are allocated to treatment groups at random, where the choice of treatment is determined by neither the patient, clinician nor any other person. Removing this choice of treatment reduces the risk of selection bias, which is often the largest source of bias in medical research. Selection bias simply refers to how doctors and patients select treatments based upon certain patient characteristics.

The *controlled* part of the name refers to two integral components of high-quality trials. The first is that there is a comparable control group with which to compare the intervention of interest. The second is that the trial is conducted in strict accordance with a pre-defined study protocol.

Study protocols are important and are essentially a detailed instruction manual outlining how a piece of research will be conducted. The main advantages of a study protocol are that it ensures investigators stick to a pre-planned analysis of their data and in the case of multicentre research, promotes standardisation across centres. Study protocols are not unique to RCTs. It is highly recommended that all clinical research (including systematic reviews and cohort studies) should be conducted according to a pre-defined protocol. Many journals now stipulate this as a requirement for even considering a study for publication. Increasingly, study protocols are published for peer review before the study starts.

Randomised controlled trials can be grouped into two categories:

- **Explanatory trials** – An explanatory trial is designed to explain precisely how an intervention may work; in other words, it is designed to elicit mechanisms. In order to minimise variation in the experimental 'model', an explanatory trial is usually conducted using a highly homogenous group of patients with the study drug/intervention compared to a placebo.
- **Pragmatic trials** – A pragmatic trial is designed to encompass as much variation in clinical practice as possible. The study population is often highly heterogeneous in order to make the trial generalisable to the true population the intervention will be used upon in clinical practice. Often, instead of placebos, pragmatic trials compare interventions to the current standard of care. Pragmatic trials are usually large in size and conducted across multiple centres. These trials are intended to give an idea as to whether an intervention works in 'real-life', rather than a highly controlled environment.

In surgical trials, patients are typically allocated to a single treatment that does not change. This type of study is called a parallel group study (**Fig. 1.3a**). The treatment group (or groups) are compared with a control group in order to calculate an effect size for the given treatment.

A second type of allocation method involves patients receiving one treatment and then changing to a different treatment or a control treatment.

This is called a crossover design. The idea of this type of study is that each patient acts as his/her own control (**Fig. 1.3b**). When the patient crosses over to the different treatment, any alterations in the clinical outcome can then be put down to the effects of giving the new treatment or halting the old one. In surgery, this type of design is rare, as surgical intervention is typically a one-time treatment. This crossover process can be repeated several times, until the investigators are certain as to the effects of the new treatment. Crossover designs can only be used to measure particular outcomes, usually scaled measures which can occur multiple times, rather than finite categorical outcomes (e.g. mortality).

Randomisation

Randomisation allocates patients to treatment groups, without the clinician or patient choosing the treatment. Randomisation ensures treatment groups are balanced for characteristics and confounding factors, either of which may be observed (data collected upon them) or unobserved (no data collected on or not yet discovered).[12] A good example of where selection bias may arise would be studying the use of non-steroidal anti-inflammatory drugs (NSAIDs) after surgery. In observational research, it has been found the use of NSAIDs is associated with fewer surgical complications. However, in these studies, where clinicians or patients choose to take NSAIDs, the group of patients who are given NSAIDs are fitter and healthier. Therefore, the observation that patients who take NSAIDs are less likely to suffer complications is confounded. If this was a randomised trial, both treatment groups would have similar baseline characteristics due to the randomisation process, which would reduce or eliminate this confounding.

Randomisation may be performed in two different ways:

Simple randomisation

Simple randomisation methods involve allocating participants to treatment groups using techniques such as coin flipping or rolling a die. These methods do not use any pre-planned methods of allocation. The advantages of these techniques are that they are easy to use and do not require any specialist equipment or planning. The disadvantage is that these methods cannot account for more complex allocation requirements, such as multiple groups or ensuring other factors are accounted for (see 'Minimisation' below). With a large enough sample size, simple randomisation methods should result in approximately equally sized groups. However, for small trials, simple randomisation methods can lead to unequally sized treatment groups.

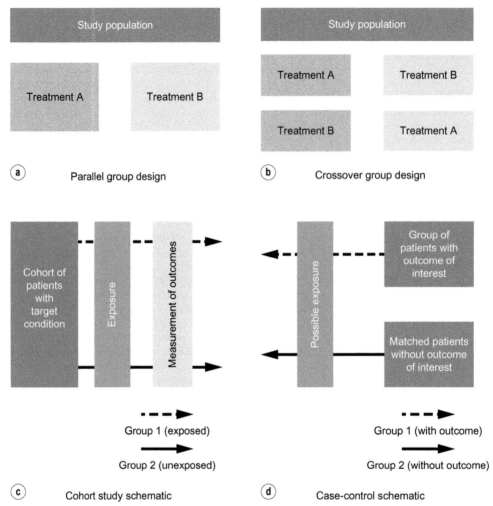

Figure 1.3 • (a) Parallel group study design; **(b)** crossover group study design; **(c)** schematic of cohort studies; **(d)** schematic of case-control studies.

Block randomisation

Block randomisation describes the process of randomising 'blocks' of patients to treatment groups, which may be based upon a specific characteristic (i.e. sex or age). Using blocks is thought to be beneficial, as it theoretically reduces differences across the treatment groups being compared. This is of particular advantage in smaller trials, where unbalanced or unequal groups cause greater problems than in trials with large sample sizes.

Randomisation can be stratified, which is a technique that first divides patients into discrete risk groups, or strata, and then randomises a patient within the given stratum to a treatment. This is a straightforward means of ensuring treatment groups are balanced for factors that may result in an increased likelihood of a given outcome occurring. For example, patients with diabetes are more likely to suffer wound infections following surgery. A trial looking at methods to prevent wound infections could use stratified randomisation to first divide patients into 'diabetic' and 'non-diabetic' strata then randomise these patients to the different treatment arms. This would therefore result in both treatment groups containing a similar number of diabetic patients, thus enabling a fairer comparison.

An extension of stratified randomisation is minimisation. Using sophisticated computer programes, randomisation procedures can be designed that take into consideration a number of different patient characteristics, a method known as 'minimisation'. This ensures treatment groups are optimally balanced for predictable potential confounders.

Blinding

Blinding is the act of disguising which treatment a participant in a research study has received. Blinding in surgical studies often proves to be difficult- or requires some flair or creativity to identify a suitable strategy for implementing blinding successfully.

Four main groups may be blinded to an intervention or an outcome:

- Patients
- Those administering the treatment, i.e. the clinical team
- Those who are measuring the effect of the treatment, i.e. observers
- Those performing the data analysis, i.e. the statistician.

In the past, where one of these groups was blinded it was classed as 'single-blind', where two groups were blinded, 'double-blind' etc. Nowadays it is best practice to specify explicitly who was blinded and what exactly was done, rather than use terminology that may be unclear without qualification.

In studies where drug administration is involved, participants and clinicians can be blinded by using placebos (i.e. 'dummy pills'). Where intravenous drugs are used, normal saline could be used as comparator for the study drug. Where intravenous fluids are coloured, black tubing could be used to mask this. If patients are receiving a different surgical procedure altogether, it can be difficult or impossible to blind patients and it is impossible to blind the surgeon to the procedure. There are, however, means to address this. Observers are often used in surgical studies because blinding patients or clinical teams is often impossible. These observers are independent from the clinical team and are employed to measure outcomes and are blinded to which intervention the patient received. One trial that used innovative methods to address difficulties in blinding was that conducted by Sihvonen et al. in Finland.[13] This trial compared arthroscopic surgery versus no surgery for degenerative meniscal tear. The intervention group received arthroscopic surgery and the control group received sham surgery. In sham surgery the patient is exposed to an environment where they believe they are undergoing surgery, however, in reality they do not receive any intervention at all. In the trial by Sihvonen et al., participants were taken into the operating theatre, draped and shown a video of arthroscopic surgery. Dressings were then placed to make it difficult to identify whether they underwent operation or not.

Sham surgery is ethically contentious, particularly with regards to procedures that must be conducted under general anaesthesia due to the associated risks of harm.

In all these cases, blinding enables the person who is assessing the outcome to judge it fairly. If the person assessing the study outcome did know which treatment the patient received, they may have preconceptions and judge the outcome in a biased way to favour one treatment over the other.

Finally, it is important to ask patients at the end of the study which treatment group they believe they were allocated to. By asking every patient this question, it enables the adequacy of the blinding to be tested.

Open-label studies

An open-label study is one where both the researchers and the patients are aware of which treatment they are receiving. They can be randomised, non-randomised and do not always require a control group.

Cluster randomisation

Some studies may randomise at the level of the hospital, rather than the patient. This can be useful when investigating healthcare processes, public health interventions or complex treatments. Cluster randomised trials (**Fig. 1.4**) have specific considerations that must be accounted for in designing the study and they are often more complex to conduct.

Some studies use methods which rely upon factors that appear to be random in order to allocate patients to treatment groups. These factors may include birthday, day of the week or even whether the patient's hospital number is odd or even. Although these may be thought to be random numbers, they are not. This is called 'pseudo-randomisation' or 'quasi-randomisation' and studies utilising this approach should not be classed as randomised trials.

Allocation concealment

Allocation concealment is often confused with blinding. It describes the principle that those determining which treatment a patient receives should not influence the selection process, either consciously or subconsciously. The classical way of addressing this is to use opaque envelopes to disguise which treatment allocation is contained in the envelope.

Phases of trials

Interventional clinical trials can be divided into four phases based on the purpose of the study.

Phase 0 trials

These trials are 'first in man' studies. Here, very small quantities of promising new compounds are given to healthy humans in a highly controlled environment. These studies aim to approximate the pharmacokinetic and pharmacodynamic properties of a drug (e.g. half-life, distribution, excretion, absorption, metabolism and potential toxicities).

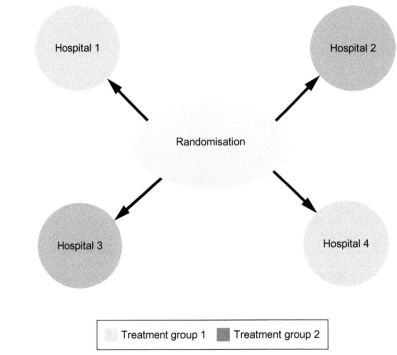

Figure 1.4 • Cluster randomisation.

Phase I trials

Phase I trials aim to assess the safety of a treatment more formally. Here a range of doses within the postulated therapeutic range are tested (this is called 'dose ranging') in a larger patient sample and the side-effects of these varying doses assessed. Usually, this sample is of healthy volunteers, but can be of those with the target condition. From these studies, the dose with the most acceptable side-effect profile is selected.

Phase II trials

In phase II trials a new treatment is administered to patients with the target condition to determine safety (i.e. side-effects) and efficacy. As these trials are designed to elucidate whether a new treatment works or not, they are usually tightly controlled and may compare the new treatment to a placebo.

Phase III trials

This is the final stage of testing prior to a new treatment being released on the open market. Phase III trials are the largest trials, where a new treatment is given to patients with the target condition. Large sample sizes are used in order to further identify rare side-effects and to accurately estimate the treatment effect of the new intervention. Often phase III trials are pragmatic, rather than mechanistic in nature to confirm the new treatment will work in the real world, rather than in more highly controlled experiments alone.

Post-marketing studies

Once the new treatment has passed national regulatory approvals, it can be sold to healthcare providers. After approval all drugs undergo monitoring for rarer side-effects and other harms that may have been missed in the initial studies. This process is called post-marketing surveillance. One well-known approach to post-marketing surveillance in the UK is the 'Yellow Card Scheme', where clinicians can report adverse events that are suspected to have been due to a specific drug.

IDEAL framework

In surgery, the IDEAL framework (Innovation, Development, Exploration, Assessment, Long-term monitoring) describes how innovations in surgery should be approached to enable direct translation to surgical care (Table 1.2).[14] It describes five stages of development which should be used to guide a new idea from conception to widespread clinical practice.

Cohort studies

In a cohort study, a population with a specific condition or a population undergoing a specific type of surgery is identified and followed over a defined period. Cohort studies are typically observational research, which means instead of

Table 1.2 • The stages of the IDEAL framework

Stage	Innovation	Development	Exploration	Assessment	Long-term monitoring
Description of stage	Proof of principle, typically done in an animal or select patient.	Refinement of idea, through practice or laboratory development	Beginning to compare refined idea to current practice to establish feasibility in clinical practice	Compares idea to current practice through well-powered study aimed to show clinical efficacy and safety	Monitors the idea in practice for long-term outcomes, safety and rare events
Type of study	Case report	Case series	Randomised clinical trial/Prospective study	Randomised clinical trial	Database

Source: McCulloch P, Altman DG, Campbell WB, et al. No surgical innovation without evaluation: the IDEAL recommendations. Lancet 2009;374(9695):1105–12.

patients being allocated randomly to treatment groups, patients and doctors are free to choose. Instead of an 'intervention', which implies patients are allocated to treatment groups, the intervention is often referred to as an 'exposure' (**Fig. 1.3c**).

As cohort studies are simply observing what happens in clinical practice they may be conducted looking forwards in time (prospective) or backwards in time (retrospective). The advantages and disadvantages of each approach are listed in Box 1.1.

Case-control studies

In a case-control study, patients are identified who have already experienced a given outcome (cases). They are compared with patients of similar characteristics who have not experienced the outcome in order to identify factors associated with the given outcome (**Fig. 1.3d**). Case-control studies are always conducted retrospectively and are common in the fields of public health and genetics. They are also useful for the study of rare diseases. The key advantages of case-control studies are that they are relatively fast to perform and inexpensive when compared with other study types. Furthermore, they do not require lengthy follow-up as the outcome of interest has already occurred.

There are several drawbacks to case-control studies. Given that they require a group of participants without the given outcome of interest as a control group, there is a high risk that selection bias could influence the results of the study. Furthermore, the design of case-control studies means that rare exposures can be missed as they lack any kind of consecutive or systematic sampling methods. Furthermore, as the study design starts with a group who already have the outcome of interest, the case-control design makes it impossible to calculate the incidence of that outcome.

Box 1.1 • Comparison of prospective and retrospective studies

Advantages of prospective	Advantages of retrospective
Real-time data collection Enables investigators to seek missing data as the patient is present during data collection Allows interventions and changes to the patient pathway to be made (in non-observational studies)	Faster, with less time required to conduct Less expensive

Disadvantages of prospective	Disadvantages of retrospective
Longer time frame More expensive Requires more staff time	Difficult to find missing data Cases may be missed more frequently May require case notes to be found Investigators assessing independent/explanatory variables may already be aware of outcome

Cross-sectional studies

Cross-sectional studies take a 'snapshot' at any one given moment in time. These studies aim to describe the entire population of interest, rather than just those who have had an outcome of interest as in a case-control study. Unlike cohort studies, all the information is gathered at once and does not necessarily take time into account, with observations being limited to one snapshot. As they sample the entire population, cross-sectional studies can be useful to estimate the point prevalence (existence) or incidence (first occurrence) of a disease. However, as cross-sectional studies collect data at one given time only, they can be susceptible to missing data or data that are unreliable.

Case series and case reports

A case report is an individual case that may be notable due to a rare condition, or a novel approach to performing a procedure. A case series refers to a collection of individual case reports. In both scenarios cases are selected by investigators. Case series and reports are considered low-quality evidence and should not be used to draw firm scientific conclusions. They can be used to present key learning points, allowing clinicians to improve their own clinical practice based upon the experience of others. As case series and reports do not contain consecutive patients nor are conducted in a scientific manner, they should not be included in systematic reviews or meta-analyses.

Single-centre or multicentre research

A further consideration in study design is whether the study was conducted at a single centre or across many centres. In surgery and other complex interventions, delivery of a surgical intervention and subsequent postoperative care can vary greatly. Conducting a study across multiple centres makes the results more generalisable as variations in practice are accounted for. Conversely, if a study is performed at a single centre there is less variation and hence the results may be less generalisable to patients elsewhere.

Finding the evidence

Identifying useful studies to answer a clinical query can be difficult. As of 2016, more than 26 million scientific papers were contained within the PubMed database alone. Knowing where to start and how evidence is organised can make the process of finding relevant literature more straightforward.

Journals

Journals are the main source of scientific research in medicine. Studies are conducted, reported and submitted to journals for peer review. Journals are commonly ranked according to their 'impact factor', calculated by how many times an article published in the journal is cited. Impact factors have received a lot of attention; however, more recently this ranking system has become discredited. Other measures have been developed, including the Eigenfactor metric, which take into account the field of science, longer-term impact and fundamental differences in how disciplines cite previous work.[15]

Books

Books are another source of scientific information. They are often useful as instructional guides or for educational purposes and enable the authors to spend time developing explanations for complex topics, unlike journal articles which often carry a word limit. Often it takes years to put a book together and by the time it is published, the information contained is immediately out of date.

Conferences

Scientific conferences are where recent work is presented to an audience consisting of members of the scientific community who specialise in that given field. Conferences are where the latest research is discussed, often before the studies are published as papers in journals. This gives investigators the opportunity to obtain peer review prior to submitting for publication. Often conferences are excellent places to network and build collaborative links with other people who share similar interests in the field.

Social media

Although not strictly a source of scientific information, social media and blogging has come to the fore in recent years. Informative opinion and debate has increasingly moved to social media platforms such as Facebook and Twitter with the result that debate surrounding treatments or medical technologies is becoming increasingly accessible, particularly to patients and the public. This shift is largely positive, helping engage members of the public with healthcare decisions and innovation. However, social media and blogging is something of a double-edged sword, as articles are unmoderated and can convey unbalanced opinion, which may be misinterpreted as fact.

Medical literature databases

At present there are two main databases containing published medical literature. These databases largely contain journal articles but also hold some content published in books.

MEDLINE

MEDLINE is a medical literature database curated by the National Library of Medicine in the United States. It covers literature published from 1945 through to the present day and at present contains over 20 million citations. It uses a system called Medical Subject Headings (MeSH) to organise literature in a systematic way that can be easily queried using specific search terms (see 'MeSH Terms' below).

EMBASE

EMBASE is the larger of the two databases and as of 2016, is run by the commercial publisher Elsevier. It contains literature from 1947 to the present day, but also information from as early as 1902. At present, EMBASE contains all of MEDLINE and supplements this with additional literature from across the world. It is the largest medical database in the world, with over 29 million citations. EMBASE specialises in detailed literature on pharmacy and drug compounds which may not be contained in MEDLINE. MeSH terms can also be used when searching EMBASE, giving it compatibility with searches designed for use in MEDLINE.

Clinical trials databases

According to legislation governing clinical trials, the declaration of Helsinki and the policies of many journals, all clinical trials must be registered prior to commencement. The main purpose is to promote the publication of research trials and reduce wastage, as many trials go unpublished, particularly those with 'negative' results. It also enables researchers and patients to view ongoing studies that may be of interest and avoid duplication of the same study idea. For patients, it provides information on the latest trials for their condition. ClinicalTrials.gov is run by the National Library of Medicine in the United States.[16] This was the first and now the largest clinical trials registry. Trials conducted in any country can be registered on ClinicalTrials.gov and may include observational research.

Search clients

Search clients are tools that enable researchers to identify evidence contained within medical literature databases. There are many search clients available and the choice of client often comes down to personal preference.

PubMed

PubMed is operated by the National Center for Biotechnology Information (NCBI) and allows searching of the MEDLINE database with additional literature from the NCBI's and National Library of Medicine's own repository of articles. PubMed is a free search client and database service. The NCBI site where PubMed is located also contains a vast collection of other electronic services for conducting research, all of which are free of charge.[17]

OvidSP

OvidSP is a commercial service operated by the publisher Wolters Kluwer and allows the searching of several different medical literature databases at once, including MEDLINE and EMBASE.

Google Scholar

Google Scholar is a free-to-use search engine accessing Google's proprietary database, which includes some of MEDLINE as well as other databases. Google does not say how large the scholar database is, but it is estimated to contain over 160 million citations across multiple disciplines. Due to the way the Google search algorithm operates, it can give different results when searched in the same way as other clients.[18]

Evidence-based medicine organisations

The Cochrane Library

The Cochrane Library is where systematic reviews and review protocols are published by the Cochrane Collaboration.[19] Cochrane reviews are conducted according to strict standards and have arguably one of the toughest peer-review processes in the world. Protocols and reviews must adhere to strictly specified standards. All reviews undergo at least two rounds of peer review by clinical experts in the field and systematic review methodologists. Hence Cochrane reviews are of consistently high quality and are often the best source of information when it comes to finding evidence for a given intervention. As well as providing information on the clinical utility of a treatment, suggestions are made for future research.

Specialist registers

Other specialist registers exist, which may encompass literature that cannot be found elsewhere. Grey literature, or literature that has not been published as a full paper in a journal, is often found on such specialist registers. One example of a database that includes grey literature is the Web of Science, which catalogues many conference proceedings.[20] Other specialist registers exist for the registration of systematic review protocols and as repositories for studies concerning diagnostics.[21,22]

Constructing a systematic search

In order to identify relevant literature, a good search strategy is required. Often when conducting a search one of two things may happen. The first is that when a specific query is entered, very few studies are found. The second is the opposite, where thousands of results are generated making it difficult to find the most useful studies. To avoid these situations, a good search strategy should be both sensitive (be able to find the right information) and specific (exclude irrelevant studies).

Using the PICOS framework is an excellent place to start.

Defining search terms using PICOS

PICOS allows us to clearly define a research question and build a systematic search that will find relevant studies effectively. Thinking about each element of PICOS allows specific search terms to be identified. For the following elements of PICOS we will use the example question 'What is the effect of laparoscopic surgery on wound infection rates after appendicectomy for acute appendicitis?'

Population

Begin by defining the population of interest for your study question. This might be a group of patients with a disease, or patients undergoing a specific operation. In the case of our example, this will be patients undergoing appendicectomy. We would then find keywords related to appendicectomy or acute appendicitis, such as: 'appendicectomy', 'appendectomy' (US spelling) and 'appendicitis'.

Intervention or exposure

Identify the intervention or exposure in your research question. This will be the variable that you wish to know the effect of. In our example, it would be laparoscopic surgery, but it may be an exposure like cigarette smoking. Good keywords to use for laparoscopic surgery searches include: 'laparoscopy', 'laparoscopic', 'videoscopic', 'keyhole' and 'endoscopic'.

Comparison

The comparison is the non-exposed group we are interested in studying as a control. In the example of laparoscopic surgery for acute appendicitis, the control group would be open surgery as a contrasting surgical approach. Here, we could use keywords such as 'open', 'laparotomy', 'McBurney's', 'gridiron' or 'Lanz', which describe open incisions. As there are currently only two common approaches for appendicectomy, open or laparoscopic, specifying open surgery may not be required.

Outcomes

The effect of an intervention is usually measured by multiple outcomes. Specifying outcomes in a search can also substantially reduce the number of irrelevant studies, although this should be balanced against the likelihood of missing important studies that may not mention outcome measures explicitly in the title or abstract. In our case, we could use terms such as 'wound infection', 'dehiscence', 'surgical site infection' or 'SSI'.

Study design

The study design can also be specified, which is particularly useful in topics with much observational evidence. If we wanted only to find randomised trials, we could find these using specific terms such as 'randomised', 'randomized', 'trial' or 'randomly'. The Cochrane collaboration has a series of terms that allow these terms to be filtered.[11]

Combining terms

The first step to a successful search is to use the right types of search terms. Broadly speaking there are three types of search term; text words (.tw), MeSH terms (.sh or [MeSH]) and Boolean operators (usually AND, OR, IF, NOT). Text words are terms that do not correspond to MeSH key terms and describe the study and topic being searched. MeSH terms allow the simultaneous and structured searching of many text words at once. Boolean operators combine text words and MeSH terms together in order to construct searches.[23]

Another consideration is variation in language. Although medical studies are overwhelmingly published in the English language, they may be written using UK or US English. Therefore, take care when searching for a word that can be spelt with a US variation. This is of particular concern when searching for words like 'randomised' (which in US English is 'randomized') or appendicectomy (in US English 'appendectomy').

Often the most difficult part of searching is to combine all the relevant terms together. Cochrane reviews tend to use numbered lists of keywords, which when combined produce an effective search. Box 1.2 shows how a systematic search may be constructed using the example of open versus endovascular aortic aneurysm repair.

Boolean operators

Boolean operators are terms that tell the search engine how to handle search terms. In PubMed, the Boolean operators AND, OR and NOT are used frequently. These are quite self-explanatory

Box 1.2 • Building a search strategy for aortic aneurysm repair

Terms	Rationale
1. Aortic Aneurysm, Abdominal	MeSH term for abdominal aortic aneurysms
2. AAA.tw	Abdominal Aortic Aneurysm is frequently abbreviated to 'AAA'
3. Endovascular Procedures	MeSH term for endovascular procedures
4. EVAR.tw	Endovascular aneurysm repair is frequently abbreviated to 'EVAR'
5. Open repair.tw	Open repair is one of the treatments we are interested in, however there are no MeSH
6. Vascular Grafting	terms to describe an open approach specifically!
7. 1 OR 2	MeSH term for vascular surgical procedures involving vessel repair
8. 3 OR 4	Search for either the aortic aneurysm MeSH term or the AAA acronym
9. 5 OR 6	Search for either the Endovascular procedures MeSH term or the EVAR acronym
10. 7 AND 8 AND 9	Search for either open repair text word or vascular grafting MeSH term
	Combines all the above terms together

This search brings up several thousand results. We are only concerned with finding the best randomised controlled trial evidence for this. To do this we can add a clinical trials filter (adapted from Cochrane Collaboration) to our search:.

1. randomized controlled trial
2. controlled clinical trial
3. randomized
4. randomly
5. trial
6. groups
7. 11 OR 12 OR 13 OR 14 OR 15 OR 16
8. animals [mh] NOT humans [mh]
9. 18 NOT 19 (N.B. this is a double negative)
10. 10. 10 AND 19

This now gives us a much narrower collection of studies which primarily contain evidence from randomised trials.

terms, which when used effectively can increase the effectiveness of a search greatly:

- Appendicitis OR Appendicectomy – to find studies concerning appendicitis or appendicectomy
- Appendicitis AND Appendicectomy – to find studies where appendicectomy took place for appendicitis
- Appendicectomy NOT Appendicitis – to find studies discussing appendicectomy only, not necessarily relevant to appendicitis.

Wildcards

Wildcards enable searches to be performed where the exact spelling of a term is not known, or there are known variations to it. The symbol denoting a wildcard varies by search client used. In PubMed it is the * symbol. An example would be to find all studies that discuss anything to do with appendix, appendicectomy or appendicitis, regardless of spelling. To do this, the term 'Append*' would be entered into the search engine. Note this example would also bring up studies to do with anything that began with 'Append'. Nevertheless, wildcards are useful when used in combination with multiple other terms, or for a quick search.

Critical appraisal

When reading a clinical research study the results should not be taken at face value immediately. In order to interpret the results and their applicability, we must consider the study and its conduct. To do so, it is useful to have a systematic approach with which to appraise a paper and an understanding of where sources of systematic error commonly arise.

Systematic approaches for critical appraisal

The most important segments of a research paper are how it was conducted (methods) and the findings. Results should not be interpreted without consideration of the study methods. Applying the 'PICOS' approach at each stage is a useful means of structuring a critical appraisal (**Fig. 1.5**).

Formal critical learning and appraisal tools exist, which are readily available as electronic resources on the Internet. The Oxford Critical Appraisal Skills Programme and the Cochrane Collaborative's electronic learning packages are useful and provide more details.[24,25]

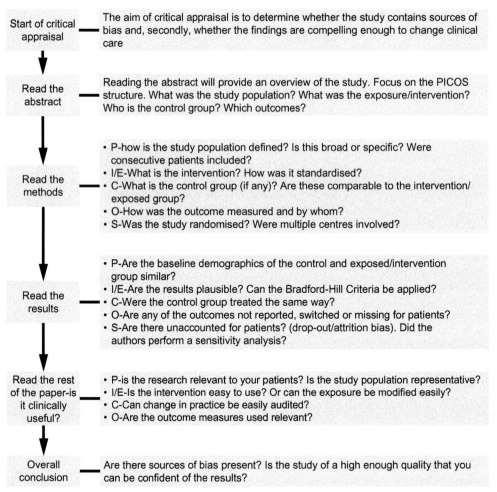

| Start of critical appraisal | The aim of critical appraisal is to determine whether the study contains sources of bias and, secondly, whether the findings are compelling enough to change clinical care |

| Read the abstract | Reading the abstract will provide an overview of the study. Focus on the PICOS structure. What was the study population? What was the exposure/intervention? Who is the control group? Which outcomes? |

| Read the methods | • P-how is the study population defined? Is this broad or specific? Were consecutive patients included?
• I/E-What is the intervention? How was it standardised?
• C-What is the control group (if any)? Are these comparable to the intervention/exposed group?
• O-How was the outcome measured and by whom?
• S-Was the study randomised? Were multiple centres involved? |

| Read the results | • P-Are the baseline demographics of the control and exposed/intervention group similar?
• I/E-Are the results plausible? Can the Bradford-Hill Criteria be applied?
• C-Were the control group treated the same way?
• O-Are any of the outcomes not reported, switched or missing for patients?
• S-Are there unaccounted for patients? (drop-out/attrition bias). Did the authors perform a sensitivity analysis? |

| Read the rest of the paper-is it clinically useful? | • P-is the research relevant to your patients? Is the study population representative?
• I/E-Is the intervention easy to use? Or can the exposure be modified easily?
• C-Can change in practice be easily audited?
• O-Are the outcome measures used relevant? |

| Overall conclusion | Are there sources of bias present? Is the study of a high enough quality that you can be confident of the results? |

Figure 1.5 • Process of critical appraisal using PICOS.

Bias

Bias occurs when systematic error is introduced into a study. Bias has the potential to influence the outcomes of a study and produce misleading results. In order to limit bias, we must understand where it may arise and identify techniques that can reduce the risk of bias. There are over 30 different types of bias, but the following are the most important to surgical research. (See **Fig. 1.6** for an overview.)

Types of bias

Selection bias

Selection bias arises where individuals are selected to treatment groups based upon their individual or disease characteristics, thus creating systematic differences between groups.[26,27] This may arise either where randomisation has not been performed adequately in interventional studies,

or in observational studies where treatment is decided by patients and clinicians. Randomisation is the only method by which selection bias can be reliably eliminated. An example of selection bias would be in lung cancer surgery, where there is a choice between videoscopic assisted thoracoscopic (VATS) lobectomy for removing a tumour, or using stereotactic ablative radiotherapy (SABR). As VATS lobectomy is a major operation, those patients who have many comorbidities are likely to have adverse outcomes. Therefore, if we compared VATS lobectomy and SABR in an observational study, there would be a selection bias as the groups would have different clinical characteristics.

Some statistical methods, known as 'methods for causal inference' are designed to reduce the effects of selection bias upon an analysis. A popular method for reducing the influence of selection bias in observational studies is regression, where the outcomes are adjusted for important confounding factors. A more recent development gaining popularity is propensity-score matching. Here computer algorithms are used to

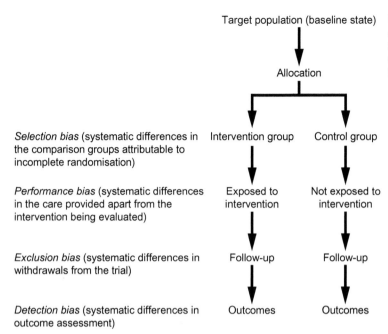

Target population (baseline state)

Allocation

Selection bias (systematic differences in the comparison groups attributable to incomplete randomisation)

Intervention group　　　Control group

Performance bias (systematic differences in the care provided apart from the intervention being evaluated)

Exposed to intervention　　　Not exposed to intervention

Exclusion bias (systematic differences in withdrawals from the trial)

Follow-up　　　Follow-up

Detection bias (systematic differences in outcome assessment)

Outcomes　　　Outcomes

Figure 1.6 • Overview of bias. Adapted from T Greenhalgh. How to read a paper: the basics of evidence-based medicine, 4e. London: BMJ Books, 2010.

match treated patients to patients in the control group, based upon characteristics that may influence which treatment group they are allocated to. The computer algorithm then weights the analysis towards patients who are most similar to one another, thereby generating a fairer experiment which compares patients like for like.

Responder bias

Responder bias describes situations in which study participants are led toward giving a specific answer. Responder bias affects surveys, questionnaires and interviews. An example of responder bias would be where a surgeon asks a patient 'were you satisfied with the treatment you received?'. In this example, the patient may feel compelled to state they were satisfied in order to be polite toward the surgeon who provided their care. Another example might be the use of leading questions, or multiple choice answers in interviews or questionnaires. Careful design of studies can eliminate responder bias.

Reporting bias

The selective reporting of information available in a study is known as reporting bias. Authors may omit to report outcomes that do not fit with preconceived ideas or the author's desired message. Reporting bias is such a major issue in medical literature that a taskforce has been set up to promote improved reporting. The 'Enhancing the QUAlity and Transparency Of health Research' (EQUATOR) network publishes checklists which state specific items that should be reported in scientific papers.[28] Many journals now require adherence to the EQUATOR network

guidelines to even consider a paper for publication. Reporting checklists exist for nearly every type of study, from randomised trials to studies of diagnostic accuracy. Good reporting facilitates critical appraisal and makes it simpler for subsequent systematic reviews and meta-analyses to be performed. One example of this is the CONsolidated Standards of Reporting Trials 2010 (CONSORT) checklist, which is the reporting checklist concerning parallel group randomised controlled trials[29] (Box 1.3). It consists of 25 items that should be explained in detail within the study report. Other common checklists include the Strengthening the Reporting of Observational studies in Epidemiology (STROBE, for cohort studies)[30] and Preferred Reporting Items for Systematic Reviews and Meta-Analyses (PRISMA, for systematic reviews).[31]

These checklists, however, do not eliminate all issues surrounding reporting bias. Where studies fail to incorporate the collection of these outcomes into their design, this is also considered as a form of reporting bias. To address this, recent work has culminated in the production of 'core outcome datasets'. These datasets, decided on by experts in the given field, consist of important and relevant outcomes which should always be reported.[32–34]

The publication of a study protocol or prior registration of a research study on a trials registry (such as ClinicalTrials.gov) also helps reduce selective reporting. Stating which outcomes will be reported prior to the study makes researchers more accountable to do so. Journal editors, reviewers and readers can use the protocol to compare to the final study report in order to identify any deliberate reporting bias.

Title and abstract

	1a	Identification as a randomised trial in the title
	1b	Structured summary of trial design, methods, results, and conclusions (for specific guidance see CONSORT for abstracts)

Introduction

Background and objectives	2a	Scientific background and explanation of rationale
	2b	Specific objectives or hypotheses

Methods

Trial design	3a	Description of trial design (such as parallel, factorial) including allocation ratio
	3b	Important changes to methods after trial commencement (such as eligibility criteria), with reasons
Participants	4a	Eligibility criteria for participants
	4b	Settings and locations where the data were collected
Interventions	5	The interventions for each group with sufficient details to allow replication, including how and when they were actually administered
Outcomes	6a	Completely defined pre-specified primary and secondary outcome measures, including how and when they were assessed
	6b	Any changes to trial outcomes after the trial commenced, with reasons
Sample size	7a	How sample size was determined
	7b	When applicable, explanation of any interim analyses and stopping guidelines
Randomisation		
Sequence generation	8a	Method used to generate the random allocation sequence
	8b	Type of randomisation; details of any restriction (such as blocking and block size)
Allocation concealment mechanism	9	Mechanism used to implement the random allocation sequence (such as sequentially numbered containers), describing any steps taken to conceal the sequence until interventions were assigned
Implementation	10	Who generated the random allocation sequence, who enrolled participants, and who assigned participants to interventions
Blinding	11a	If done, who was blinded after assignment to interventions (for example, participants, care providers, those assessing outcomes) and how
	11b	If relevant, description of the similarity of interventions
Statistical methods	12a	Statistical methods used to compare groups for primary and secondary outcomes
	12b	Methods for additional analyses, such as subgroup analyses and adjusted analyses

Results

Participant flow (a diagram is strongly recommended)	13a	For each group, the numbers of participants who were randomly assigned, received intended treatment, and were analysed for the primary outcome
	13b	For each group, losses and exclusions after randomisation, together with reasons
Recruitment	14a	Dates defining the periods of recruitment and follow-up
	14b	Why the trial ended or was stopped
Baseline data	15	A table showing baseline demographic and clinical characteristics for each group
Numbers analysed	16	For each group, number of participants (denominator) included in each analysis and whether the analysis was by original assigned groups

Box 1.3 • The CONSORT checklist for reporting randomised controlled trials—cont'd

Outcomes and estimation	17a	For each primary and secondary outcome, results for each group, and the estimated effect size and its precision (such as 95% confidence interval)
	17b	For binary outcomes, presentation of both absolute and relative effect sizes is recommended
Ancillary analyses	18	Results of any other analyses performed, including subgroup analyses and adjusted analyses, distinguishing pre-specified from exploratory
Harms	19	All important harms or unintended effects in each group (for specific guidance see CONSORT for harms)
Discussion		
Limitations	20	Trial limitations, addressing sources of potential bias, imprecision, and, if relevant, multiplicity of analyses
Generalisability	21	Generalisability (external validity, applicability) of the trial findings
Interpretation	22	Interpretation consistent with results, balancing benefits and harms, and considering other relevant evidence
Other information		
Registration	23	Registration number and name of trial registry
Protocol	24	Where the full trial protocol can be accessed, if available
Funding	25	Sources of funding and other support (such as supply of drugs), role of funders

Source: Schulz KF, Altman DG, Moher D. CONSORT 2010 statement: Updated guidelines for reporting parallel group randomised trials. Int J Surg. 2010;115(5):1063–70.

Attrition bias

Attrition bias occurs when there are systematic differences in withdrawals between study and control groups within research studies. This can be due to missing outcome data from participants withdrawing from the study, or due to the investigators excluding cases. In either situation, it must be ensured that there are no underlying reasons for this to occur which may lead to bias. If there are differences between groups with regards to drop-outs or exclusions, there should be a high index of suspicion for attrition bias.

If there are more participants withdrawing from a treatment group, it may indicate that the treatment is causing harm, is ineffective, or is poorly tolerated by the study participants. To detect this effect, an intention-to-treat (ITT) analysis should be performed. ITT analysis includes all participants allocated to a treatment or control group, regardless of whether they have withdrawn from or adhered to the intervention. This analysis presents a better 'real-world' measure of clinical effectiveness.

Per-protocol, or efficacy, analyses look at how effective the treatment was in the patients who completed the treatment course. This provides an estimate as to how effective the treatment is in those patients who adhere to it. Ideally, a study will first perform an intention-to-treat analysis, followed by an efficacy analysis. Doing so provides both a measure of real-world clinical effectiveness and a measure of how effective the treatment is for adherent patients.

Performance bias

Performance bias describes a phenomenon in which those administering an intervention or aftercare are aware of the treatment group the patient is allocated to and consciously or subconsciously alter their behaviour.

An example of this may be where a new surgical operation is being tested. If the staff involved in the postoperative care are aware of the treatment the patient received, they may unknowingly provide different care across groups, thus leading to results that misleadingly favour one treatment over another.

There are two methods to minimise the effects of performance bias. The first is to ensure all care providers are blinded to the treatment group allocation as far as possible. An example of where this may be difficult is in studies of laparoscopic versus open surgery; creative methods using large bandages or dressings may be required to cover the abdomen of a patient to disguise surgical scars.

The second method is to use a clearly defined pathway of care which should be adhered to in the study protocol. Note that studies which stipulate close protocol adherence often create a lot of work for clinical staff and can be difficult to achieve in many healthcare settings.

Recall bias

Recall bias is systematic error caused by difficulties a patient may have in recalling an event accurately. This is of particular concern in the retrospective determination of a particular outcome. An example may be conducting a telephone survey of patients who have undergone surgery to ask if they suffered a wound infection. If a study contacted patients at 30 days following surgery, the patient would be likely to recall whether they had a wound issue or not. If the study, however, contacted patients 2 years after the index operation, recalling details would be far more difficult and subject to recall bias.

Observer bias

This is where an individual determining a study outcome introduces bias, either consciously or subconsciously, by altering their judgements based on knowledge of treatment group allocation. An example is in studies assessing surgical site infection. If the individual assessing the wound is aware of the treatment group allocation of the patient, the assessment of the outcome may be prejudiced and favour one treatment over another. The only means of adequately addressing observer bias is to use a blinded design, where observers are unaware as to the treatment group allocation. Often in surgical studies this cannot be a member of the surgical team, as they are already aware of the group allocation given they performed the intervention. In this case, an independent blinded observer should assess the study outcomes to minimise the influence of observer bias.

Publication bias

Similar to reporting bias, publication bias involves the selective reporting of research. Publication bias, however, occurs when a study goes unpublished. This may be for many reasons including failure to recruit participants, patients coming to harm leading to the study being terminated early, and results that were not as expected or hoped (particularly 'negative' results). Studies that show 'positive' results, where there are statistically significant correlations between interventions or exposures, are more likely to be published than those that do not.

Thorough systematic reviews attempt to identify publication bias. Investigators of reviews search clinical trials registers, conference abstracts and other sources in order to ascertain whether additional research studies have been performed, but remain unpublished. It is also possible to determine statistically whether there are likely to be unpublished studies using meta-analysis techniques. Funnel plots show the effect size of each study against a measure of precision (**Fig. 1.7**). Where publication bias exists, the expected distribution of studies showing effects both greater and less than the mean effect is absent, and the plot is asymmetric. This suggests expected 'negative' studies are absent. The use of protocols published prior to a study taking place and registration of studies on clinical trials databases ensure investigators can be held accountable for unpublished work.

Judging the risk of bias

There are formal, validated tools to help researchers systematically assess bias in research studies. These tools ensure that a uniform approach is taken and studies are directly comparable. One popular tool for appraising the risk of bias in non-randomised research is the Newcastle–Ottawa scale. The Newcastle–Ottawa scale covers the domains of Selection, Comparability, Exposure and Outcome. Using the tool investigators make judgements as to the quality of the piece of research across these specific domains. Other available tools include

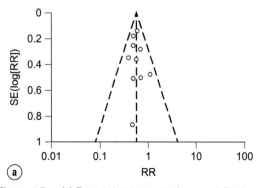
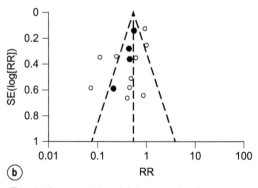

Figure 1.7 • (a) Funnel plot demonstrating no publication bias. The plot is symmetrical. **(b)** Asymmetrical funnel plot demonstrating the presence of publication bias, with outlying dots indicating studies with apparent bias. The solid dots indicate where we may expect studies to lie (within the dotted funnel).

the Cochrane Collaboration's tool for appraisal of randomised controlled trials and observational appraisal tool (ROBINS-I).[35]

For making judgements on the overall findings of a systematic review and assessing the strength with which a recommendation can be made, there exists another set of criteria known as 'GRADE' (Grading of Recommendations Assessment, Development and Evaluation).[10] This set of criteria aim to summarise the findings of a systematic review based upon more than just the quality of evidence contained within the review itself. GRADE considers five domains:

1. Risk of bias – was there bias across the included studies that may influence the results of the review?
2. Imprecision – if further studies were done, could they plausibly change the results of the review?
3. Indirectness – are the results of the review applicable to clinical practice?
4. Inconsistency – were included studies consistent (in agreement) across the review?
5. Publication bias – was there publication bias present and if this were not present would it change the results of the review?

After analysing the review's findings across the five domains, an overall grade rating is awarded. This can be up- or downgraded based on these five domains. There should be one GRADE rating awarded per outcome reported in the review:

- High quality – it is highly likely that the results of the review lie very close to the true value.
- Moderate quality – it is likely that the results of the review lie close to the true value, but further research could alter this.
- Low quality – it is unlikely that the results of the review are close to the true value and are likely to be substantially different.
- Very low quality – it is very unlikely that the results of the review are anywhere near the true value.

Simple statistics

An understanding of basic statistics is crucial to the successful interpretation of research studies. Statistical terms are often confusing and a clear understanding of the definitions and workings of statistics can make a paper clearer to read and interpret. In this section, we will provide a brief overview of statistical terms and provide straightforward explanations for frequently used techniques.

Summarising data

Often the first table contained in a study summarises the characteristics of the population included in the study. This is useful, as it enables the reader to see whether the study is applicable to the population they treat. There are three types of data variable: categorical, ordinal and continuous.

- Categorical data can take one of several defined groups which do not have precedence. Where there are two groups, the data can also be called 'binary'. An example of categorical data is gender, which usually takes the value of male or female.
- Ordinal data are similar to categorical data except they have a natural order of precedence. Ordinal data can take only the values of each group, with there being no intermediate values possible. An example of this would be in the TNM tumour staging system, where there is an order of precedence as to tumour grade, but this cannot be described on a continuous numerical system.
- Continuous data are numbers on a continuous scale. These can be in the form of whole numbers (integers) or be described as parts of a whole using a decimal format (i.e. 12.5).

Summarising ordinal or categorical data
Summarising ordinal and categorical data is straightforward. Simple counts for each group can be used and percentages calculated.

Summarising continuous data
Summarising continuous data is less straightforward than categorical or ordinal data. Continuous data follow a distribution, which describes how the data are spread across study subjects. The distribution the data follows dictates the type of average measure that is used. An average is also known as a measure of 'central tendency' as it describes the central point around which the data are distributed. The degree to which data are spread around this central point is called 'dispersion'. Where central tendency is measured using averages, dispersion is measured using values such as standard deviation or confidence intervals. When an estimate of the central tendency and dispersion are known, it is possible to interpret the distribution of continuous data.

Broadly speaking, data can follow a parametric (one with a defined shape) or non-parametric distribution (without an obviously defined shape). In statistics, most parametric data naturally follow a distribution known as the 'normal distribution' (also known as 'Gaussian'). The normal distribution follows a symmetric distribution around a central point. When plotted, the curve generated by this data looks like a bell that might be found in a church (**Fig. 1.8**).

Figure 1.8 • The normal or Gaussian distribution, an example of a parametric distribution.

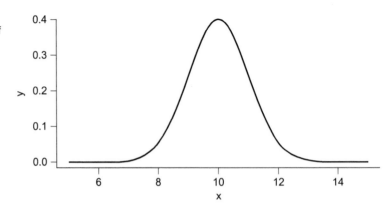

Not all data follow this exact distribution. One example is age, where conditions may affect older or younger people disproportionately. If we plotted the distribution of ages of patients at the first diagnosis of Alzheimer's disease, we would see that older patients would be more affected and hence the plot would be moved to the right-hand side. This effect is known as skew and is important to consider, as highly skewed data will require different measures to assess the central tendency and dispersion of data.

There are three types of average:

- Mean – this is calculated by adding up all the values in the data and dividing by the number of observations. This type of mean is called an arithmetic mean. There are more complex types of mean available, which include geometric and harmonic means, but these are outside the scope of this chapter.
- Median – this is the value of the middle observation when the data are ordered in ascending or descending order. For example, if there were 100 observations made on a continuous scale, the median would be the value of the 50th observation.
- Mode – this is the most common value found within the continuous dataset.

Measuring dispersion

There are four main types of measures of dispersion that are important to know about.

Standard deviation (SD or σ)

$$\sigma = \sqrt{\frac{1}{N}\sum_{i=1}^{N}(x_i - \mu)^2}$$

Where N is the number of observations, μ is the mean of all values and x is the value for each observation. The standard deviation describes the

distribution of a continuous variable around a given point. It works well if the data are parametric and are not skewed.

Confidence interval (CI)

$$95\%CI = x \pm (1.96 \times SE_x)$$

Where x is the effect size, and SE is the standard error of the effect size. A confidence interval describes the certainty of a treatment effect.

Interquartile range (IQR)

$$IQR = Q3 - Q1$$

Where $Q1$ is the value of the 25th centile contained within the data and $Q3$ is the 75th centile. This is a common way to describe non-parametric data (i.e. data that do not follow a normal distribution).

Range

$$Range = Maximum\,Value - Minimum\,Value$$

This describes the overall spread of values within a dataset. It is useful for both parametric and non-parametric data.

When a continuous variable is normally distributed (it's always wise to plot it first to check!) and not highly skewed, central tendency can be summarised using the arithmetic mean and dispersion can be summarised using a standard deviation or confidence interval.

In the case where a continuous variable does not follow a normal distribution or is highly skewed, the median or mode should be used in place of the mean. Dispersion is then conventionally presented using the interquartile range or ranges.

Missing data

Dealing with missing data is important, as missing data may lead to biased results. Missing data on explanatory variables (such as age, gender, disease type etc.) should not be simply excluded from an analysis if there are accompanying outcome data present. To do so would be to introduce attrition bias. Data can be missing due to the following reasons:

- Missing not at random (MNAR) – here data are missing for a reason. This may be due either to factors that have been collected in the study (observed), or for reasons that data have not been collected for (unobserved).
- Missing at random (MAR) – here data are missing, but the reason why can be fully accounted for using factors that have already been collected (observed).
- Missing completely at random (MCAR) – here data are missing completely independently (e.g. a blood sample was dropped).

Missing data should never be ignored. There are several means of dealing with missing data, which often include imputing an estimated value for the missing variable.

Treatment effect

The treatment effect (also known as effect estimate or effect size) describes the influence of the intervention or exposure being studied on the outcome of interest. The treatment effect measures the average difference in outcomes between the group who received the intervention or exposure and the control group. It can be measured using statistical methods and is usually presented alongside a confidence interval to demonstrate the level of uncertainty surrounding the estimate. Other measures may also be used, such as absolute risk reduction or number needed to treat.

Risk

Risk is defined as the probability of an outcome occurring in a given population. There are two types of risk measurement used in clinical research: absolute risk and relative risk. Absolute risk measures the actual probability within a population. Relative risk is a measure of the probability of an outcome occurring in one treatment group versus another; this is sometimes known as a risk ratio. An absolute risk reduction describes how good or bad one treatment is versus another.

$$Absolute\ risk = \frac{Number\ of\ events\ of\ interest}{Number\ of\ participants\ in\ population}$$

Absolute risk reduction (ARR)

$$= \frac{Number\ of\ events\ of\ interest\ in\ exposed\ group}{Number\ of\ participants\ in\ exposed\ group}$$
$$- \frac{Number\ of\ events\ of\ interest\ in\ unexposed\ group}{Number\ of\ participants\ in\ unexposed\ group}$$

Relative risk (risk ratio)

$$= \frac{Absolute\ risk\ of\ an\ event\ occurring\ in\ exposed\ group}{Absolute\ risk\ of\ an\ event\ occurring\ in\ unexposed\ group}$$

Odds

Odds are defined as the ratio of an event occurring versus an event not occurring in a given population or study group. For example, if in a population of 100 patients undergoing liver surgery, 25 develop complications, the odds of a complication occurring would be 1 to 3.

The 2 x 2 table, risk ratios and odds ratios

For calculating odds and risk it is useful to consider a 2×2 table:

	Exposure Yes	Exposure No
Outcome Yes	A	B
Outcome No	C	D

Using the 2×2 table, absolute risk can be expressed as:

Absolute risk of Outcome 'Yes' in exposed group
$$= \frac{a}{a+c}$$

Absolute risk of Outcome 'Yes' in unexposed group
$$= \frac{b}{b+d}$$

To calculate a risk ratio, we would calculate the absolute risk for both groups and divide one by the other. Alternatively, based upon a 2×2 table, a risk ratio may be expressed as:

$$Risk\ ratio\ of\ Outcome\ 'Yes' = \left(\frac{a}{a+c}\right) \div \left(\frac{b}{b+c}\right)$$

Using the 2 x 2 table, the odds of outcome 'Yes' occurring in the exposed group would be expressed as $\frac{a}{c}$ and for outcome 'Yes', in the unexposed group $\frac{b}{d}$.

To calculate an odds ratio, we would calculate this using the following formula:

$$Odds\ Ratio\ (OR) = \frac{a}{c} \div \frac{b}{d}$$

Due to mathematical convention, when two fractions are divided sequentially, this is the same as multiplying them once. Therefore, an odds ratio may be also expressed as:

$$Odds\ Ratio\ (OR) = \frac{ad}{bc}$$

If an odds ratio or a risk ratio is greater than one, the outcome of interest is more likely to occur with the exposure. If the odds ratio or risk ratio takes a value less than one, the outcome of interest is less likely to occur with the exposure. If the odds or risk ratio is close to one, the outcome of interest does not alter with the exposure.

The difference between the risk ratio and the value 1 is also known as the risk difference. An example of this would be for a risk ratio of 0.8. If we subtract 0.8 from 1, we are left with 0.2. Therefore, we can say there is a 20% relative risk reduction between the treatment groups.

Risk ratio versus odds ratio

Although they may appear similar in numerical format, there are clear distinctions to be made between odds ratios and risks ratios.

Odds can be converted to risks and vice-versa; however this is not a straightforward process as their relationship depends upon the event rate for the outcome of interest. For common outcomes, odds ratios can be very different from risk ratios and should not be confused. Odds ratios do not translate well to describing risk either as they are not immediately intuitive.

Hypothesis testing

Statistical tests are used to reject study hypotheses. There are two types of study hypotheses:

* The null hypothesis is that there is no difference between treatments or exposed groups. It further stipulates that any observed differences may be due to error.
* The alternative hypothesis is that there is a difference between treatments or exposed groups. This is opposite to the null hypothesis.

A hypothesis in this sense can only be rejected or fail to be rejected and never fully accepted, as there is hypothetically always a chance that the observations are due to error. Statistical testing aims to reject the null hypothesis in order to demonstrate that there is a significant difference between treatment groups.

Association and causation

Perhaps one of the most important skills when interpreting statistics is to discern association from causation. The objective of most medical studies is to identify or postulate as to why a particular result is observed (or in some cases, not observed).

Distinguishing causation from association is particularly important in observational research. If there is a relationship or correlation between two variables, statistically significant or not, these variables are said to be associated. We cannot directly infer that the variables have a cause-and-effect relationship, as the observation may be simply due to chance or bias. Interventional studies, where an experiment is constructed to minimise sources of bias and error are more likely to establish causality. This is a particular strength of the randomised controlled trial design.

According to the Bradford–Hill criteria, an observation is likely to be causal if the following are fulfilled:

* Strength of association – the larger the effect size of associated variables, the more likely there is a causal effect present. Unless an obvious confounding factor is unaccounted for.
* Consistency – if multiple, independent studies find the same association in different populations, this increases the likelihood of an effect being present.
* Specificity – if there is a very specific association between one group of patients and the exposure of interest it is likely to be causative.
* Temporality – if the outcome occurs following the exposure within a plausible timeframe, causality is more likely to be present.
* Biological rationale – if there is a 'dose–response' relationship between the exposure and the outcome, this makes causality more likely. For example, the higher the dose of antibiotics a patient receives, the greater the chances of developing *Clostridium difficile* pseudo-membranous colitis.
* Plausibility – if there is a clear explanation between a cause and an observed effect, causality is more likely. For example, oranges are fruit high in vitamin C, therefore children

who eat more oranges are less likely to suffer from scurvy.

- Coherence – if the observations of a clinical research study tie in with the findings of a laboratory study, causality is more likely.
- Analogy – when a result is observed, other analogous (similar) or confounding factors should be taken into consideration. If when these factors have been taken into consideration, the observed result persists, causality is more likely.

Statistical significance

Statistical significance is a concept that is often misunderstood by scientists and clinicians alike. When considering significance there is one question that should be asked: is the finding clinically significant?

Statistical significance can be described as the level at which the probability of a test reaches an acceptable level at which the null hypothesis can be rejected. Often this is described using a P-value, which describes the probability of an observation being down to chance (i.e. a P-value of 0.05 means there is a 1 in 20 probability the observed association is due to chance).

The P-value has become synonymous with statistical significance over the past hundred years. It was invented in the 20th century by Ronald Fisher, an eminent frequentist statistician. Fisher arbitrarily selected 0.05 as an example to illustrate the use of the P-value and since then it has stuck.

Adjusting for confounding factors

In well-conducted randomised studies, both treatment groups should contain patients with similar characteristics and be reasonably balanced. In observational studies, however, due to a lack of randomisation, patient groups are likely to be unbalanced. In order to account for this imbalance and address the possible source of selection bias that accompanies this (as imbalance is likely to be due to clinical treatment decisions), these factors can be adjusted for using regression methods.

Example studies

The following studies are excellent examples for applying the principles of evaluation described above.

MRC-CLASICC

This study looked at whether laparoscopic surgery for colorectal cancer was equivalent to open surgery. The study began in 1996 when there was genuine uncertainty as to whether laparoscopic colorectal surgery was safe and effective.[36]

The study demonstrated that for colonic resection for cancer, laparoscopic surgery was as safe as open surgery. The authors went on to publish data on both the short- and long-term outcomes. In conjunction with several other trials, this study paved the way for the implementation of routine laparoscopic colorectal surgery.

EVAR-1

This is a randomised comparison of open abdominal aortic aneurysm repair versus endovascular repair, published in 2004.[37,38] The study took patients who were eligible for either open or endovascular repair and randomised them to either treatment. At this time, EVAR was relatively new and the benefits of the technique were yet to be fully established.

The EVAR-1 trial found no difference in all-cause mortality or quality of life and found EVAR to be more expensive than open repair with a higher complication rate. The trial demonstrated open repairs were in fact better for patients who could opt for either approach, thus clarifying the role of open surgery. Secondly, it enabled research into the EVAR technique to become focused on patients who were unfit for open approaches, thus enabling surgeons and commissioners to provide the best outcomes and utilisation of clinical resources.

ProtecT

This was a study of surgery versus radiotherapy versus surveillance for localised prostate cancer.[39] The use of prostate specific antigen (PSA) testing for the detection of prostate cancer is controversial. When PSA is elevated and cancer is detected, it is uncertain as to whether there is benefit to treating tumours detected in this way.

The 10-year results of the ProtecT study found that survival following treatment of PSA-detected local prostate cancer did not differ between treatment groups. Surgery and radiotherapy were found to have lower rates of disease progression; however, these had associated risks. The implications of this study pose a dilemma for men with localised prostate cancers: the choice between surveillance or a radical intervention with urinary, sexual and bowel function complications, both of which have similar long-term survival outcomes.

Key points

- In research, formulating a good study question will help both you and others understand your work. The PICOS (Population, Intervention, Comparison, Outcomes, Study design) framework should be used to help achieve this.
- Prior to undertaking a research study, a thorough systematic review is key to identifying relevant studies and will help in developing a research question that addresses weaknesses in the literature. This should be thought through carefully to maximise the number of relevant studies included. There are numerous sources of evidence that should be considered.
- Good design is key to a successful and high-impact study. If methodological flaws are present, this will affect both where it is published and whether it will change clinical practice or not.
- Ensuring research is as applicable as possible to the real world will help clinicians interpret it easily and apply it to their patients faster. Means of doing this include conducting pragmatic trials or performing the research in multiple centres.
- Research should be reported as per standards outlined by the EQUATOR network. These guidelines outline the key elements required to allow research to be assessed for quality, interpreted and used in future studies successfully.
- It is important to understand the differences between association and causation. If there is an association between an explanatory (independent) variable and an outcome (dependent) – it must be determined whether this is a causal relationship or not. There are several ways of doing so; however, in medicine the most common way of demonstrating causality is through a randomised controlled trial (RCT).
- Statistical analyses should be pre-planned. Any kind of power calculation should be pre-planned and based on existing literature. Where statistical tests are used, the underlying data should meet the assumptions required for the specific test. Finally, regression models can be used to account for confounding factors by adjusting for them.

Medical research and challenges

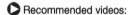 Recommended videos:

- The story of 200 years – how evidence came to the fore – https://www.youtube.com/watch?v=Qxx14RCxblg
- Challenges in surgical research – https://www.youtube.com/watch?v=-jQIBiVTpCk

---

🌐 Full references available at **http://expertconsult.inkling.com**

Appendix

Further reading

The details below provide references to sources of further information, particularly those accessible through the Internet. It must be remembered that there are rapid changes in the material available online and Internet addresses are liable to change. Several of these sources provide extensive links to other sites.

Books

DV Swinscow, MJ Campbell. *Statistics at square one*. 11e. London: BMJ Books; 2002. pp. 158. ISBN 0-7279-1552-5.

T Greenhalgh. *How to read a paper: the basics of evidence-based medicine*. 4e. London: BMJ Books; 2010. ISBN 0-7279-1552-5.

Websites

CASP (Critical Appraisal Skills Program)
http://www.casp-uk.net/

Centre for Evidence-based Medicine, established in Oxford
http://www.cebm.net

Centre for Evidence-based Mental Health –
http://www.cebmh.com

NIHR Health Technology Assessment Programme
http://www.hta.ac.uk/

NHS Centre for Reviews and Dissemination University of York –
http://www.york.ac.uk/inst/crd/

National Institute for Health and Research
http://www.nihr.ac.uk/

NHS Evidence
https://www.evidence.nhs.uk/

The Cochrane Collaboration
http://www.cochrane.org/
Cochrane Collaboration Handbook
http://www.cochrane-handbook.org/
Good Clinical Practice Training Course – many providers, however, the National Institute for Health Research (NIHR) has a good scheme
http://www.nihr.ac.uk/our-faculty/clinical-research-staff/learning-and-development/national-directory/good-clinical-practice/

Journals

British Medical Journal (BMJ)
http://www.bmj.com/
Journal of the American Medical Association (JAMA)
http://jamanetwork.com/journals/
The Lancet
http://www.thelancet.com
British Journal of Surgery
http://www.bjs.co.uk
HPB
http://onlinelibrary.wiley.com/journal/10.1111/(ISSN)1477-2574
Colorectal Disease
http://onlinelibrary.wiley.com/journal/10.1111/(ISSN)1463-1318
Surgical Endoscopy
http://www.springer.com/medicine/surgery/journal/464
World Journal of Surgery
http://www.springer.com/medicine/surgery/journal/268

Databases

PubMed
http://www.ncbi.nlm.nih.gov/pubmed/
Google Scholar
http://www.scholar.google.co.uk
Internet access to the Cochrane Library and databases
http://www.thecochranelibrary.com/view/0/index.html
PROSPERO – worldwide prospective register of systematic reviews
http://www.crd.york.ac.uk/prospero/
ClinicalTrials.gov
https://clinicaltrials.gov/

Sources of guidelines and integrated care pathways

AHRQ (Agency for Healthcare Research and Quality) – provides practical healthcare information, research findings and data to help consumers
http://www.ahcpr.gov/
Evidence Based Practice Centres – developed in conjunction with the AHRQ
http://www.ahcpr.gov/clinic/epc/
National Institute for Health and Care Excellence (NICE)
http://www.nice.org.uk/
Scottish Intercollegiate Guidelines Network (SIGN)
http://www.sign.ac.uk

2

Perioperative care and enhanced recovery

Kristoffer Lassen

Introduction

Updated guidelines focus on comprehensive protocols for each step of the perioperative 'journey' in various abdominal procedures.[1-8] Several reviews confirm an association between the use of an enhanced recovery protocol (ERP) and improved outcomes in abdominal surgery.[9-12] While some results indicate gains from adhering to specific protocols (e.g. Enhanced Recovery After Surgery (ERAS) guidelines) and aiming for an optimal compliance,[13,14] others suggest that it is the use of a protocol in itself that is useful.[10] Comparison with historical controls is the study design used most frequently, but a host of confounding factors exist. As a complex intervention with outdated or contaminated control groups, this is a difficult issue to assess in a controlled manner and poorly suited for randomised design.[15] Nevertheless, the common theme behind these potentially conflicting views is the message that the efforts of the surgeon and anaesthetist do not start and stop solely with the operation itself. Optimal risk reduction through preoperative preparation and prehabilitation as well as structured evidence-based care encompassing every aspect of the postoperative period is crucial to minimise morbidity and mortality following major surgery. The modern surgical intervention begins some 4 weeks prior to the operation and continues for several weeks thereafter.

Before the operation

The first encounter with the patient is crucial for several reasons. Confidence has to be established; it is the first opportunity to educate the patient for the operation ahead; and it is an opportunity to improve his or her risk profile. For those with cancer, there is often the added consideration of timing of surgery, particularly if neoadjuvant therapy is required.

Patient counselling

Patient counselling is about more than explaining the operation and the probable outcome – including any risk of complications. It is the key opportunity to make sure the patient realises what the perioperative course will entail and what his/her daily targets should be in terms of mobilisation, drinking, eating and so forth.[1,3,4,6,7] If his/her expectations are based on stories of a parent's operation in 1967, they might expect to be hospitalised for 3 weeks following a hemicolectomy and to be bed-bound for the first week with an indwelling nasogastric tube. If these are their expectations you will have a tough time on the evening of the operation encouraging them to drink and to get out of bed. Achievable targets for each day following the operation should be stated and also provided in writing with easy-to-understand drawings. The patient's own part in his/her recovery should be emphasised. This area is poorly suited for a randomised trial[15] and it would be unethical to attempt one. It is, however, an intervention with collateral benefits and without known side-effects, although it requires some extra time.

✓ Preoperative counselling is strongly recommended and details about risk reduction, the operation and the postoperative course should be covered.

Preoperative nutrition and immunonutrition

Preoperative weight loss is a robust and strong risk factor for adverse surgical outcomes. Weighing the patient and comparing the results to patient-reported pre-morbid weight is sufficient and as a predictor probably as valid as more complex nutritional risk assessment tools. Even as little as 5% weight loss is a significant risk factor.[17] While preoperative dietary interventions can help the patient to regain lost weight before surgery, it is less clear whether this affects postoperative risk or is merely alleviating symptoms. Intravenous nutrition, enteral tube feeding and oral supplements (sip feeds) have all been evaluated as interventions to attenuate patient risk for complications following major surgery and in general they are recommended.[18] Numerous studies suggest a beneficial effect, but double-blinded trials with adequate control groups are few.[18] Importantly, providing nutrition is a stable intervention that can be blinded and placebo-controlled in randomised controlled trials (RCTs) and in conditions suitable for optimal design we should accept nothing less.[15] It appears prudent to provide nutritional support to grossly malnourished patients, orally if possible; enteral if oral is not feasible; and parenteral if the gut is not working. For patients with only mild malnutrition, the rationale is mainly supported by uncontrolled or open-label trials or trials measuring surrogate endpoints.[18] Weight gain is achieved consistently in these studies, but lowered postoperative risk has not been documented in a reproducible manner.

Additional provision of immune-enhancing formulas like arginine or glutamine has been supported by several trials and international guidelines.[18] Immunonutrition (IN) is particularly aimed at reducing infectious complications. However, there are few double-blinded trials with isonitrogenous control groups measuring clinical outcomes. The most recent ERAS guidelines do not recommend the routine use of immunonutrition,[6,19] and several recent high-quality trials in high-risk patients have failed to show any benefit.[20–22]

✔✔ There is currently no good evidence to support routine provision of preoperative nutritional support in patients who are not grossly malnourished.
✔✔ Immunonutrition is not recommended.

Cessation of smoking

Smoking negatively affects oxygen delivery to peripheral tissues, as well as those involved in an anastomosis. While chronic obstructive pulmonary disease (COPD), and risk of bronchial adenocarcinoma and cardiovascular disease will remain unchanged following 3 weeks of cessation from smoking, increasing evidence suggests that oxygen delivery and pulmonary function can both be improved by smoking cessation over as little as 3–4 weeks.[23,24] Even in cancer surgery, where delaying the operation will not be done lightly, allowing 4 weeks of complete cessation from smoking is probably wise in high-risk patients or planned high-risk anastomoses in, e.g., low rectal, oesophageal or pancreatic head resections. It is a cheap and well-understood intervention and it places the patient in the centre of the efforts to reduce risk.

✔✔ Patients should stop smoking for at least 3 weeks prior to major surgery.[23,24]

Prehabilitation

Impaired functional capacity in elderly cancer patients is multifactorial and constitutes a risk during major surgery. Some of the causes are cardiovascular disease, COPD, lean muscle wasting and other elements of cachexia. Prehabilitation, which aims to increase functional capacity in patients with impaired functional capacity, hinges on the issue of whether elderly and frail patients can benefit from short-term exercise to such an extent that risk is reduced. Again, the presence of cancer – as is often the case – will usually not allow for extended periods of intervention. Cardiopulmonary function tests have been shown to correlate closely with risk for major morbidity following surgery,[25] and interestingly, Dunne and colleagues have shown that a short-term, hospital-based exercise programme does indeed improve cardiopulmonary function for patients at risk.[26] However, hospital-based daily training programmes may have suboptimal compliance,[26] and may not be feasible to implement. It remains to be seen what can be achieved with short-term, home-based, intensified exercise programmes supervised by e.g. physiotherapists. Although a direct effect on major morbidity has not been demonstrated, a reasonable interpretation of available data suggests patients at risk will benefit from dedicated prehabilitation.

✔ Patients at risk should be instructed to exercise at home or at a facility on a daily basis up to the day before surgery.

Antithromboembolic drugs in the perioperative period

An increasing number of patients take an increasing variety of antithrombotic drugs for primary or secondary prophylaxis. Due to uncertain enteral absorption and risk of intra- or postoperative bleeding, these drugs are transiently withheld during the perioperative period for a duration dependent on the type of surgery. Perioperative prophylaxis with low molecular weight heparin (LMWH) or unfractionated heparin (UFH) varies depending on the indication for the patient's use of prophylaxis, the drug in question and the magnitude of increased risk pertaining to the operation. Most departments will have access to national guidelines for each drug under several indications and most cardiology departments will issue additional guidelines for prevention of thromboembolic complications to coronary stents. The following section is intended as an overview and the reader is strongly advised to consult national and local guidelines for details.

Vitamin-K antagonists (VKA)

Warfarin. Antidotes for reversal in the emergency setting include vitamin-K, fresh-frozen plasma and prothrombin complex concentrate (PCC). In the elective setting, warfarin is usually withheld for 3–5 days prior to major surgery. Depending on the risk of thromboembolic events balanced against the risk of bleeding during or after surgery, bridging therapy with LMWH/UFH may be indicated. Warfarin is usually resumed the evening after surgery if haemostasis is adequate.

Direct oral anticoagulants (DOAC)

These are relatively new drugs.[27] Importantly, they have no direct antidote, but PCC will reduce active bleeding. Their half-life increases significantly with impaired renal function and this has clinical implications, as surgery is usually acceptable after a cessation of one half-life. In such cases it will be important to measure renal function (creatinine and glomerular filtration rate [GFR]), and INR/APTT (international normalised ratio/activated partial thromboplastin time), and identify time for last dose taken.

Dabigatran. If INR/APTT is elevated, consider PCC. Normal APTT suggests low or no drug action. Emergency surgery should be delayed if possible to one half-life from latest dose. For scheduled major surgery there should be a 48 hours suspension period (with normal renal function) and 96 hours if GFR is 30–50 mL/min.[27] Restart dabigatran on postop day 1–3 depending on haemostasis and indication. Consider LMWH in the intervening period.

Rivaroxaban. Effect cannot be measured by INR/APTT, consider PCC for reversal. For emergency and scheduled major surgery, as for dabigatran.

Apixaban. Again its effect cannot be measured by INR/APTT, consider PCC. For emergency and scheduled major surgery, as for dabigatran.

Anti-platelet drugs

Acetylsalicylic acid (ASA, aspirin). Unless high risk of bleeding is anticipated in areas where surgical control is difficult, aspirin does not need to be discontinued before surgery.[28]

Clopidogrel, ticagrelor, prasugrel. Dual anti-platelet medication (aspirin + clopidogrel, ticagrelor or prasugrel) is prescribed following insertion of coronary artery stents. Duration is usually 6 weeks for bare-metal stents (BMS), and 6–12 months for drug-eluting stents (DES). Abrupt cessation of these drugs represents a significant risk for thrombosis, hence replacement therapy (LMWH) must be used in the perioperative period. Clopidogrel should be discontinued at least 5–7 days before any planned, major surgery;[29,30] ticagrelor somewhat less,[31] but prasugrel should be discontinued at least 7 days before.[30] Whether bridging anticoagulation (LMWH/UFH) is indicated should be assessed for individual patients.

Immediate preoperative period

The patient is usually admitted to the hospital the afternoon before or, increasingly, on the day of surgery. This is the last opportunity to identify any unforeseen deterioration in the patient that could make surgery hazardous and to check that all preparations to reduce risk are in place as planned.

Preoperative bowel preparation

Traditionally, procedures to empty the large bowel before surgery have been a pillar of preoperative preparation for colorectal procedures, with the intention of reducing the bacterial load in the colon and hence risk for infectious complications. Traditional per oral, or mechanical, bowel preparation implies intake of large amounts of fluids together with osmotic and laxative agents that induce diarrhoea. The risk of severe fluid shifts is substantial, especially for elderly and frail patients, and the procedure is quite burdensome. Modern guidelines and reviews have failed to identify significant benefits and balancing against the unwanted consequences, have largely advised against it.[1–8,32] Bowel preparation has, however, received some renewed interest in combination with repeated doses of per oral antibiotics aiming at a more complete decontamination of the large bowel. Recent data indicate that such a combination does lower complication rates in colorectal surgery,[33–35] but high-quality evidence is lacking. Two of the most recent publications are observational studies,[33,35] and a 2016 meta-analysis of seven RCTs found that only three had blinded outcome assessors.[34] The main benefit demonstrated is reduction in superficial incisional surgical site infections (SSIs) (and not organ/space SSI or deep incisional SSI). This is a weak outcome in open-label trials, as a robust definition is lacking.

Mechanical preparation (with or without decontaminating antibiotics) or enemas will be necessary in selected colorectal operations. Identifying small and ill-defined lesions during surgery might require careful palpation or intraoperative colonoscopy, both requiring an empty bowel. Furthermore, the use of diverting ileostomies to protect an ultra-low rectal anastomosis is meaningless if the colon is not emptied preoperatively.

✔✔ There is no strong evidence to support routine preoperative bowel preparation before major colonic (non-rectal) abdominal surgery.

Prevention of thromboembolic events

Patients undergoing major abdominal surgery have a significantly increased risk of thromboembolic complications, either in the form of deep venous thromboembolism (VTE) or pulmonary embolism (PE). Patients are often elderly, have malignant disease, are immobilised for some time, are exposed to fluid shifts and temporary dehydration and many have coexistent conditions like atrial fibrillation (AF) or congestive heart failure. The thromboembolic events may be asymptomatic or symptomatic and this makes interpretation of available data difficult. In addition, many of the earlier trials were conducted in environments where patients were immobilised for many days, limiting the generalisability (external validity) of the results in modern settings. It is a general consensus that patients undergoing major surgery should receive prophylaxis with LMWH for the days they have impaired level of mobility and suffer altered physiology from anaesthesia and surgery.[1,3–7] There are some other issues that are still under debate. A recent Cochrane review suggests that UFH is equal to LMWH,[36] and UFH has the advantage of not being dependent on renal function. Several studies support the use of intermittent pneumatic compression stockings in high-risk patients.[37] Of note: 'high-risk' in this review mainly refers to major orthopaedic surgery,[37,38] and the relevance in major abdominal surgery is less certain. It would, however, appear prudent to use such devices in patients under very high risk in major abdomino-pelvic surgery

as well, as side-effects are negligible. Extending thromboembolic prophylaxis beyond the hospital stay has also been advocated, especially in high-risk patients like those undergoing hip replacement surgery.[39] NICE Guidelines from 2012 also support extended prophylaxis for abdominal surgery,[40] citing a 2009 Cochrane review.[41] This Cochrane review, again, includes four RCTs published between 1998 and 2006, of which two were stopped prematurely due to lack of funding. Meta-analysis has demonstrated a benefit of extended prophylaxis for 28 days both for overall VTE and even symptomatic VTE. These trials were, however, conducted in an era where laparoscopic colorectal surgery and enhanced recovery protocols were just beginning to gain acceptance, and postoperative routines were probably different from those of today – even in Denmark and Sweden.[42] Data from a recent open-label RCT support the use of extended prophylaxis even following laparoscopic colorectal resections, but the benefit was almost exclusively on asymptomatic VTE and there was no pulmonary embolism in either group.[43] In conclusion, the clinical benefit of extended prophylaxis beyond discharge in fully mobilised patients without disseminated malignancy remains unproven.[44,45] Patients with pancreatic cancer and patients receiving neoadjuvant chemotherapy have been identified at risk for VTE even prior to surgery and a low threshold for deep vein ultrasonography could be considered.[46]

✔✔ VTE prophylaxis using UFH or LMWH is strongly recommended in all patients undergoing major abdominal or pelvic surgery (whether laparoscopic or open) and should be continued until the patient is mobile.

Preoperative fasting

Following fatal aspirations in the early days of anaesthesia, an extensive period of preoperative fasting has been a part of perioperative care for over a century. Modern evidence-based guidelines now recommend that patients be fasted for 6 hours for solid food and 2 hours for clear drinks before induction of anaesthesia.[1–5,7,8]

Preoperative carbohydrate loading

The theoretical concept of saturating the liver's glycogen storage capacity prior to surgery is appealing, as even overnight fasting will to some extent deplete these stores.[47] Intake of carbohydrate-rich fluids on the night before, and on the morning of surgery, has been shown to attenuate postoperative insulin resistance.[48] Being reasonably cheap and safe, they have been recommended in modern guidelines,[2,5] but significant impact on complications after surgery has not been demonstrated.[49]

Antibiotic prophylaxis

In this context, antimicrobial/antibiotic prophylaxis is designating a one-shot, preoperative administration of antibiotics to achieve a systemic level of appropriate drugs during surgery and lower the risk of SSIs. Systemic antibiotic prophylaxis is recommended by a host of perioperative guidelines.[1-8] The magnitude of risk reduction for SSI will depend on the 'a priori' risk of the patient and the type of operation. Patients undergoing contaminated or potentially contaminated operations should receive systemic prophylaxis. The rapidly increasing use of laparoscopy for several types of operations probably lowers the risk of SSI,[50] and extrapolation of evidence from open surgery might not be appropriate. The choice of drugs will vary according to profile of drug resistance and national guidelines should be consulted. Drugs that are recommended for therapeutic settings should not be used as prophylaxis to avoid selection of resistant bacterial strains. Antibiotic prophylaxis in scheduled surgery represents huge numbers of doses provided and this will spur ecological and economical concerns.

Intraoperative care

Preventing postoperative nausea and vomiting (PONV)

Nausea and vomiting postoperatively are more feared than pain.[51] Risk factors include female sex, non-smoking status and history of motion sickness (or PONV), and scoring systems are available.[52] Patients at risk should receive adequate prophylaxis with dexamethasone and/or serotonine receptor antagonists and/or droperidol.[4,5,53] Anaesthesia by propofol and remifentanyl is probably indicated for individuals at high risk.[4,5] Several other newer agents are emerging and for individuals at risk, a multimodal approach should be employed.[54]

Postoperative analgesia

Pain is an inevitable consequence of surgery, but modern analgesia can attenuate this to a level where most patients can ambulate almost immediately after the operation without too much discomfort. The aim should be complete analgesia at rest and only mild pain upon movement. Aiming for complete analgesia also upon movement is likely to lead to high doses of drugs that may again cause counterproductive sleepiness, nausea and contribute to delayed gut function recovery.

Thoracic epidural

The thoracic epidural catheter has been the keystone of multimodal pain management after surgery in ERAS for three decades. A functional epidural combining local anaesthetic and opioid provides excellent pain relief and attenuates the physiological stress-response to surgical trauma by neuroaxial blockade.[55] A recent meta-analysis suggested a beneficial effect on morbidity and mortality,[56] but most of the included trials were conducted in pre-ERAS environments and the role of epidural analgesia as mainstay today is being disputed.[57,58] While epidural infections or haematomas are rare, they may have disastrous consequences. Almost 30% of epidurals have been documented to have suboptimal function, even in high-volume centres.[59] Hypotension following vasodilatation and impaired mobility are other undesirable side-effects that must be weighed against the perceived benefits. Furthermore, many patients experience some degree of 'withdrawal pain' when weaned from epidural analgesia. This pain may be easily controlled by opiates, but the timing is unfortunate as it hits the patient when on the verge of becoming fully mobilised and increasing to a full solid diet. The increasing use of minimally invasive surgery will further reduce the demand for epidural analgesia.

Transverse abdominal plane blocks

These blocks can be arranged in several fashions, usually by a small-bore catheter positioned just superficially to the external oblique fascia, with disposable systems delivering a constant dosage of an anaesthetic. They have some of the benefits of an epidural and fewer side-effects, but they must be applied correctly either intraoperatively or guided by ultrasonography.

Intravenous analgesia

Patient controlled intravenous analgesia (PCA) with opioids is the modern modification of the oldest analgesic modality. It provides a baseline infusion rate with a possibility for a patient-activated boost. PCA remains the fallback option for failed peripheral blocks, as it is easy to set up. Opioid effect may vary however, and accumulated doses affect gut motility, mobilisation and appetite. Continuous infusion of the local anaesthetic lidocaine is receiving increasing attention,[60–62] and may attenuate surgical stress besides boosting the PCA analgesic combination.[61] Another drug group gaining renewed interest are beta-blockers. Besides their well-established cardiovascular effects, they appear to have an intriguing potential as an adjunct in the treatment of postoperative pain.[63,64]

Oral non-opioid analgesics

Non-steroidal anti-inflammatory drugs (NSAIDs) provide excellent analgesic effect for moderate pain and have served as valuable opioid-sparing adjuncts for decades. A possible association with increased rates of anastomotic failures has spurred several studies with conflicting results,[65–68] but high-quality trials are lacking. It is probably prudent to use them with caution in patients with freshly created anastomoses until more data are available. For patients with adequate liver function, paracetamol/acetaminophen is safe and can reduce opioid requirements.

Access and incision

The laparoscopic revolution has significantly impacted on patient recovery, most importantly through attenuated stress-response and reduced pain. While there is an obvious reduction in tissue damage through minimal access surgery, the differences in functional recovery (pain, gut function, mobilisation, length-of-stay) compared to modern ERAS-era open surgery, are much smaller than was previously assumed. Functional recovery is an outcome with high risk of observer bias in open-label trials, but it has received most of the attention. As surgical technique is skill-dependent with a learning curve and hard to blind in trials, this issue is not well suited for randomised design (RCTs).[15] Observational data (non-randomised, prospective cohort studies) are weakened by the possibility of selection bias and publication bias. Importantly, while dedicated centres can boast length-of-stay of 23 hours after laparoscopic colectomy,[69] and 48 hours after open resection,[70,71] these figures are applicable to only a tiny minority of patients. We know far too little about how the vast majority of our patients are faring and data on short-term outcome following different access modalities must be viewed with a high degree of

caution. The modern surgeon should master both techniques and choose the one that is best suited to the patient and the operation.

Perioperative fluid balance, blood pressure, oedema and diuresis

Ensuring adequate oxygen supply to crucial tissues is the core task of intraoperative and immediate postoperative care and is heavily dependent on the patient's fluid balance. The newly created anastomosis is at the periphery of the circulatory bed and has had parts of its natural blood supply severed. Its perfusion is vital to the success of the operation, but at present impossible to assess directly. Among the surrogate markers of tissue perfusion used are peripheral oxygen saturation in the capillaries of the fingers, blood pressure, central venous pressure (CVP) and urine output, as an assumed reflection of renal perfusion. In the presence of some degree of systemic oedema, which is almost invariably the case, the gut is also likely to be oedematous which in turn will compromise local perfusion and hence oxygen delivery. The challenge is to avoid oedema and optimise stroke volume in the well-oxygenised patient.

Intraoperative fluid balance

In the intraoperative period it is important that fluid management is appropriate, to ensure optimal organ perfusion, whilst avoiding fluid overload which can lead to gut oedema and contribute to ileus. It is well recognised that traditional monitoring of arterial and central pressures gives a poor indication of intravascular filling.

A number of techniques are now available intraoperatively for estimation of cardiac output and fluid responsiveness, and provide welcome additional information on which to base intraoperative fluid therapy.

Minimally invasive monitors include arterial pulse contour analysis, which can provide data on stroke volume and variations in pressures and stroke volume when the patient is mechanically ventilated, allowing an estimate of intravascular volume status. Another technique used relatively widely is transoesophageal Doppler, which monitors velocity of blood flow in the descending thoracic aorta from which stroke volume and cardiac output can be calculated.

These are dynamic monitors allowing the anaesthetist to provide a fluid challenge either by placing the patient head-down or by infusing a given volume of fluid and assessing the response.

Algorithms have been published suggesting goals for fluid therapy intraoperatively based on these measurements of stroke volume. A number of studies suggest that application of these may benefit patients by optimising the volume of intraoperative fluid given.[72] Trials evaluating restrictive fluid regimens or the use of goal directed therapy have often been compared to obsolete regimens and almost exclusively included ASA I and II patients.[1,4,74] Data for high-risk patients are lacking. This is an important limitation of these trials, as one must assume that the fittest patients probably have significant safety margins, will cope well with quite poor fluid regimens and may not be in need of any optimisation.[75] As emphasised by recent guidelines, it is probably important to offer ASA III and IV patients a dedicated and optimised fluid guidance led by an experienced anaesthetist to ensure optimal tissue oxygenation.[1,4,76]

Postoperative fluid balance

The impact of surgery and anaesthesia has severe effects on most aspects of the patient's physiology. For most of the first day and night, normal homeostatic mechanisms are blocked or overridden; positive pressure ventilation, intravenous infusion of litres of fluids, bleeding and epidural blocking of peripheral regulation of vascular resistance are just a few of the challenges. Unfortunately this often leads to a situation on the first morning after surgery where the patient weighs several kilos more than the morning of surgery, a sure sign of fluid accumulation. Blood pressure is variable or low, or maintained by vasopressors – especially in patients with epidurals. Urine output is poor. All this can and should be avoided by better per- and immediate postoperative fluid management.

In the immediate postoperative period fluid status is measured less effectively than intraoperatively and the result is a tendency to treat hypotension and low urine output with large volumes of fluids.[73] As hypotension is a recognised side-effect of epidural analgesia and low urine output a part of the physiological response to trauma, fluids exceeding maintenance volumes are unnecessary and probably harmful. At the same time, splanchnic hypovolaemia must be avoided.

Frank postoperative hypotension implies inadequate peripheral perfusion. At what level an individual patient has a clinically significant hypotension is difficult to assess and depends on habitual blood pressure and medication. Significant hypotension must be treated and experimental data indicate that blood pressure should be increased with vasopressors even if these drugs cause some vasoconstriction.[77] If normotension cannot be restored, epidurals should be discontinued and replaced with intravenous analgesics.

Fluids are a medication with side-effects. The surgeon prescribing them must know the sodium and chloride content of the formulas prescribed and the daily needs of the patient.[78] Balanced fluids should be used in place of 0.9% saline,[79] and high chloride content is probably not beneficial.[80] It is also worth recalling that infusion of sodium- and chloride-containing fluids is much harder to reverse than judicious use of vasopressors.

Attempts at correcting low urine output with bolus infusions of fluid are unnecessary and probably counterproductive.[81,82] We don't know if the low output is caused by renal hypoperfusion at all – or, if so, whether fluids will increase perfusion. The gain from an additional litre of fluid may be a negligible change in CVP or vasopressor dosage but the only foreseeable clinical result is overhydration and oedema.

Postoperative care

Nasogastric drainage

The nasogastric (or after gastrectomies: the nasojejunal) drainage tube has been another of the hallmarks of traditional postoperative care. They were believed to be crucial to remove gastrointestinal secretions thereby reducing the risk of aspiration, passage of fluids across a freshly created anastomosis and/or intestinal ileus. Up to a decade ago they could be left in for a week following hemicolectomy.[42] Recent data have shown convincingly that they are unnecessary and even harmful and modern guidelines unanimously advise against routine use.[1-8] A minority of patients will suffer gastric emptying problems following surgery, mostly following Whipple's procedure and partial gastrectomy. These are fewer than previously suggested and may need nasogastric (NG) tube insertion on-demand in selected cases.[4] Oesophageal resections pose specific challenges with a positive pressure environment for a denervated gastric conduit frequently resulting in conduit dilatation and risk of aspiration. Decompression NG tubes should not be removed in these patients without the responsible surgeons being consulted. However, the default routine, in all but oesophageal resections, should be to remove the tube before leaving theatre.

Glycaemic control

The trauma of surgery usually induces a phase of insulin resistance that again leads to poorly controlled serum-glucose levels. Patients at risk who undergo major operations frequently exhibit temporary features of type-II diabetes and an increased susceptibility to infectious complications has been suggested. Reduced rates of infections in critically ill patients intensively treated with insulin were shown in a large trial from 2001,[83] but this has not been reproduced and there are no data to support such treatment outside of the ICU.[84] Modern guidelines suggest glycaemic control well within safety limits to avoid hypoglycaemia.[5]

Abdominal drains

This issue is yet another of the traditional pillars being challenged by modern routines.[1–8] A functioning drain that produces copious volumes of amylase-rich content following a pancreatic resection will appear a success when it dries up after a week without any further intervention. This is not often the situation. A variety of drain types and calibres, passive or with suction, all have a tendency to become clogged or dislodged or kinked, and they are usually painful for the patient. A dry drain is either a signal that the patient is doing well, or that the drain is doing badly. There are other – and better – ways of telling the former. Even for pancreatic surgery, where routine use of drains has been studied extensively,[4] robust conclusions are wanting in spite of stratifying patients according to duct calibre and gland texture or volume. The jury is still out regarding the correct cut-off, but pancreatic resections and urology aside,[1,4] the tendency is to use them less and less in straightforward cases. The development of interventional radiology in recent decades has played a part in relinquishing previous practices of routine drainage: wide availability of modern ultrasound- or CT-guided drainage procedures means that most abscesses, bilomas, haematomas or other fluid accumulations may be drained percutaneously on demand with a small-bore drain that may later be up-sized if necessary.

Stimulation of bowel movement

Some degree of gut paralysis (ileus) will follow any abdominal operation, but the spectrum of clinical conditions is considerable. The small bowel may regain function almost immediately; the remnant stomach after Whipple's procedure will sometimes need a week or more. Following a large bowel resection, ileus is common and the typical duration is 1–3 days. The symptoms are vomiting or gastric distension needing decompression by tube, abdominal distension, nausea and pain. On top of a major operation, it is a very uncomfortable situation. When duration exceeds a few days, the condition impedes mobilisation, halts intake of food and drink and causes anxiety – to both patient and surgeon. Stimulating return of gut function after surgery is a key target for perioperative care. The following options may be considered.

The strategy should be multimodal. Comprehensive protocols, like modern enhanced recovery guidelines,[1–8] have focused extensively on these strategies. It is highly likely that the sum of many small adjustments of the perioperative pathway acting in concert will shorten the duration of postoperative gut paralysis to a minimum.

- Early oral intake of food and drink is thought to aid in stimulating bowel movement, but this is hard to prove scientifically as the intervention itself becomes the target. It is, however, likely that vagal stimulation by smell, taste, chewing and swallowing helps stimulate bowel movement.

- Chewing gum has been proposed as a cheap and safe way of achieving the same stimulation of vagal reflexes even in patients who do not yet have appetite for eating. However, the effect of postoperative chewing of gum has been evaluated in several trials and the results are conflicting.[85] If all other measures have been applied (enhanced recovery protocols), additional effect of chewing gum has not been proven.[85]

- Optimal fluid balance avoiding both hypovolaemia and gut oedema.[86]

- Epidural analgesia with local anaesthetics in combination with low doses of opioids was for decades a cornerstone of modern regimens.[2,5] The 'opioid-sparing' effect of the epidural was considered a crucial part of the enhanced recovery protocol. The increased use of laparoscopy, comprehensive protocols, modern opioids with fewer motility-blocking effects and other non-opioid analgesic drugs have caused a shift in interest away from the routine use of epidural analgesia.

- Minimally invasive surgery (i.e. laparoscopy) causes less gut manipulation and less tissue trauma and is hence associated with shorter duration of postoperative ileus.

- Several pharmaceutical interventions have received considerable attention, but the magic drug remains elusive. Alvimopan is a partial μ-receptor antagonist available in the USA. The effect on gut function postoperatively has been evaluated in several studies with conflicting results,[87–90] and additional benefit for patients already treated by modern, enhanced recovery routines is disputed.[91,92] Alvimopan is currently not available for routine use in Europe.

- Magnesium oxide (laxative) was an integral part of the first ERAS guidelines mainly aiming at open colonic surgery.[2] A placebo-controlled trial conducted for colonic surgery in the context of modern enhanced recovery principles failed to confirm a beneficial effect.[93]

✓✓ There is no compelling evidence that any single intervention to stimulate gut activity can be recommended, but a multimodal approach as suggested in ERAS guidelines will reduce the duration of postoperative gut dysfunction.

Postoperative artificial nutrition

It is important to distinguish oral intake, i.e. eating, which is the volitional and natural intake of ordinary food, from enteral nutrition. Enteral nutrition is a non-volitional, artificial way of providing nutrients through tube or catheter. Nil-by-mouth implies that the patient does not eat or drink, regardless of whether enteral tube feeding is provided or not. The enteral versus parenteral nutrition controversy of the 1990s obscured this distinction and wrongly grouped enteral nutrition with natural oral diet.[94]

With the exception – again – for patients undergoing oesophagectomy, all patients should have their NG tubes removed and be offered drink and food without delay postoperatively, as soon as they are fully awake and not bothered by nausea. Oral intake at will has been a part of colorectal and liver guidelines for a decade or more.[2,5,8] Oral diet at will is now also recommended for gastrectomies and pancreaticoduodenectomies (Whipple's resections).[4,6] Care is required following Whipple's resections as some patients may also have a problem with gastric motility. This means that they need to be well counselled about their altered physiology and digestion. They should be advised to begin carefully and increase according to tolerance.[4,6]

Some patients will need enteral tube feeding or parenteral nutrition, but – save oesophagectomies – this is the exception. Even patients who have undergone emergency surgery for obstruction or perforation will generally tolerate food within 2–4 days. Artificial nutrition becomes an option in a patient who cannot eat. This might be due to rare cases of delayed gastric emptying, long-standing gut paralysis, reoperations, complications, unconscious patients etc.

Routine provisions of hypercaloric supplements to patients who are eating have been evaluated in colorectal surgery. Beneficial effects on surrogate endpoints like hand grip strength or insulin resistance are regularly demonstrated,[95] but effects on robust clinical endpoints have not been convincingly shown. One trial showed an impressive reduction from 9 to 6.5 days length of stay (LoS), but without any difference in hand grip strength or time to return of gut function.[96] Such findings must be viewed with caution as bias is highly probable and must be confirmed or refuted by placebo-controlled double-blinded trials with an iso-nitrogenous control. Neither post-discharge oral supplements[97] nor intense dietary advice to patients at risk have been shown to confer benefit.[98]

✓✓ All patients – save those undergoing oesophagectomy – should as a routine have their NG tube removed as they leave theatre and be offered to drink and eat on demand.

Early and scheduled mobilisation

Mobilisation prevents loss of lean muscle and thromboembolic complications. Being independently mobile is an inherent part of the composite process we call functional recovery. It is probably easier to achieve independent mobilisation if there are set targets to be met and when the patient has a schedule to adhere to.[2,5] There are no RCTs to prove this, but it is a concept unsuited for this methodology and probably unethical to attempt it!

Key points

- The perioperative period starts at the moment surgery has been decided and ends when the patient's functional recovery is complete.
- The entire period is a target for the care-giving professionals to make surgery safer and to enhance recovery.
- The surgeon and the anaesthetist have complementary expertise and should cooperate in risk assessment, optimisation and prehabilitation.
- Perioperative care can be broken down to a set of care items and many of these are now corroborated by strong evidence.
- Enhanced recovery protocols are compiled sets of care items that will standardise the patient journey and improve recovery.

⊕ Full references available at **http://expertconsult. inkling.com**

Key references

1. Cerantola Y, Valerio M, Persson B, et al. Guidelines for perioperative care after radical cystectomy for bladder cancer: enhanced Recovery After Surgery (ERAS((R))) society recommendations. Clin Nutr 2013;32(6):879–87. PMID: 24189391.
   Evidence-based perioperative care guidelines issued by the ERAS Society for a range of surgical specialities – see other key references listed below.

3. Gustafsson UO, Scott MJ, Schwenk W, et al. Guidelines for perioperative care in elective colonic surgery: Enhanced Recovery After Surgery (ERAS(R)) Society recommendations. Clin Nutr 2012;31(6):783–800. PMID: 23099039.

4. Lassen K, Coolsen MM, Slim K, et al. Guidelines for perioperative care for pancreaticoduodenectomy: Enhanced Recovery After Surgery (ERAS(R)) Society recommendations. Clin Nutr 2012;31(6): 817–30. PMID: 23079762.

6. Mortensen K, Nilsson M, Slim K, et al. Consensus guidelines for enhanced recovery after gastrectomy: Enhanced Recovery After Surgery (ERAS(R)) Society recommendations. Br J Surg 2014;101(10):1209–29. PMID: 25047143.

7. Nygren J, Thacker J, Carli F, et al. Guidelines for perioperative care in elective rectal/pelvic surgery: Enhanced Recovery After Surgery (ERAS) Society recommendations. Clin Nutr 2012;31(6):801–16. PMID: 23062720.

3

Organisation of emergency general surgical services

Simon Paterson-Brown

Introduction

Emergency general surgery remains a significant part of the work of all general surgeons and not surprisingly contributes to the majority of the morbidity and mortality of general surgery as well as hospital resources. This has now been recognised by many Colleges, specialist associations and hospitals so that emergency patients are increasingly being managed by a multidisciplinary emergency team in emergency wards and supported by appropriate resources. This is unfortunately not yet widespread and much work is still to be done and the increasing expense of healthcare in general and surgical services in particular has a major influence on how future services will be provided. This is particularly apparent when comparing high-, middle- and low-income countries where the mortality from emergency surgery is three times higher between the low- and high-income countries.[1] When the American College of Surgeons National Surgical Quality Improvement Project examined the results of emergency appendicectomy, cholecystectomy and colorectal resections in 95 hospitals between 2005 and 2008,[2] they found that the risk of severe morbidity or death was 3.7% in the 30788 appendicectomies performed, 6.37% in the 5824 cholecystectomies and 41.56% in the 8990 colorectal resections. Interestingly, they also identified that in 7–10% of hospitals good or bad performance could be generalisable across these three procedures, suggesting that there are 'best' and 'worst' practices to be identified. A more recent study, again from the USA,[3] examined 421476 patients who required emergency general surgery between 2008 and 2011. This study identified the seven most common

procedures that represented 80% of activity, 80% of the mortality, 79% of the morbidity and 80% of the costs as: partial colectomy, small-bowel resection, cholecystectomy, operative management of peptic ulcer disease, lysis of peritoneal adhesions, appendicectomy and laparotomy.

Reduced length of stay and improvements in patient care are not surprisingly associated with earlier and better clinical decision-making, prompt and appropriate surgery, along with reductions in re-admissions and later requirements for surgery. This is made possible by separating emergency and elective surgical care,[4] which has now become commonplace in the UK and increasingly worldwide. In many places this has been facilitated by regional reorganisation of surgical services. In the USA and Canada there is now a specialist association of Acute Care Surgery (http://www.aast.org/AcuteCareSurgery). The variation worldwide in operative experience for trainees in general surgery remains a concern[5] and therefore concentrating more emergency activity in fewer hospitals, through which trainees rotate, does provide better opportunities for 'out of hours' training. Further improvements are also seen by the early assessment of patients by experienced senior surgeons with easy access to radiological investigations and operating theatres for timely surgical intervention,[4] preferably by someone with an interest in that condition.[6] The Association of Surgeons of Great Britain and Ireland (ASGBI) held a consensus meeting on the future of emergency general surgery in 2006, subsequently publishing their conclusions[7] which are summarised in Box 3.1. A subsequent survey of consultant surgeons in the UK by the ASGBI[8] reported then that: only 55% considered they were able to care well for their emergency patients; the workload was increasing with junior support decreasing; only 19% had comprehensive interventional radiology service out of hours; 55% had inadequate access to an emergency theatre; current pressure within the NHS favoured elective over emergency work; many felt they could not argue the case for change at a local level; and many felt that helpful changes would include national standards of practice and of service delivery, proper theatre access, and increased separation of elective and emergency work. As a result, and combined with the recent trend of some general surgeons wishing to pursue a dedicated subspecialist interest in emergency surgery, the ASGBI set up an Emergency General Surgery Board[9] which specifically looks at ways of improving the delivery of all aspects of emergency general surgery and supporting those who provide this care.

There remains no doubt as to the overall need to improve emergency general surgical provision. The results of an audit of 367,796 emergency general surgical operations for higher-risk surgical conditions (average national 30-day mortality rate >5%) in 145 hospitals in England between 2000 and 2009 demonstrated an overall 30-day mortality of 15.6% (range 9.2–18.2%).[10] Independent risk factors between low- and high-performing hospitals included access to critical care beds and early use of computed tomography (CT). The resources available in all hospitals providing emergency surgical care and the subsequent outcomes is clearly an important issue and is confirmed by another study undertaken during a similar time period (2005–2010), which again looked at the higher-risk emergency general surgical patients.[11] This study demonstrated a mortality for all patients admitted (not just undergoing emergency surgery) between 1.6% and 8% and again showed a significant difference between hospitals based on their staffing and infrastructure, the lowest mortality rates being observed in hospitals with higher levels of medical

and nursing staffing, and a greater number of operating theatres and critical care beds relative to provider size.

Separation of elective and emergency surgery

Where in the past the continuity of care for surgical patients was maintained by the 'middle grade' surgical team, current rotas are now primarily of a shift pattern where the maximum time worked per week is around 48 hours and as a result consultants find they rarely work with the same trainees,[12] and the continuity of care is reduced.[13] One solution to this problem was the introduction of the 'surgeon of the day', first suggested in 1995,[14] and then fully implemented in Edinburgh, UK, as the 'emergency team' in 1997.[15] With this system, the whole surgical team (consultant and supporting junior staff) have no elective commitments for their time on-call, and, although unfortunately shift working remains essential in many countries due to restricted working hours, the same trainees take part in the emergency team for extended periods of time, thus re-introducing the old 'team' structure. Their subsequent attachment to elective activity then no longer suffers from the disruption associated with intermittent on-call shifts, a state of affairs that enhances both emergency and elective training opportunities. This 'emergency team' system, with various adaptations according to local requirements,[16] has now been adopted in most units throughout the UK and increasingly worldwide. Two recent publications from the Association of Surgeons of Great Britain and Ireland include descriptions of the different ways that individual hospitals and regions in the UK have changed their service in order to improve the provision of emergency surgical services.[17,18] Box 3.2 provides recommendations published by the Royal College of Surgeons of England[4] for the separation of elective and emergency general surgery.

The emergency team undoubtedly improves the ability of the consultant general surgeon, as well as the middle-grade team, to provide safe and effective emergency care, but requires other conditions to be met if this is to be both efficient and cost-effective, not only in terms of lost elective activity for the consultant, but also training opportunities for the surgical trainees. These include easy access to radiological imaging, a dedicated emergency operating theatre with full (and senior) anaesthetic support available 24 hours each day,[19] enough surgical admissions to make the system worthwhile, and a distinct and dedicated admission area for emergency patients to be assessed. This is particularly useful in the assessment of patients with equivocal clinical signs, such as in early appendicitis, where the

Box 3.2 • Summary of recommendations for separation of emergency and elective surgical care[4]

1. A physical separation of services, facilities and rotas works best, although a separate unit on the same site is preferable to a completely separate location.
2. The presence of senior surgeons for both elective and emergency work will enhance patient safety and the quality of care, and ensure that training opportunities are maximised.
3. The separation of emergency and elective surgical care can facilitate protected and concentrated training for junior surgeons providing consultants are available to supervise their work.
4. Creating an 'emergency team', linked with a 'surgeon of the week', is a good method of providing dedicated and supervised training in all aspects of emergency and elective care.
5. Separating emergency and elective services can prevent the admission of emergency patients (both medical and surgical) from disrupting planned activity and vice versa, thus minimising patient inconvenience and maximising productivity for the hospital. The success of this will largely depend on having sufficient beds and resources for each service.
6. Hospital-acquired infections can be reduced by the provision of protected elective wards and avoiding admissions from the emergency department and transfers from within/outside the hospital.
7. The improved use of IT (information technology) solutions can assist with separating workloads (for example, scheduling systems for appointments and theatres, telemedicine, picture archiving and communication systems, etc.), although it is recognised that developments in IT for the NHS are generally behind schedule.
8. High-volume specialities are particularly suited to separating two strands of work. Other specialities can also benefit by having emergencies seen by senior surgeons – this can help to reduce unnecessary admissions, deal with ward emergencies and facilitate rapid discharge.

value of 'active observation' with reassessment after 2–3 hours by the same surgeon, repeated thereafter as necessary, is well established.[20]

> ✔✔ Emergency general surgery should be provided by a team that is free of elective commitments. All emergency general surgical patients should be admitted to a single dedicated admission area within the hospital where they can be assessed and reviewed by the admitting surgical team. This should be supported by easy access to an emergency operating theatre and appropriate and timely radiological investigations.[4,7]

Subspecialisation in emergency general surgery

Along with the recognition that emergency surgery deserves more attention and support has also come the recognition that specialist conditions are often better treated by surgeons with a particular interest and experience in that sub-speciality. This has of course been recognised for some time in the elective performance of a number of surgical procedures, including oesophagectomy, gastrectomy, abdominal aortic aneurysm repair, lung lobectomy, cardiac surgery and colectomy,[21,22] and although mainly thought to be related to hospital and surgeon volumes,[23] specialisation of the surgical team also appears to be an important factor.[24] However, there are now data available to support similar improvements in patient

outcomes for emergency conditions, such as acute gallstone disease,[25,26] and acute colorectal disorders.[27] This is not surprising considering the subspecialisation that has occurred in elective general surgery over the last decade,[28] with consultant surgeons now being expected to deal with surgical conditions in the emergency situation which they rarely, or no longer, see in their elective practice.

Reports of the separation of upper and lower elective and emergency gastrointestinal (GI) services in one region of Scotland have been encouraging. Not only has there been a significant increase in the number of patients with acute gallstone problems undergoing same-admission laparoscopic cholecystectomy,[29] there have also been improvements in the management of perforated duodenal ulcers[30] and acute diverticulitis where patients have a lower mortality and fewer stomas.[31] The challenge now is for all those surgeons involved in the development and provision of emergency surgical care to produce on-call rotas that allow, where possible, patients with specific subspeciality conditions to be treated and operated upon by surgeons with a specific interest in that area. This will undoubtedly involve reorganisation of regional emergency surgical services, bringing together a wider group of surgeons for the on-call rota, with the ability to provide both upper and lower GI cover. The political hurdles of closing or downgrading emergency services in some hospitals in order to provide these larger emergency surgical units in other hospitals must not be underestimated. However, they must be overcome if the undoubted improvements in patient care associated with dedicated emergency surgical services delivered by surgical teams with appropriate subspeciality expertise are to be realised, while at the same time providing robust junior doctor rotas that comply with the appropriate working time directives.

Process and facilities

For an emergency team system to work efficiently patients must have rapid access to diagnostic blood tests and appropriate imaging, which should include plain and contrast radiology, both diagnostic and interventional (percutaneous drainage and angiography), ultrasound (US) and computed tomography (CT). There is increasing use of Interventional Radiology networks as not all hospitals receiving emergencies have this expertise, similarly with the provision of interventional endoscopy for gastrointestinal bleeding. These and other diagnostic modalities are discussed in more detail in Chapter 11. However, it is essential that where possible appropriate use is made of the diagnostic investigations available. It has been known for many years that plain radiography evaluated by senior radiologists substantially enhances senior surgical assessment of patients with acute abdominal pain, resulting in reduced surgical admissions.[32] This can now be moved on to include CT reporting. A recent UK audit of emergency abdominal CT for acute abdominal pain examined the diagnostic accuracy of the reporting in 4931 patients, approximately half surgical and half non-surgical.[33] In the surgical group 36/132 patients who had a major discrepancy in the provisional report were considered to have come to harm: delay in diagnosis, delay in surgery, inappropriate surgery and unnecessary further investigations. The risk of major discrepancies was reduced by on-site consultant reporting, as compared to off-site reporting.

There remains some controversy as to whether admission during the week or at weekends alters risk of mortality in surgical patients. One very large study that retrospectively examined 14,217,640 patients admitted to NHS England hospitals as an emergency between 2009 and 2010 observed 187,337 in-hospital deaths within 30 days.[34] This study included all patients from all specialities and noted the risk of death was higher following admission at the weekend. Another study focusing on 294,602 emergency general surgical patients during a similar time period in England also demonstrated a small but significant increase in mortality for those patients admitted over the weekend,[11] suggesting that it may be the potential resource difference which was important. When day of the week for elective colorectal resections is examined

there again appears to be a difference in mortality for patients operated on a Friday compared to Monday through Thursday,[35] but when examined in more detail the difference appeared to be due to patient-related factors rather than anything about their care. Another study found a difference in mortality according to day of operation, being worse at weekend, but not day of admission.[36] However, these findings have not been confirmed by a smaller study published recently which looked at 50 844 general surgical patients in Scotland who underwent emergency surgery between 2005 and 2007 and were followed up until 2012.[37] This study failed to demonstrate any difference in either short- or long-term mortality according to whether the surgery took place during the week or at the weekend. The jury is therefore probably still out on the significance of mortality according to day of admission or day of surgery, due to a number of confounding variables which include degree of emergency, type of surgery and whether the surgery is carried out during the day or night. Suffice to say that we would all hope that patients would get the same care whichever day they were admitted or operated upon and it is the responsibility of the local healthcare managers and surgical teams to ensure that this is possible. Resources will undoubtedly be one of the issues and these studies do suggest that where similar staffing structures and standards exist between midweek care and that at weekends, mortality is lower than where they are not.

Many of these studies led directly to the first National Emergency Laparotomy Audit (NELA)[38] which was carried out on around 20,000 patients in 192 NHS hospitals in England and Wales. The aim of the audit was to examine how many patients received what was considered to be the recommended standard of care based on accepted guidelines (see Box 3.3).

The first NELA report[38] demonstrated an overall mortality of 11.7% and not surprisingly there was a wide variation in reaching the above targets in many hospitals. The second NELA report[39] measured similar but more refined standards of care as shown below, in 186 hospitals and in the region of 23,000 patients, with a slightly lower mortality of 11.1%. The revised standards of care are shown in Box 3.4.

Again there was a wide variation between hospitals in their ability to reach these standards but a general overall improvement was seen. What seems clear from all these data and studies is that the delivery of emergency general surgical care must be separated from elective activity, delivered by a dedicated multidisciplinary team with appropriate resources that include access to beds, radiology, critical care and fully staffed operating theatres.

All these studies have resulted in further attempts to improve the outcomes for emergency abdominal surgery. One recent report implemented an acute high-risk abdominal surgery (AHA) protocol

1 Before surgery
- Clinical review and formulation of a care plan by a consultant surgeon soon after admission to hospital.
- Ready availability of diagnostic investigations to help define the need for and type of surgery.
- Formal assessment of a patient's risk of death and complications.
- Prompt administration of antibiotics where there is evidence of infection.
- Prompt access to an operating theatre.

2 During surgery
- Direct care by a consultant surgeon and consultant anaesthetist.

3 After surgery
- Planned admission to critical care for patients when the estimated risk of death exceeds 5%.
- Review of patients older than 70 years by specialists in Medicine for Care of the Older Person.

Box 3.4 • Revised standards of care for managing emergency general surgical patients who require laparotomy as defined in the second NELA

1 Timeliness of care
- Review by a consultant surgeon within 14 hours of admission.
- Prompt administration of antibiotics (when indicated).
- CT scans reported by a consultant radiologist before surgery.
- Access to theatres without delay.

2 Appropriate level of care guided by assessment of risks of complications and death
- Documented assessment, before surgery, of the risks of surgery.
- Review before surgery by consultant surgeon and anaesthetist for high-risk patients.
- Presence of consultant surgeon and anaesthetist in theatre for high-risk patients.
- Admission to critical care after surgery for high-risk patients.
- Input from Elderly Medicine specialists in the care of older patient.

involving: continuous staff education; consultant-led attention and care; early resuscitation and high-dose antibiotics; surgery within 6 hours; perioperative stroke volume-guided haemodynamic optimisation; intermediate level of care for the first 24 hours after surgery; standardised analgesic treatment; early postoperative ambulation and early enteral nutrition.[40] This protocol was used for 600 patients and the outcome compared with 600 historical controls. The unadjusted 30-day mortality rate was significantly higher at 21.8% in the control cohort compared with 15.5% in the intervention cohort. The 180-day mortality rates were also significantly higher at 29.5% compared to 22.2%, respectively. Another study involved the introduction of an emergency laparotomy pathway quality improvement care (ELPQuiC) bundle into four hospitals in England.[41] The care bundle consisted of: initial assessment with early warning scores, early antibiotics, interval between decision and operation less than 6 hours, goal-directed fluid therapy and postoperative intensive care. There was an associated increase in the numbers of lives saved per 100 patients treated in all hospitals, from 6.47 in the baseline interval (299 patients) to 12.44 after implementation (427 patients), with an overall risk of death reduced from 15.6% to 9.6%.

What also has to be remembered is that many emergency operations in hospital relate to complications from elective surgery, so there needs to be a robust system in every hospital for managing such patients. What has been clearly demonstrated in colorectal surgery is that failure to rescue patients with complications is a valuable marker as to the overall standard of care of that unit/hospital.[42] The management of such patients is often complex and high risk, and provides further support for the overall view that consultant surgeons need to be available 7 days a week.[43] This needs to be arranged between colleagues and teams if the high standards of care demonstrated in some units are to be mirrored in every hospital. The paper from the Academy of Medical Royal Colleges[43] provides very clear standards for consultant-delivered care across the board in all specialities, not just surgery:

Standard 1: Hospital inpatients should be reviewed by an on-site consultant at least once every 24 hours, 7 days a week, unless it has been determined that this would not affect the patient's care pathway.

Standard 2: Consultant-supervised interventions and investigations along with reports should be provided 7 days a week if the results will change the outcome or status of the patient's care pathway before the next 'normal' working day. This should include interventions which will enable immediate discharge or a shortened length of hospital stay.

Standard 3: Support services both in hospitals and in the primary care setting in the community should be available 7 days a week to ensure that the next steps in the patient's care pathway, as determined by the daily consultant-led review, can be taken.

Emergency general surgery 'Hot Clinics'

Over the past few years many attempts have been made to try to increase consultant involvement in emergency general surgery care and especially the early decision-making. While it has been shown to help the overall outcome for emergency surgery, as demonstrated by the NELA audits,[38,39] there have been fewer data to say whether similar improvements are associated with early patient assessment at the time of presentation. While this has clear implications on resource, if it results in a significant reduction in inappropriate admission to hospital and earlier decisions for appropriate investigations and/or surgery then it might provide overall value for money. As a result, the surgical unit in Bradford, UK, introduced a general surgical 'Triage Unit' or 'Hot Clinic',[44] to facilitate early senior surgical assessment. Early results have shown reduced admissions and better scheduling of urgent surgical procedures, such as drainage of abscesses and acute cholecystectomies. Such a clinic allows a number of activities to occur: general practitioners to refer directly to a consultant surgeon for a quick assessment; a quicker review of patients with acute abdominal pain in the emergency department; and senior review the following day of patients sent home during the night. Such a clinic must have easy access to radiological investigations (US, CT and MRCP as required), bed space for short-term observation and review, as well as both nursing and trainee doctors' support. Once set up, the workload can be quite substantial but one recent study demonstrated admission rate can be reduced from 85% to 48% and overall length of stay of emergency patients from 64 to 49 hours.[45] Such a service is also a very good place for teaching of undergraduates and foundation doctors, with protected exposure to emergency patients directly supervised by a consultant surgeon.

Summary

There is no doubt that the delivery of emergency general surgical care has improved significantly over the past 5 years or so, supported by the Colleges, Associations and individual hospitals. Efficiencies in delivery have been assisted by regional reorganisation of services, separation of elective and emergency surgical services and, in some units, dividing upper and lower GI care. Provision of acute receiving wards and observation facilities greatly helps such service delivery along with senior-surgeon-delivered 'Hot Clinics'. Resources in each hospital must be put in place to facilitate the optimum management of emergency general surgical patients and these need to include the bundles of care and protocols associated with improved outcomes discussed earlier. These include: early consultant assessment and decision-making as well as direct involvement in emergency surgery; ready access to appropriate investigations including CT with consultant radiologist reporting; and appropriate use and access to critical care beds. The ideal service model may not yet have been reached, but at least many units are now well on the way to such a situation and their support in helping other units move in the same direction is essential if we are to deliver the type of emergency general surgical care which we would all like to receive for ourselves and our family.

Key points

- Regular reassessment of patients admitted with acute abdominal pain is essential and facilities should be provided so that emergency patients are kept in an area of the hospital where regular review is facilitated. Introduction of a consultant-led 'Hot Clinic' further facilitates this process, reduces hospital admissions and speeds up decision-making.
- The ability to provide adequate emergency surgical care, with careful observation, reassessment and early access to the operating theatre, is best provided by dedicated emergency surgical teams without elective commitments.
- Swift access to investigations and an emergency theatre is an essential requisite for the appropriate management of patients with acute abdominal pain.
- Although emergency subspecialisation has great attractions for the overall care of the emergency patient with complex problems, this area of development will depend very much on local resources, requirements and workload.

⊕ Full references available at **http://expertconsult. inkling.com**

Key references

4. The Royal College of Surgeons of England. Separating emergency and elective surgical care: recommendations for practice. 2007. [Online] https://www.rcseng.ac.uk/search/#SearchTerm=separating emergency and elective surgical care 2007.

Strong support and recommendations for the separation of emergency and elective surgical care.

7. Association of Surgeons of Great Britain and Ireland. Emergency general surgery: The future. A consensus statement. June 2007. http://asgbidocuments. surgicalmembershipportal.co.uk/Consensus%20 Statment/egs_statement_july07_.pdf.

This consensus statement provides details of the current problems in the provision of emergency general surgery and recommendations for improving practice.

4

Patient assessment and surgical risk

Chris Deans

Introduction

Surgical risk is an estimation of the likelihood of an adverse event occurring as a consequence of a patient undergoing a particular surgical procedure or intervention. Patient assessment is a process that attempts to quantify this risk for an individual patient. The ability to undertake individualised assessment to determine surgical risk for a patient is fundamental to modern surgical practice. It informs decision-making by both surgeon and patient and facilitates the process of informed consent. It is important to remember that risk is not only associated with surgical procedures, but includes other treatments or investigations that may pose a particular risk to the patient, for example performing a colonoscopy or interventional radiological procedure. The risks of not performing a particular procedure or intervention should also be considered and the possible implications for the patient of not undertaking a procedure should be part of any informed consent process (Box 4.1).[1] Individualisation of surgical risk is fundamental to informed consent for every patient.

Why assess surgical risk?

Estimation of surgical risk is important for several reasons. Firstly, as already stated, determining a

patient's risk influences surgical decision-making and, in turn, facilitates informed consent. This process underpins the choice of treatment options for individual patients. Secondly, identifying higher-risk patients allows appropriate pre-emptive measures to target particular areas of concern and optimise the patient in the perioperative period (see also Chapter 2). This process may also help anticipate potential adverse events. A further positive effect of this process is to aid case mix adjustment. There is increasing public availability of surgical activity/outcome figures (or 'league tables'), which may include crude mortality or complication rates. Case mix adjustment allows units with a greater proportion of high-risk patients to compensate for any differences in their figures compared to national outcomes and allow meaningful comparison of data against national audits. This is an important aspect of future quality assurance (Box 4.2).

How can we assess surgical risk?

Determination of surgical risk is complex and is influenced by many variables. However, the process may be simplified by thinking of the assessment according to two main factors – the patient, and those related to the surgical procedure itself. **Procedural-related risks** are generally easier to quantify where national, local and even individual complication rates may be known. The introduction of national and regional audit programmes in some specialities, as well as improved quality of data collection in local departments, have enabled a better understanding of the more common risks and complications associated with many surgical procedures. However, procedural-related risk will also depend on additional factors, such as the urgency and duration of the procedure, volume of blood loss and type of surgery undertaken. The UK National Institute for Health and Care Excellence (NICE) has attempted to stratify surgical procedures into different grades of severity in an effort to provide guidance on the use of preoperative investigations and estimate perioperative risk (Table 4.1).[2]

Patient-related risk factors are less easy to quantify. They may be broadly divided into either subjective or objective factors. Subjective risk assessment includes patient history, clinical examination, pattern recognition, accumulated clinical experience and 'the end of the bed test'. Objective risk assessment includes formal laboratory results and assessment of comorbidity and physiological function through further investigation. Patient factors will be influenced by the 'fitness' of the patient (functional/performance status), age, comorbid illness, the underlying disease process and nutritional status, as well as many other inter-related variables.

Several risk prediction models and scoring systems have been developed in an attempt to help measure surgical risk. In addition, techniques to formally quantify patient fitness (functional assessment), such as exercise testing, and measurements of serum biomarkers have also been introduced specifically to predict perioperative risk, with varying success. This chapter will discuss some of the scoring systems and functional assessment tools that may be used for patient assessment and estimation of surgical risk. These may be broadly classified into risk prediction models (general and specific), functional assessment tools and novel biomarkers.

Estimation of surgical risk

Clinical assessment

It is the role of the surgeon as a clinician to undertake a thorough clinical assessment of every patient in order to identify individual characteristics of the patient's comorbidity and underlying disease process that may influence surgical risk. Only then may a fully informed decision be made regarding treatment choices for individual patients. Some patient factors may be clearly identifiable, such as the presence of ischaemic heart disease or obesity, whereas others may not yet have been diagnosed. A thorough history and examination should be undertaken and targeted investigations requested based on the clinical findings. More challenging patients should involve consultation with colleagues and other clinicians as part of the wider multidisciplinary team – for example, obtaining a cardiology review or asking for an anaesthetic opinion. In difficult cases a second opinion may be sought from an independent source. The experienced clinician's 'gut instinct' or 'surgical intuition' can be more effective than formal risk prediction models in identifying the patient with a poor prognosis in the context of a particular procedure, especially in the elective setting.[3,4] However, there is also epidemiological evidence suggesting that clinicians often fail to identify patients at high risk of complications and as a result do not allocate them to the appropriate level of perioperative care.[5]

Risk prediction models and scoring systems

Attempts to improve the accuracy of estimation of risk and to provide a more robust quantitative assessment have led to the development of several scoring systems and risk prediction models.[6] Many of these are freely available online or through mobile applications (listed in Box 4.3). These tools have been developed to calculate estimated morbidity and mortality rates for individual patients prior to the proposed intervention. It should be noted that there

Table 4.1 • Examples of surgical procedures by severity grading (NICE)

Grade 1	Grade 2	Grade 3	Grade 4
Upper gastrointestinal endoscopy	Haemorrhoidectomy	Amputation	Gastrectomy
Vasectomy	Varicose vein surgery	Mastectomy	Colectomy
Tooth extraction	Adenoidectomy	Thyroidectomy	Renal transplant
Excision skin lesion	Reduction of dislocated joint	Prostatectomy	Hip replacement

Source: National Institute for Health and Care Excellence, NICE Guideline [NG45], April 2016.

P-POSSUM/O-POSSUM-CR-POSSUM/V-POSSUM – http://www.riskprediction.org.uk/
Surgical Risk Calculator – http://riskcalculator.facs.org/RiskCalculator/PatientInfo.jsp
Surgical Outcome Risk Tool – http://sortsurgery.com
Revised Cardiac Risk Index – http://www.mdcalc.com/revised-cardiac-risk-index-pre-operative-risk/

is no perfect tool, that the models available must not be used to guide decision-making in isolation and that there is no substitute for the combination of objective markers with surgical experience and intuition. Furthermore, the models available pertain to populations rather than individual patients, and therefore have limitations that need to be recognised before using them to inform surgical risk assessment. For example, the mortality rate for a surgical intervention in a particular population may be 5%, but for the individual patient it can only be 0% or 100%. As such these models should be considered as tools to aid risk stratification for a patient, rather than providing an individual risk profile.

The scoring systems available usually incorporate physiological and comorbidity data that have been selected using logistical regression techniques in a large database of patients, which may not be similar to the local population. A coefficient may be assigned in order to weight the variables and the resulting equation provides a numerical indication of risk for the patient, although it is frequently more meaningful to the operating surgeon.

Ideally, the patients in the database on which the scoring system is developed and validated should be similar to the individual patient in question. However, publication bias may mean that only the best outcome data are published. While this has inherent flaws, it may also be viewed as an opportunity to benchmark one's own results against those from other centres.

Finally, the accuracy of predictive models is dynamic and they should be retested periodically against an evolving surgical patient population. When accuracy deteriorates, models should be revised and updated.

POSSUM

The Physiological and Operative Severity Score for the enUmeration of Mortality and morbidity (POSSUM) was first described in 1991.[7] Designed as a scoring system to estimate morbidity and mortality following a surgical procedure and, by including data on the patient's physiological

condition, it provides a risk-adjusted prediction of outcome. This facilitates more accurate comparison of hospital or surgeon performance and it can be used as an audit and clinical governance tool. However, the model involves inclusion of operative variables, such as volume of blood loss and the presence of peritoneal soiling, which precludes its use in the preoperative setting to inform the consent process. Despite this, POSSUM is the most widely applied, validated, surgical risk scoring system in the UK and has been modified by several authors to provide speciality-specific information.

The original POSSUM score was developed after initially subjecting 62 parameters to multivariate analysis in order to determine the most powerful outcome predictors. Twelve physiological and six operative parameters were identified, and each of these factors weighted to a value of 1, 2, 4 or 8 to simplify the calculation. It was re-evaluated in 1998 in Portsmouth, UK by Whiteley et al., who reported concerns that it overestimated mortality in their patients, particularly in the lowest risk group.[8] The POSSUM formula was modified to create the Portsmouth predictor equation for mortality (P-POSSUM; Box 4.4). The modified formula fitted well with the observed mortality rate; however, it still overestimates mortality in low-risk groups, the elderly and in certain surgical subspecialities.[9] The latter finding has prompted the development

Box 4.4 • Variables used in the calculation of the P-POSSUM score

Physiological variables
Age
Cardiac disease
Respiratory disease
Electrocardiogram (ECG)
Systolic blood pressure
Pulse rate
Haemoglobin concentration
White cell count
Serum urea concentration
Serum sodium concentration
Serum potassium concentration
Glasgow Coma Scale (GCS)

Operative variables
Operation severity class
Number of procedures
Blood loss
Peritoneal contamination
Malignancy status
Urgency

P-POSSUM formula
$\text{Ln } R/1 - R = -9.065 + (0.1692 \times \text{physiological score}) + (0.1550 \times \text{operative severity score})$

of speciality-specific POSSUM for major elective surgery.

CR-POSSUM (colorectal)

The value of POSSUM and P-POSSUM in predicting in-hospital mortality was examined in patients undergoing colorectal surgery in France. Both POSSUM and P-POSSUM overestimated postoperative death in elective surgery and the authors concluded that it had not been validated in France in the field of colorectal surgery.[10] The original POSSUM score and P-POSSUM were derived from a heterogeneous population of general surgical patients. Subgroup analysis of high-risk colorectal surgery patients found that the models underpredicted death in the emergency patients.[11] There was also a lack of calibration at the extremes of age in both emergency and elective work. This resulted in remodelling of the POSSUM score for colorectal surgery patients and led to the development of the Colorectal-POSSUM model (CR-POSSUM). The CR-POSSUM model was superior to the P-POSSUM model in predicting operative mortality in a study involving almost 7000 patients undergoing emergency and elective colorectal surgery in the UK.[12] External validation of CR-POSSUM was derived from three multicentre UK studies involving a total of 16 006 patients and CR-POSSUM was superior in predicting postoperative death.[13]

However, a recent systematic review pooled data from 18 studies to compare the accuracy of POSSUM, P-POSSUM and CR-POSSUM in predicting postoperative mortality for patients undergoing colorectal cancer surgery.[14] This study reported greater predictive accuracy for the P-POSSUM model compared with CR-POSSUM. These conflicting data may represent the limitations associated with risk models which may lose accuracy when applied to different patient populations. For example, a study from the Netherlands on patients undergoing elective sigmoid resection for either carcinoma or diverticular disease demonstrated that CR-POSSUM overpredicted mortality in the patients with malignant disease and underpredicted it in patients with benign disease. However, in the whole group CR-POSSUM predicted postoperative mortality accurately.[15]

O-POSSUM (oesophagogastric)

A UK study of 204 patients demonstrated that POSSUM did not accurately predict morbidity and mortality in patients undergoing oesophagectomy.[16] A dedicated oesophagogastric model (O-POSSUM) developed in a study population of 1042 patients was described in 2004. The O-POSSUM model used the following independent factors: age, physiological status, mode of surgery, type of surgery

and histological stage. It provided a more accurate risk-adjusted prediction of death from oesophageal and gastric surgery for individual patients than P-POSSUM.[17] However, to date there have been several conflicting studies examining the predictive value and accuracy of O-POSSUM. A Dutch study of 663 patients undergoing oesophagectomy in a tertiary referral centre (in-hospital mortality 3.6%) demonstrated that O-POSSUM overpredicted in-hospital mortality threefold and could not identify those patients with an increased risk of death.[18] This was supported by similar studies from both the UK and Hong Kong, which found that P-POSSUM provided the most accurate prediction of in-hospital mortality and O-POSSUM again overpredicted mortality, particularly in patients with low physiological scores and in older patients.[19,20] A recent systematic review comparing P-POSSUM with O-POSSUM, which included data from 10 studies, concluded that P-POSSUM was the most accurate predictor of postoperative mortality and O-POSSUM consistently overestimated postoperative mortality in gastro-oesophageal cancer patients.[21]

In summary, the data reported in the original study to construct O-POSSUM have not been validated in other centres. It may be that individual units have to modify the O-POSSUM model to take account of local factors.

V-POSSUM (vascular)

V-POSSUM was devised for use specifically in patients undergoing arterial surgery. One study examined the records of 1313 patients and added 'extra items' to the original POSSUM dataset, although this did not appear to significantly improve the accuracy of prediction.[22] The model has, however, been used in further studies and has been modified further to take account of only the physiology component of the score, with improved prediction accuracy (V-POSSUM physiology only). However, a recent UK study involving almost 11 000 patients undergoing elective abdominal aortic aneurysm repair evaluated the accuracy of five risk prediction models, including V-POSSUM.[23] V-POSSUM performed poorly, with the Medicare and Vascular Governance North West (VGNW) models demonstrating the best discrimination, leaving the authors to conclude that V-POSSUM should not be used for risk prediction for these patients. Neither the V-POSSUM nor P-POSSUM models appear to be accurate in predicting mortality in the context of ruptured abdominal aortic aneurysms (RAAAs).[22] In a larger comparison of P-POSSUM, RAAA-POSSUM, RAAA-POSSUM (physiology only), V-POSSUM and V-POSSUM (physiology only) models in 223 patients with RAAA (in-hospital mortality was 32.4%), only V-POSSUM and P-POSSUM (physiology only) demonstrated significant lack of fit.[24]

A recent evaluation of V-POSSUM in New Zealand has indicated that it is a useful tool not only in the assessment of outcome, but of longitudinal surgical performance in major vascular surgery. Major vascular procedures ($n = 454$) were prospectively scored for V-POSSUM over a 10-year period. There was a trend towards improved surgical performance over time, with a drop in the observed-to-predicted mortality ratio. This novel role has not yet been tested using other POSSUM models, but there may be potential to use them to evaluate training and performance in other surgical subspecialities.[25]

✔ POSSUM is the most widely applied, validated, surgical risk scoring system currently used in the UK. The original POSSUM equation has been modified in an effort to increase its accuracy as a risk prediction tool for in-hospital surgical mortality. Of these, P-POSSUM is the most widely used and validated general modification. Speciality-specific POSSUM has been developed for use in colorectal, oesophagogastric and vascular patients, with some improvement in risk stratification. The available data suggest that the various POSSUM models have a tendency to overestimate mortality rates. Despite these limitations, the POSSUM models provide a useful tool for risk assessment, audit and comparing outcomes between different units and within the same unit over time. However, due to the variables included in the calculation, POSSUM cannot be used in the preoperative setting to inform risk.

ASA

In 1963 the American Society of Anesthesiologists (ASA) adopted a five-point classification system for assessing the physical status of a patient prior to elective surgery. A sixth category was added later (Box 4.5).

Box 4.5 • ASA classification

1. A normal healthy patient
2. A patient with mild systemic disease
3. A patient with severe systemic disease
4. A patient with severe systemic disease that is a constant threat to life
5. A moribund patient who is not expected to survive without the operation
6. A declared brain-dead patient whose organs are being removed for donor purposes

Note: If the surgery is an emergency, the ASA grade is followed by 'E' (for emergency), for example '3E'. Category 5 is always an emergency so should not be written without 'E'.

The ASA grade is a combination of the subjective opinion of the anaesthetist taken in conjunction with a more objective assessment of the patient's general fitness for surgery, and is used routinely in most centres in the UK. There are a number of studies assessing the utility and accuracy of the ASA grade in determining surgical risk and, as anticipated given the nature of this scoring system, the literature is conflicting.

One study of 113 anaesthetists in the UK demonstrated such marked variation in the inter-individual assessment of 10 hypothetical patients that the authors concluded that the ASA grade should not be used on its own to predict surgical risk.[26] A further study of 97 anaesthetists demonstrated that the agreement for the assessment of each hypothetical patient varied from 31% to 85%. The overall correlation was only fair, and the inter-observer inconsistency was similar to that in a study from 20 years previously.[27]

However, the largest study to date is more encouraging.[28] Of 16 227 patients undergoing elective surgery over a 5-year period, 215 died within 4 weeks of operation. There was a significant correlation between perioperative mortality and the ASA grade. The mortality was lowest (0.4%) when the ASA grade was less than or equal to 2 and increased up to 7.3% in ASA grade 4 patients. The authors concluded that perioperative mortality can be predicted using the ASA grade. The ASA classification is now incorporated into many other risk prediction models.

✔ The ASA classification remains a quick, simple, widely used and reasonably accurate assessment of surgical risk in both the elective and emergency settings.

Surgical Mortality Probability Model and Surgical Risk Scale

The Surgical Mortality Probability Model (SMPM) was derived from retrospective data analysis of almost 300 000 patients using the American College of Surgeons National Surgical Quality Improvement Program (ACS NSQIP) Database.[29] The primary outcome was 30-day mortality for patients undergoing non-cardiac surgery. The model identified three risk factors – ASA status, emergency or elective surgery and surgery risk class – as the main determinants of outcome. Points are allocated in accordance with these three factors and predicted 30-day mortality is calculated from the total score (Table 4.2). Patients with a total risk score less than 5 had a predicted mortality of less than 0.5%, whereas a risk score greater than 6 predicted a mortality of more than 10%. Other models, such as the Surgical Risk Scale,

Risk factor	Points
ASA	
I	0
II	2
III	4
IV	5
V	6
Procedure severity	
Low	0
Intermediate	1
High	2
Urgency	
Elective	0
Emergency	1
Total points	**Mortality risk**
0–4	<0.5%
5–6	1.5–4%
7–9	>10%

The SMPM was developed to predict 30-day mortality for patients undergoing non-cardiac surgery. The model utilises three risk factors (ASA status, severity of procedure and urgency of the procedure). A score is awarded for each variable and the mortality risk is calculated form the total score.

have identified the same three factors as the main determinants to predict surgical outcome: namely complexity of procedure (minor, intermediate, major, major-complex), urgency of procedure (elective, urgent, emergency) and ASA grade.[30] A recent systematic review highlighted P-POSSUM and the Surgical Risk Scale as the most accurate tools to predict outcome in patients undergoing major abdominal surgery.[31]

✔ The Surgical Risk Scale and P-POSSUM model were identified as the most accurate tools for predicting postoperative outcome in a recent systematic review. The Surgical Risk Scale uses only three simple variables: complexity of surgery, urgency and ASA grade.

Surgical Risk Calculator

This model, first published in 2013, was also derived from the ACS NSQIP database and has recently been re-calibrated following analysis of data from almost 3 million patients.[32,33] The latest version of this model uses 21 predictors to estimate risk for 11 separate adverse outcomes. The authors

claim improved and highly accurate estimation of risk for these adverse outcomes. Time will tell if they are correct.

Surgical Outcome Risk Tool

The Surgical Outcome Risk Tool (SORT) was developed from analysis of 19 000 patient outcomes in the UK.[34] This model aims to estimate risk of death at 30 days and utilises six variables including the three already described (ASA, complexity of procedure and urgency) in addition to patient age, surgical risk speciality (thoracic, gastrointestinal or vascular surgery) and presence of malignancy. The addition of these three variables demonstrated improved accuracy in predicting 30-day mortality compared with the Surgical Risk Scale (area under receiver operator curve 0.91 vs. 0.88).

Surgical Risk Preoperative Assessment System (SURPAS)

The most recently published risk prediction model has been developed with the aim of producing a simplified model using as few variables as possible incorporating data that is readily available.[35] The SURPAS model has been developed from the American College of Surgeons National Surgical Quality Improvement Program (ACS NSQIP) database of over 2 million patients. The model has been designed to predict 30-day mortality and risk of six common postoperative complications, such as renal failure and respiratory infection. The authors identified eight predictive variables (compared with 24 variables included in the original NSQIP model) that provide comparable risk prediction without the additional requirement for laboratory data. Four of these variables are patient-related factors and the four are related to the type of operative procedure (Table 4.3). Once again, three recurrent variables are identified: ASA, urgency and complexity of procedure. The authors claim that this simpler model provides comparable risk prediction to more complex models and this new model is applicable to a broad range of surgical patients without the requirement for speciality-specific models. Future validation studies will be required to support these claims.

✔ The two most recent risk prediction models produced from the UK (Surgical Outcome Risk Tool – SORT) and the USA (Surgical Risk Pre-operative Assessment System – SURPAS) have been developed with the aim of simplicity and ease of use. These parsimonious models promise accurate risk prediction using a few readily available predictor variables.

Table 4.3 • The Revised Cardiac Risk Index: six risk factors to predict mortality and cardiovascular complications following surgery

Risk factor	Number of risk factors	Risk of death/ myocardial infarction
Major (high risk) surgery	0	0.4%
History of ischaemic heart disease	1	1%
History of heart failure	2	2.4%
History of cerebrovascular disease	3	5.4%
Diabetes requiring insulin treatment		
Serum creatinine concentration >177 µmol/L		

Other risk prediction models

There are many other published risk prediction models that have not been presented here for reasons of brevity. Some of these have been designed to predict specific complications. The Revised Cardiac Risk Index (RCRI) was developed to predict risk for cardiac complications in major elective non-cardiac surgery.[36] The risk of myocardial infarction and cardiac death can be predicted according to the number of risk factors that are present (Table 4.4, **Fig. 4.1**).

Many other models have been disappointing when validated against external patient populations. The inability of these models to reproduce initial predictive accuracy has resulted in many failing to gain widespread acceptance. It is fair to say that at present there is no single model that can accurately

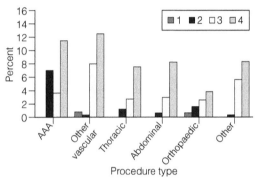

Figure 4.1 • Risk of major cardiac complications predicted by the Revised Cardiac Risk Index according to type of surgical procedure performed. The greater the number of risk factors present, the greater the risk of complications, irrespective of the type of surgery undertaken. Reproduced from Lee TH, Marcantonio ER, Mangione CM, et al. Derivation and prospective validation of a simple index for prediction of cardiac risk of major noncardiac surgery. Circulation 1999;100(10):1043–9. With permission from Wolters Kluwer Health.

predict surgical risk for all patient populations. Weblinks to access many of the risk models described in this chapter are shown in Box 4.3.

Functional assessment

Assessment of exercise capacity provides useful information about the functional status of a patient and their response to physiological stress. This information can then be used to inform an assessment of how the patient might respond to surgical stress and may therefore be used to predict perioperative risk. Patients with higher exercise tolerance usually have lower risk. Evaluation of exercise capacity may be subjective or objective, where formal exercise testing is performed.

Subjective assessment of exercise tolerance can usually be undertaken by asking some simple

Table 4.4 • Examples of common activities and their metabolic equivalents (METs)

Activity	MET value
Watching television	1
Showering	2
Playing the piano	2.3
Washing the dishes	2.5
Playing snooker	2.5
Walking the dog	3
Slow ballroom dancing	3
Lawn bowls	3
Moderate housework	3.5
Climbing two flights of stairs	4
Golf (using an electric cart)	3.5
Golf (carrying clubs)	4.3
Mowing the lawn	5.5
Moderate swimming	5.8
Jogging	7
Running (10 minute/mile pace)	9.8

questions to assess the functional capacity of the patient. Determination of how many stairs a patient can climb before stopping due to limitation by symptoms, or how far they can walk on the flat without stopping, are commonly employed questions. There is evidence to suggest that these simple assessments of exercise capacity correlate with surgical risk. In a study of 600 patients undergoing major non-cardiac surgery, serious postoperative complications, especially cardiac complications, were twice as common for those patients unable to climb two flights of stairs preoperatively.[37] Inability to climb two flights of stairs was associated with a positive predictive value of 82% for the development of cardiopulmonary complications in patients undergoing major thoracic and abdominal surgery and stair-climbing ability was inversely related to duration of hospital stay.[38]

Exercise capacity may also be measured objectively. Metabolic equivalent of tasks (METs) is a measure of energy expenditure related to physical activity. One MET may be considered as the resting metabolic rate (RMR) and is defined as energy consumption at a rate of 3.5 mL O_2 per kg per minute. Physical activities may be measured as a ratio compared to the RMR. For example, ironing clothes is equivalent to 1.8 METs and climbing two flights of stairs is equivalent to 4 METs. Some further examples are given in Table 4.5. This process may then be used to identify patients with reduced exercise capacity who may benefit from a more objective assessment of their functional status. A full list of physical activities and the MET equivalents can be found at the web address listed in reference.[39]

Cardiopulmonary exercise testing (CPEX)

Cardiopulmonary exercise testing (CPEX) is an objective measurement of cardiorespiratory function for the assessment of surgical risk. In 1993 Older et al. performed CPEX testing among a group of elderly patients undergoing major surgery. An anaerobic threshold (AT) of less than 11 O_2 mL/min/kg was associated with a mortality rate of 18%

compared with a mortality rate of less than 1% for those patients with an AT greater than 11 O_2 mL/min/kg.[40] Subsequent studies confirmed that an AT of less than 11 O_2 mL/min/kg was associated with increased hospital mortality following major elective abdominal and vascular surgery.[41,42] CPEX testing was also predictive of longer-term outcome. In a study of 102 patients undergoing elective abdominal aortic aneurysm repair, CPEX testing was not only predictive of 30-day mortality, but was also predictive of longer-term survival at 30 months.[42]

Other studies have identified alternative values for the optimal discriminatory anaerobic threshold. In patients with a low functional capacity (less than 7 METs), a lower AT value was associated with increased likelihood of postoperative complications and the optimal AT threshold was 10.1 O_2 mL/min/kg.[43] An AT cut-off of 11 O_2 mL/kg/min was found to be a poor predictor of postoperative cardiopulmonary morbidity for patients undergoing oesophagectomy for cancer.[44] However, this study did confirm an association between lower exercise capacity and risk of complications, without defining a specific alternative AT threshold for this group of patients.

A recent systematic review examined the role of CPEX testing to predict outcome in patients undergoing major abdominal surgery.[45] The review identified variable prediction accuracy depending on the patient group. CPEX was accurate in predicting 90-day survival and morbidity in liver transplant patients and patients undergoing pancreatic surgery, but was poor at predicting risk for bariatric, upper GI and colorectal patients. The authors concluded that CPEX testing has a role in certain patient groups, such as liver transplant patients, and different AT thresholds are required for different patient groups.

The optimal AT threshold value is generally accepted at 11 O_2 mL/min/kg.[46] This correlates closely to 4 METs (14 O_2 mL/min/kg) and, in turn, the ability to climb two flights of stairs. Stair climbing therefore has the potential to be used as a screening tool for the identification of patients who would benefit from further assessment by CPEX testing.

Limitations of CPEX testing relate to the process of conducting the test itself. Patients are required to exercise, usually on a cycle ergometer, and full assessment may be limited by physical ability rather than limitations due to cardiorespiratory function – for example, patients with arthritis or amputees. Another potential limitation of CPEX testing relates to availability and cost. The equipment and expertise to perform the test are not widely available in the UK at present. Despite these limitations, CPEX testing is becoming an increasingly adopted tool

Table 4.5 • Eight predictive variables included in the Surgical Risk Preoperative Assessment System (SURPAS) prediction model

Patient variables	Operative variables
Age	Urgency
ASA	Primary surgeon speciality
Presence of systemic sepsis within 24 hours	Inpatient versus outpatient procedure
Functional health status	Relative value unit[a]

[a]Relative value unit is a Medicare reimbursement tariff and is an indirect measure of complexity of the operative procedure

for preoperative assessment of higher-risk patients undergoing major surgery.

✅ Cardiopulmonary exercise testing (CPEX) is the 'gold standard' measure of cardiorespiratory function. An anaerobic threshold (AT) less than 11 O_2 mL/min/kg has been associated with increased risk of postoperative complications and mortality in some patient groups, although the exact threshold AT value may need to be modified for different patient groups or different surgical procedures. CPEX testing requires specialist equipment and expertise to perform, and it is not widely available in the UK at present, but it is likely to be increasingly used for assessment of perioperative risk in selected high-risk patient populations.

Other objective measures of exercise capacity

The incremental shuttle walk test (ISWT) requires the patient to walk between two markers placed 10 metres apart within a set time period. This time period becomes progressively shorter, requiring more effort from the patient to make the distance within the shorter time. The test stops when the patient cannot reach the end of the 10-metre course within the given time. The ISWT has been shown to correlate with measured oxygen consumption in patients with cardiac and chronic lung disease.[47] A small study investigated the ability of ISWT to predict 30-day mortality following oesophagogastrectomy.[48] No patients with a walk distance greater than 350 metres died in the postoperative period, while patients who did not achieve the threshold of 350 metres had a 30-day mortality of 50%. Distance achieved on the shuttle walk test was compared with CPEX measurements in a study of 50 patients undergoing abdominal surgery. All patients who walked in excess of 360 metres had an anaerobic threshold (AT) greater than 11 O_2 mL/min/kg.[49] It was also noted that some patients who walked less than 360 metres may also have had satisfactory CPEX results, suggesting that the ISWT was good at identifying patients with a good AT, but could not accurately identify those who had a poor anaerobic threshold (i.e. a good positive predictive value, but poor negative predictive value). These data suggest that the ISWT may be used as a screening tool to identify patients who may then benefit from more formal exercise testing with CPEX.

The 6-minute walk distance is another standardised assessment tool for estimation of exercise capacity. The AT determined by CPEX testing was compared with maximum distance achieved during the 6-minute walk test in a study of 110 patients awaiting major general surgery. Patients who completed in excess of 563 metres during the 6-minute test had an AT greater than 11 O_2 mL/min/kg and those who managed less than 427 metres had an AT less than 11 O_2 mL/min/kg.[50] The authors recommended that those patients who completed 563 metres did not require formal exercise testing, whereas those who could not manage more than 427 metres should undergo CPEX assessment. There was 'clinical uncertainty' in those patients who walked between 427 and 563 metres, requiring consideration of other clinical risk factors in the decision-making process.

The timed stair-climbing test involves timing how long it takes a patient to walk down then up a single flight of seven steps. The patient's pulse and blood pressure are measured before and immediately after the activity. On multivariate analysis the time taken to perform the stair climb test was the single strongest predictor of postoperative complications in 264 patients undergoing elective abdominal surgery.[51]

✅ The incremental shuttle walk test (ISWT), the 6-minute walk test and the timed stair climb are simple tools to assess exercise capacity objectively. They are indirect tests of oxygen consumption and have been shown to correlate with formal exercise testing values (CPEX). The main value of these tests is to identify higher-risk patients who may benefit from formal exercise testing.

Frailty

Frailty is a clinical syndrome characterised by reduction of physiological reserves due to the ageing process. Frailty is associated with increased risk of adverse outcomes following surgery. It is estimated that frailty is present in 10% of people over 65 years of age and up to half of patients over 85 years. In an ageing population surgeons need to be aware of this clinical syndrome, understand how outcomes may be adversely affected and know how to identify it. Several tests for frailty are available, but the Edmonton Frail Scale (EFS) is the most widely used for surgical assessment. This is a simple scoring system that assesses cognition, nutrition and functional status.[52] An EFS score of seven or more was not only associated with increased risk of complications following elective surgery, but also a lower chance of being discharged home in patients over 70 years of age.[53] Inability to return to a previous level of function is an important consideration for elderly patients contemplating surgery and a method of assessing this risk is vital for the consenting process.

Sarcopenia and body composition analysis

Sarcopenia is a clinical syndrome characterised by the loss of lean body mass as a result of ageing. The reduction in skeletal muscle is associated with loss of strength and functional capacity. Cachexia is a similar syndrome also associated with loss of skeletal body mass that is associated with disease states (most notably cancer) but has different pathophysiology. Both syndromes are refractory to conventional treatments such as nutritional supplementation, may lead to progressive functional decline and are associated with poor treatment outcomes and prognosis. Both conditions may be difficult to recognise in obese patients who may nonetheless meet the criteria for sarcopenia or cachexia despite a high body mass index (sarcopenic obesity).

Sarcopenia is identified through measurement of muscle mass and by assessing muscle strength and function. Muscle strength is most commonly measured using hand-grip strength and functional performance is determined by methods already described in this chapter, such as timed stair climb. Morphometric parameters may be measured from routine computed tomography (CT) and magnetic resonance imaging (MRI) imaging using computer software programs to calculate lean body mass and visceral adipose tissue from cross-sectional images generated at L3 level. A standardised lumbar skeletal muscle index (LSMI) is generated following adjustment for patient height. Studies have demonstrated association of sarcopenia with increased risk of postoperative complications in patients undergoing oesophagogastric surgery and colorectal surgery.[54–56] The strongest associations were between reduced lean body mass and increased rates of pulmonary complications and wound infections. A systematic review of patient outcomes following gastrointestinal surgery identified that sarcopenia was associated with increased rates of immediate postoperative complications as well as adverse longer-term prognosis and outcomes.[57] This information is clearly important in selecting treatment options for patients with confirmed sarcopenia.

Although the syndrome of sarcopenia is not fully reversible there is some evidence to suggest that early identification of these patients with focused attention on nutritional and functional (physical) support may reduce mortality rates and length of stay following surgery.[58] Trials adopting a multimodal approach addressing exercise, nutrition

✅ Sarcopenia, characterised by reduced lean body mass, is associated with higher rates of postoperative complications and poorer outcomes following surgery. Reduced skeletal muscle mass is most easily measured by CT or MRI and is an indirect measure of reduced muscle strength and function. Trials to investigate potential therapeutic strategies to ameliorate the adverse effects of sarcopenia are ongoing.

and anti-inflammatory treatment strategies (MENAC Trial) are ongoing.[59]

Biomarkers

There is emerging evidence that estimation of serum biomarkers in the preoperative period may assist risk stratification for patients undergoing surgery. 'Routine' biomarkers, such as serum creatinine, albumin and HbA1c, are routinely performed preoperative laboratory tests that provide information on organ function and are often incorporated into risk prediction models – for example, P-POSSUM. 'Novel' biomarkers are measured with the specific aim of improving outcome prediction accuracy. Brain natriuretic peptide (BNP) and C-reactive protein (CRP) are the most promising biomarkers for risk assessment. Both of these markers mainly target cardiovascular complications. BNP is released from cardiac ventricles in response to excessive stretching and elevated serum concentrations are correlated with prognosis in heart failure.[60] Elevated preoperative serum concentration of BNP (>40 pg/mL) was associated with an increased risk of death and perioperative cardiac events in a study of 204 patients undergoing non-cardiac surgery.[61] A further study of 190 patients undergoing elective non-cardiac surgery also identified elevated serum NT-proBNP (a co-secretory product of BNP) as an independent predictor of postoperative cardiac complications.[62] A recent meta-analysis examined the value of preoperative serum BNP concentrations for predicting postoperative mortality and cardiac complications following vascular surgery.[63] The authors concluded that elevated BNP concentrations were predictive of adverse outcome, but there was wide variation in the serum concentration of BNP chosen as the threshold for discrimination (range 35–100 pg/mL). The optimal discriminatory concentration remains unknown and it is likely that threshold values may vary depending on the patient group under investigation.

CRP is a marker of systemic inflammation and serum concentrations are associated with atherosclerotic disease and adverse outcomes in cancer. A preoperative serum CRP concentration greater than 6.5 mg/L was associated with increased 30-day mortality and postoperative cardiac complication rates in a study involving 592 patients undergoing vascular surgery (odds ratio 2.5; 95% confidence interval 1.5–4.3).[64] Moreover, this association was independent of serum BNP concentration and other established cardiac risk factors. The association between elevated CRP and adverse perioperative outcome may be due, in part, to a correlation between markers of systemic inflammation and exercise capacity. Elevated serum CRP concentrations have been demonstrated to be inversely correlated with VO_2 max in male subjects without evidence of coronary heart disease.[65] Further study is required to determine the true value of these serum biomarkers in risk assessment for surgical patients.

In updating this chapter there have been very few additional publications relating to advances in the study of biomarkers to predict surgical outcomes and quantification of risk. This is somewhat surprising given the importance of this field and the lack of established measures. In an age of developing personalised treatments for patients perhaps future advances will incorporate patient genotyping to predict an individualised patient risk.

Communicating risk

The use of risk prediction models, scoring systems, exercise tests and serum biomarkers as adjuncts to decision-making is an increasingly important part of surgical practice. This information must then be communicated effectively to the patient to allow fully informed choice. UK General Medical Council guidance on this issue states that informed decisions require clear, accurate information about the risks of any proposed investigation or treatment and should be presented in a way patients can understand. The amount of information about risk that the clinician should share with patients will depend on the individual patient and what they want, or need, to know. Discussions with patients should therefore focus on their individual situation and risk.[1] In the UK, this discussion has been altered profoundly following a Supreme Court ruling in the case of *Montgomery* v. *Lanarkshire Health Board*.[66] The case removed the longstanding legal precedent on consent from the 'reasonable doctor' to the 'reasonable patient' test. In essence it is now the duty of the clinician to ensure that all risks, however small, are conveyed to a patient if

> ✓ Brain natriuretic peptide (BNP) and C-reactive protein (CRP) are the most promising biomarkers for risk assessment. Elevated preoperative serum concentrations have been associated with increased risk of mortality and cardiac complications in surgical patients; however, the optimal threshold cut-off value remains unknown. The real value of serum biomarkers may lie in the selection of patients into high- or low-risk groups and therefore help identify which patients merit further assessment.

deemed of significance to that patient – i.e. what a reasonable person in the patient's position would wish to know. This ruling now makes discussions about risks (and alternatives) considerably more challenging.

In communicating risk there are several techniques to impart the concept of how likely it is that the patient will have a complication of the procedure, or die as a result of it. These broadly fall into using numerical data or descriptive details of risk. As always, this communication must be tailored to the needs and expectations of the individual patient and it is likely that a combination of these techniques will be most appropriate.

Percentages alone are often not well understood, and as they apply to a population rather than an individual patient, they may be misleading. Odds, relative risk and absolute risk may be too complex, but quoting for example 'a 1 in 10 or 1 in 100 chance' may be helpful. Using relativity (comparison with a concept the patient understands) or examples ('of the last 50 patients this has happened to …') may also clarify the concept of surgical risk to the patient.

To complicate matters further, there is marked variation in perception of risk and decision to operate among even experienced surgeons. Seven hundred and sixty-seven surgeons were asked to review four clinical scenarios and assess the risk of various procedures and state whether they would advise proceeding to surgery.[67] The decision to operate varied from 49% to 85% and was based on a wide variation in the interpretation of risk.

Finally, it is worth remembering that the perceived surgical risk that concerns the surgeon is not necessarily what the patient is worried about. Assessing, discussing and communicating risk has the primary aim of allowing patients to understand what may happen to them, and to help them make an informed choice about investigation or therapeutic options. However, this process of discussion, coupled with careful documentation, affords the surgeon some protection against litigation.

Key points

- Estimation of surgical risk is vital to inform treatment decision-making and facilitate informed consent, anticipate potential complications and target aspects of care to optimise the patient, and allow meaningful comparison of clinical outcomes, audit and quality assurance.
- Determination of surgical risk is complex, but may be more simply considered in terms of *patient-related* risks and *procedural-related* risks.
- Patient-related risk factors will be influenced by patient age, comorbidity, the underlying disease process, nutritional status and the performance status of the patient.
- Procedural-related risk factors include the grade of severity of the procedure planned, urgency of the procedure, volume of blood loss and other technical aspects.
- Risk prediction models and scoring systems (such as POSSUM, ASA and the Revised Cardiac Risk Index) have been developed in an attempt to improve risk prediction. These tools work best for patient populations (groups) rather than individual patients, and therefore their main value is for audit purposes and comparing outcomes between different units and within the same units over time. There is no perfect risk prediction model.
- Assessment of functional capacity may be undertaken simply by the use of simple screening questions. More objective measurements may be performed by using standardised walking tests or CPEX testing.
- Serum biomarkers, such as BNP and CRP, may have a future role in identifying high-risk surgical patient groups, who may then benefit from more detailed assessment.
- Estimation of surgical risk should include a thorough clinical assessment, an assessment of the functional capacity of the patient (through simple questions relating to METs) and should take into account the severity of the surgical procedure proposed. If this process identifies the patient to be at high risk, then further testing should be considered – for example, objective exercise testing (CPEX).

⊕ Full references available at **http://expertconsult. inkling.com**

Key references

9. Wakabayashi H, Sano T, Yachida S, et al. Validation of risk assessment scoring systems for an audit of elective surgery for gastrointestinal cancer in elderly patients: an audit. Int J Surg 2007;5(5):323–7. PMID: 17462968.
   Modification of the original POSSUM score led to the development of the P-POSSUM risk score. The modified formula fits better with observed mortality rates; however, it still overestimates mortality in low-risk groups, the elderly and in certain surgical subspecialities.

28. Prause G, Ratzenhofer-Comenda B, Pierer G, et al. Can ASA grade or Goldman's cardiac risk index predict perioperative mortality? A study of 16,227 patients. Anaesthesia 1997;52(3):203–6. PMID: 9124658.
   This is the largest study investigating ASA classification and assessment of surgical risk. This study reports a significant correlation between perioperative mortality and the ASA grade. Mortality was lowest (0.4%) when the ASA grade was less than or equal to 2 and increased up to 7.3% in ASA grade 4 patients. The ASA classification is now incorporated into many other risk prediction models.

30. Sutton R, Bann S, Brooks M, et al. The Surgical Risk Scale as an improved tool for risk-adjusted analysis in comparative surgical audit. Br J Surg 2002;89:763–8. PMID: 12027988.
   This study reports on the development of a new risk score: the Surgical Risk Scale. This novel model identified three factors as the main determinants to predict surgical outcome: namely complexity of procedure (minor, intermediate, major, major-complex), urgency of procedure (elective, urgent, emergency) and ASA grade. A main advantage to this model lies in its simplicity.

31. Moonesinghe SR, Mythen MG, Das P, et al. Risk stratification tools for predicting morbidity and mortality in adult patients undergoing major surgery: qualitative systematic review. Anesthesiology 2013;119(4):959–81. PMID: 24195875.
   This recent systematic review highlights P-POSSUM and the Surgical Risk Scale as the most accurate tools to predict outcome in patients undergoing major abdominal surgery.

34. Protopapa KL, Simpson JC, Smith NC, et al. Development and validation of the Surgical Outcome Risk Tool (SORT). Br J Surg 2014;101(13):1774–83. PMID: 25388883.

The Surgical Outcome Risk Tool (SORT) was developed from analysis of 19 000 patient outcomes in the UK. This model aims to estimate risk of death at 30 days following surgery. This tool utilises six variables: ASA, complexity of procedure, urgency, age, surgical risk speciality (thoracic, gastrointestinal or vascular surgery) and the presence of malignancy. The combination of these six variables demonstrated improved accuracy at predicting 30-day mortality.

35. Meguid RA, Bronsert MR, Juarez-Colunga E, et al. Surgical Risk Preoperative Assessment System (SURPAS): III. Accurate preoperative prediction of 8 adverse outcomes using 8 predictor variables. Ann Surg 2016;264(10):23–31. PMID: 26928465.

The SURPAS model has been developed from the American College of Surgeons National Surgical Quality Improvement Program (ACS NSQIP) database of over 2 million patients. The authors identified eight predictive variables (compared with 24 variables included in the original NSQIP model) that provide comparable risk prediction without the additional requirement for laboratory data. The authors claim that this simpler model provides comparable risk prediction to more complex models and this new model is applicable to a broad range of surgical patients without the requirement for speciality-specific models.

45. Moran J, Wilson F, Guinan E, et al. Role of cardiopulmonary exercise testing as a risk-assessment method in patients undergoing intra-abdominal surgery: a systematic review. Br J Anaesth 2016;116(2):177–91. PMID: 26787788.

This systematic review examined the role of CPEX testing to predict outcome in patients undergoing major abdominal surgery. The review identified variable prediction accuracy depending on the patient group. CPEX was accurate in predicting 90-day survival and morbidity in liver transplant patients and patients undergoing pancreatic surgery, but was poor at predicting risk for bariatric, upper GI and colorectal patients. The authors concluded that CPEX testing has a role in certain patient groups, such as liver transplant patients, and different AT thresholds are required for different patient groups.

51. Reddy S, Contreras CM, Singletary B, et al. Timed stair climbing is the single strongest predictor of perioperative complications in patients undergoing abdominal surgery. J Am Coll Surg 2016;222(4):559–66. PMID: 26920993.

On multivariate analysis the time taken to perform the stair climb test was the single strongest predictor of postoperative complications in 264 patients undergoing elective abdominal surgery.

57. Wagner D, DeMarco MM, Amini N, et al. Role of frailty and sarcopenia in predicting outcomes among patients undergoing gastrointestinal surgery. World J Gastrointest Surg 2016;8(1):27–40. PMID: 26843911.

A systematic review of patient outcomes following gastrointestinal surgery identified that sarcopenia was associated with increased rates of immediate postoperative complications as well as adverse longer-term prognosis and outcomes.

5

Perioperative and intensive care management of the surgical patient

Katherine McAndrew
Maurizio Cecconi
Andrew Rhodes

Introduction

The incidence of death directly attributable to anaesthesia has decreased significantly over the last few decades. In the 1950s a number of studies demonstrated that the postoperative mortality solely associated with anaesthesia was approximately 1 in 2500[1-3] and by 1987, in the Report of a Confidential Enquiry into Perioperative Deaths (CEPOD),[4] this cause of death had fallen to 1 in 185 000. While patient outcomes have improved, the European Surgical Outcomes Study in 2012 (EuSOS) found an overall mortality rate of 4% in patients undergoing non-cardiac surgery throughout Europe,[5] perhaps higher than might be expected. This chapter deals with the perioperative and intensive care management of these patients with a specific focus on how to ensure that each patient has adequate cardiovascular performance for their needs during the perioperative period, in order to reduce their risk of complications and death.

Postoperative critical care is a key factor in the improvement of outcome for surgical patients, particularly those who are at high risk of postoperative morbidity and mortality. Thus, postoperative critical care admission should always be considered when the preoperative physiological condition of the patient suggests that there is a reasonable probability or risk of postoperative complications and organ dysfunction. In order to provide this postoperative critical care it is necessary to be able to identify these high-risk patients preoperatively.

How big is the problem?

It is estimated that over 300 million operations take place globally per year and these growing numbers of patients need to be cared for in an appropriate setting.[6] A high-risk group of patients was identified from the UK population who accounted for over 80% of all deaths but only 12.5% of procedures. Despite high mortality rates, fewer than 15% of these patients were admitted to the Intensive Care Unit (ICU) and the highest mortality rate (39%) was found in patients who required ICU admission following initial care in a ward environment.[7] These findings have recently been confirmed, with only 5% of all patients being admitted to ICU electively after their procedure.[5] Unplanned admissions were associated with a higher mortality and 73% of those who died were not admitted to ICU at any stage.

Recent data have suggested that there continues to be a problem with the allocation of critical care resources to those most at need following elective surgery. However, availability of critical care beds remains limited, with an average of 2.8 critical care beds per 100 acute care beds across Europe.[5] This varies considerably between countries, with Germany having 6.9 times the number of critical care beds per head of population that Portugal has.[8] Studies have demonstrated the paucity of both ICU and HDU beds in the UK[9-11] and found that patients were often admitted later and with a worse severity of illness.

Repeated publications by the National Confidential Enquiry into Postoperative Deaths (NCEPOD) have cited inadequate preoperative preparation, inappropriate intraoperative monitoring and poor postoperative care as contributing causes of perioperative mortality. The most recent[12] NCEPOD Report (Knowing the Risk) suggests that patients in the UK often die after surgery because they are not given the level of care they are entitled to or could reasonably expect. In this latest report less than half of the patients actually received the care that the advisors felt was the minimal acceptable standard. As far back as 1996, the Department of Health issued guidelines as to which patients should be admitted to critical care units. In particular, they suggested that postoperative patients who needed close monitoring for more than a few hours after surgery should be admitted. However, the great variation in underlying pathology and premorbid physiology of these patients makes it very difficult to provide hard-and-fast rules as to which patients will benefit from perioperative admission to either ICUs or high-dependency units (HDUs).

✔✔ Patients who need close monitoring for more than a few hours after surgery should be admitted to a critical care unit.[13]

Why do patients die after surgery?

Major surgery is associated with a significant stress response[14] that is vital for the body to recover and heal from the surgical trauma. This response manifests in many different ways, but a common delineating pattern is one of a hyperdynamic circulation with increased oxygen requirements postoperatively.[15] If the body is unable to increase the cardiac output in response to the surgical stress, then the increased need for oxygen cannot be met and the patient develops tissue dysoxia and cellular dysfunction. This has been described by some authors as an acquired oxygen debt,[16] which if left results in organ failure and death. The important point to recognise is that the normal response to surgery is to increase the cardiac output and the delivery of oxygen to the tissues. Any patient who, for whatever reason, is unable to develop this response is at higher risk of subsequent complications.

What is a high-risk surgical patient?

The challenge is the early identification of patients who are at a high risk of postoperative complications and death, and this is vital in order to ensure that correct care and therapy are initiated

at an optimal time in order to reduce the associated morbidity and mortality.

The number of patients with diabetes, heart failure and obesity continues to grow, along with the challenges of the ageing population, adding to this high-risk demographic.

On the whole, this patient group is characterised by undergoing major surgery whilst having concurrent medical illnesses that limit their physiological reserve to compensate for the stressful situation. Well-validated risk assessment scores such as P-POSSUM are commonly used to evaluate patient risk and may guide further preoperative assessment (see also Chapter 4). It has been suggested that elective surgical patients can be assessed by cardiopulmonary exercise testing,[15,17,18] in which a strong correlation has been demonstrated between anaerobic threshold and postoperative outcome. The anaerobic threshold is the point where aerobic metabolism fails to provide adequate adenosine triphosphate and anaerobic metabolism starts to reduce the resultant deficit. The threshold is determined by monitoring inhaled and exhaled levels of oxygen and carbon dioxide during escalating levels of exercise. This provides an objective measure of physiological reserve. However, it must be remembered that complex cardiopulmonary testing in patients who have established poor cardiorespiratory reserve is only of use if used to target preoperative preparation and these patients must have specific optimisation of their comorbidities prior to surgery whenever possible. This requires that patients booked for elective surgery have all their comorbidities treated and investigated to ensure best possible physiological status prior to surgery. This is also the opportunity to consider if surgical intervention is the best course of action in view of the risk of the potential adverse outcomes. A full and truthful risk assessment should be undertaken and the patient fully involved in the decision to proceed to surgery. A national report published in 2011 suggested that only 7.5% of patients at high risk of death or severe complications were given any indication of their risks of mortality and morbidity prior to surgery.[12]

Variables associated with postoperative complications and death

Several authors[19,20] have examined the prognostic ability or power of many variables that can be monitored in the postoperative setting. One group[7] found that none of the routinely measured variables such as heart rate, blood pressure, central venous pressure, urine output or any marker of acid–base status was able to predict subsequent postoperative complications. The variables independently associated with subsequent significant complications were the central venous oxygen saturation and the cardiac index. This association between oxygen flux in the perioperative period and subsequent complications is not new and is essentially the same as work published by Shoemaker et al.[16] some 30 years previously, when they identified the key variables as being cardiac index, oxygen delivery and oxygen consumption. It was from this body of work that the theories surrounding the targeting of oxygen delivery to values of over 60 mL/min per m² in the perioperative period to improve patient outcome originated.

The role of the splanchnic circulation

There is some evidence that the splanchnic circulation has a role in the pathogenesis of postoperative morbidity and mortality. It has been shown that increasing global tissue oxygen delivery increases splanchnic oxygen delivery,[21–23] and in the early stages of shock any inadequacy of tissue oxygen delivery predominantly affects the splanchnic circulation.[24] The splanchnic circulation is particularly sensitive to hypoperfusion states, and the reduction in flow to the splanchnic bed is out of proportion to the overall reduction in cardiac output and is usually the last major system blood flow to recover when the hypoperfusion state improves.[25–27] It is thought that this splanchnic hypoperfusion leads to disruption of the enteric mucosal barrier with translocation of endotoxins and micro-organisms into the systemic circulation.[28–31] This translocation initiates a cytokine pathway, increasing the risk of sepsis and organ failure. This risk of splanchnic hypoperfusion and translocation increases with age, the urgency of the surgery and the preoperative presence of bowel obstruction. The translocation of bacteria and endotoxins induces cytokine release by tissue macrophages, activates the complement and coagulation systems, and produces a proinflammatory state. These cytokines themselves can impair oxygen delivery to the splanchnic circulation, further increasing translocation.

Strategies to improve outcomes

The overall postoperative standard of care has improved significantly through the use of education and quality improvement initiatives, such as the National Emergency Laparotomy Audit (NELA) (see also Chapter 3). Care bundles are frequently utilised as a way to improve the consistent delivery of appropriate care following certain procedures and a specific 'care bundle' delivered to emergency laparotomy patients resulted in a 25% reduction in crude mortality, with up to 35% reduction in higher-risk patients.[32]

The concept of augmenting cardiac output in the perioperative period to improve the outcome of surgical patients has been described by many authors as 'optimisation' or 'goal-directed therapy'. The main aim of all optimisation strategies for high-risk patients has been to ensure that the circulatory status is adequate for the needs of the patient in the perioperative period. This has been achieved with a number of differing protocols utilising different time periods, resuscitation endpoints and pharmacological agents, with almost all smaller studies having led to an improved outcome. The OPTIMISE trial, published in 2014, attempted to determine whether these benefits could be reproduced on a larger scale. Initial analysis found no clear reduction in complications or mortality. However, after incorporating the results into an updated systematic review and meta-analysis, there remains evidence of clinically significant reductions in both these outcomes. The OPTIMISE II trial should provide further clarity on the benefits of cardiac output-guided haemodynamic therapy treatment algorithms.[33]

✔✔ The OPTIMISE trial demonstrated that algorithm-based goal-directed therapy probably reduces the risk of postoperative morbidity and mortality. The OPTIMISE 2 trial will provide more information on the potential benefits.[33]

Oxygen delivery

In order to understand the rationale behind many of the protocols that have been utilised in the perioperative setting, it is vital to appreciate the important variables that determine oxygen delivery: haemoglobin concentration, arterial oxygen saturation and cardiac output. It therefore becomes clear that in order to ensure that an adequate volume of oxygen is delivered to the body's vital organs, the haemoglobin concentration (Hb), the arterial saturation of haemoglobin with oxygen (S_aO_2) and the cardiac index must all be at a satisfactory level. Maximising all three of these variables to clinically acceptable levels is the aim of resuscitation in any given patient, although not always achievable. The Hb level is governed by the clinical situation as well as the underlying pathophysiological process, but many experts aim to keep the Hb level above 7–8 g/dL in a stable perioperative setting.[34–37] The S_aO_2 is usually targeted to be 94–98% (or 88–92% in those at risk of type 2 respiratory failure)[38] with increased inspired oxygen and/or continuous positive airways pressure

(CPAP) if necessary, so the main variable that can be manipulated is the cardiac output. There is a growing understanding that atelectasis in the postoperative period is not just associated with hypoxaemia but also with a proinflammatory response that potentiates tissue injury. As a result the use of CPAP, or other non-invasive positive pressure ventilation (NIPPV) therapy, has the potential to improve many physiological parameters without serious side-effects in certain high-risk groups of patients.

✅ Intraoperatively, the use of lung protective ventilation utilising low tidal volumes, recruitment manoeuvres to open collapsed alveoli and moderate levels of PEEP to prevent further collapse has improved patient outcomes.[39]

Postoperatively, studies suggest NIPPV can reduce pneumonia and the need for intubation, but the data remain limited.[40,41] High-Flow Nasal Oxygen Therapy has similar efficacy to NIPPV in preventing postoperative atelectasis and may be more comfortable to some patients.[42]

Cardiac output can be increased with several easy-to-use protocols. The targeting of cardiac index does necessitate the measurement and monitoring of this variable, which nowadays can be done relatively non-invasively. Once measured, if the cardiac output is perceived to be too low, then it is increased with intravenous volume therapy and then, if it has still not improved sufficiently, pharmacologically, using appropriate cardiovascular pharmaceutical agents that will improve cardiac output.

Measurement and monitoring of cardiac output

There are a variety of technologies available to monitor cardiac output. In the past, pulmonary artery catheters were used, which enabled a thermodilution curve to be constructed across the right ventricle thus enabling cardiac output to be calculated from the Stewart–Hamilton equation. In recent times this tool is rarely used due to a lack of evidence demonstrating a beneficial effect on outcome and the perceived invasiveness of its approach. Many devices and techniques are now available that can provide the same information in a less invasive fashion. Oesophageal Doppler analysis of the descending aorta has been widely described in the perioperative period, while titrating therapy with pulse power analysis has recently been shown to reduce length of stay and postoperative complications. Completely non-invasive methods utilising bioreactance are becoming available, although evidence is conflicting with regards to their accuracy.[43–46]

Fluid resuscitation

It is important to recognise that the aim of management is to give the right amount of fluid at the right time. There is evidence that excessive fluid administration is detrimental in critically ill and postoperative patients and it is likely that inappropriate volume overload has just as many detrimental effects as inadequate volume resuscitation. The 2011 NCEPOD report[12] shows that mortality is related to fluid management, with mortality being only 4.7% in patients receiving adequate preoperative fluids as compared to 20.5% and 33.3%, respectively, in those patients who received either inadequate or excessive pre-operative intravenous fluid. This mandates the need to monitor very carefully fluid administration in critically ill or high-risk patients where simple measures or markers of preload status are often inadequate. Defining the endpoint at which filling is optimal and the need for inotropic therapy begins is difficult. A plateau in the stroke volume, the flow correction time as determined by oesophageal Doppler and the stroke volume variation (with the pulse pressure analysis) can all be used to define the endpoint.

✅✅ The British Consensus Guidelines on Intravenous Fluid Therapy for Adult Surgical Patients (GIFTASUP) state that 'in high-risk patients treatment with intravenous fluid and inotropes should be aimed at achieving predetermined goals for cardiac output and oxygen delivery' in order to improve outcome.[47] It is important that whatever endpoints of resuscitation are chosen, they are reached with the minimal amount of volume and inotropic therapy possible.

Delirium as a postoperative complication

The number of people aged over 75 is projected to increase by 89.3% by 2039.[48] Elderly patients are at high risk of delirium and a recent paper has suggested that prophylactic low-dose dexmedetomidine significantly decreases the occurrence of delirium during the first 7 days after surgery in those aged over 65 years.[49] Whilst this is not routine practice, it highlights the ongoing areas of research aimed at improving overall post-surgical outcomes in the high-risk surgical patient.

Conclusions

This overview of the literature relating to the high-risk surgical patient and current improvements associated with goal-directed therapy leads to some inevitable conclusions:

1. There is good evidence to suggest that patients with poor cardiorespiratory reserve have a higher mortality and complication rate when undergoing major surgery. Most of these patients can be identified by simple clinical methods before surgery.
2. It is likely that there are significant numbers of patients undergoing different types of surgery who may be at substantial risk of developing major complications or death.
3. There is some evidence that targeted protocolised treatment for this group can improve outcome, but this is becoming less certain with improving basic standards of care.
4. It is apparent that optimising the circulation can be carried out using several different techniques and at different times (i.e. preoperatively, intraoperatively and postoperatively).
5. The decision to operate on high-risk patients should be made at consultant level and should involve surgeons as well as those who will provide the intra- and postoperative care (anaesthetists and critical care consultants).
6. An assessment of mortality risk should be made explicit to the patient and recorded clearly on the consent form and in the medical notes.
7. Appropriate intraoperative physiological monitoring is required for all high-risk patients and NICE Medical Technology Guidance 3 relating to cardiac output monitoring should be applied.[50]

✓✓ There are very good evidence-based recommendations on the CardioQ-ODM oesophageal Doppler monitor for people having major or high-risk surgery.[50]

8. All hospitals undertaking surgery for high-risk patients should have facilities to provide perioperative goal-directed monitoring and therapy and the hospital should analyse the volume of work they undertake to ensure they have sufficient capacity of facilities to be able to accommodate all the patients they treat. This should be assessed annually.[12]
9. The Royal College of Surgeons of England have considered the high-risk surgical patient and have made a series of key suggestions for improvement in care and outcomes.[51] These include: recommendations that all hospitals should formalise their pathways for unscheduled adult surgical care; that there should be prompt recognition and treatment of emergencies and complications to improve outcomes and reduce costs; hospitals should match theatre access to patient needs; every patient should have his/her expected risk of death estimated and documented; high-risk patients are those at greater risk of death than 5% and all should have active consultant input and be admitted to a critical care area postoperatively for at least 12 hours; surgical procedures with a risk of death greater than 10% should only be conducted under the direct supervision of a consultant surgeon and consultant anaesthetist.

Key points

- Patients with poor cardiorespiratory reserve undergoing major operations have a high postoperative complication and mortality rate. The mortality rate is much higher if these patients have emergency operations.
- These patients can be identified preoperatively by simple clinical history and examination.
- This high postoperative complication and mortality rate can be reduced by therapy aimed at enhancing the cardiorespiratory performance of these patients with poor physiological reserve during the perioperative period.
- Goal-directed therapy aims to ensure that tissue oxygen delivery is enhanced to levels shown to confer survival without postoperative complications.

Full references available at **http://expertconsult. inkling.com**

Key references

13. Department of Health. Guidelines on admission to and discharge from intensive care and high dependency units. London: NHS Executive; 1996.
A useful guide for criteria for admission to critical care units in the UK.

33. Pearse RM, Harrison DA, MacDonald N, et al. for the OPTIMISE Study Group. Effect of a perioperative, cardiac output-guided hemodynamic therapy algorithm on outcomes following major gastrointestinal surgery: a randomized clinical trial and systematic review. JAMA 2014;311(21):2181–90. PMID: 24842135.
The OPTIMISE trial demonstrated that algorithm-based goal-directed therapy probably reduces the risk of postoperative morbidity and mortality. The OPTIMISE 2 trial will provide more information on the potential benefits.

47. British Consensus Guidelines on Intravenous Fluid Therapy for Adult Surgical Patients (GIFTASUP). PMID: 19302633.
This is a useful publication in which the treatment of high-risk patients with intravenous fluid and inotropes is discussed.

50. National Institute for Health and Care Excellence. Medical technologies guidance MTG3: CardioQ-ODM oesophageal Doppler monitor. March 2011. http://www.nice.org.uk/MTG3.
Evidence-based recommendations on the CardioQ-ODM oesophageal Doppler monitor for people having major or high-risk surgery.

6

Surgical nutrition

William G. Simpson
Steven D. Heys

Introduction

Despite improved understanding of the importance of nutrition in health, up to 40% of hospitalised patients can be classified as being malnourished, and the problem is still frequently missed clinically. In patients undergoing gastrointestinal surgery, for example, the prevalence of 'mild' and 'moderate' malnutrition has been estimated to be approximately 50% and 30%, respectively.

The clinical significance of this is vitally important because when patients are malnourished, disturbances in function at the organ and cellular level can manifest as the following:

- altered partitioning and impairment of normal homeostatic mechanisms;
- muscle wasting and impairment of skeletal muscle function;
- impaired respiratory muscle function;
- impaired cardiac muscle function;
- atrophy of smooth muscle in the gastrointestinal tract;
- impaired immune function;
- impaired healing of wounds and anastomoses.

As a result of these malnutrition-induced changes, patients have an increased risk of postoperative morbidity and mortality. Furthermore, patients undergoing surgery are often fasted for varying periods of time (preoperatively and/or postoperatively). Moreover, if patients then experience postoperative complications (e.g.

sepsis), these effects may be further potentiated and the disturbances of cellular and organ function occurring in malnutrition then made even more complex.

In this chapter the following areas, which are important for surgical practice, will be outlined:

- the principles of the metabolic responses to feeding, trauma and sepsis;
- nutritional requirements for surgical patients;
- identification of patients who are malnourished or are at risk;
- nutritional support principles for surgical practice and modifications in defined common clinical situations;
- modulation of nutritional support with key nutrients – application to clinical practice.

Metabolic response to feeding, trauma and sepsis

In order to maintain the health of cells, tissues and organs, the metabolism must adapt to changes in nutritional intake, trauma and sepsis. While a detailed knowledge of complex biochemical pathways is not necessary, it is important to understand the principles of these metabolic and biochemical changes, and the metabolic response when a patient experiences trauma, undergoes surgery or develops sepsis. This forms the basis for understanding nutrition and nutritional support in critically ill patients.

Trauma

A major advance in understanding occurred more than 80 years ago when Sir David Cuthbertson described the loss of nitrogen from skeletal muscle that occurred following trauma.[1] Cuthbertson concluded that the response to injury could be considered as occurring in two phases (Fig. 6.1):

1. the 'ebb' phase, which is a short-lived response associated with hypovolaemic shock, increased sympathetic nervous system activity and reduced metabolic rate;
2. the 'flow' phase, which is associated with a loss of body nitrogen and resultant negative nitrogen balance.

These changes result in the following:
Ebb phase

- decreased resting energy expenditure;
- increased glycogenolysis;
- increased gluconeogenesis;

Flow phase

- increased resting energy expenditure;
- increased heat production, pyrexia;
- increased muscle catabolism and wasting, and loss of body nitrogen;
- increased breakdown of fat and reduced fat synthesis;
- increased gluconeogenesis and impairment of glucose tolerance.

If the changes of the 'ebb phase' are not replaced by the 'flow phase', then despite any advances in surgery, anaesthesia and intensive care support, death of the patient is the inevitable outcome.

The central nervous system and the neurohypophyseal axis play key roles in regulating these metabolic changes following trauma, utilising a range of hormones and cytokines. Afferent nerve impulses also stimulate the hypothalamus to secrete hypothalamic releasing factors that, in turn, stimulate the pituitary gland to release prolactin, arginine vasopressin (antidiuretic hormone, ADH), growth hormone and adrenocorticotrophic hormone (ACTH). The changes in hormone concentrations in plasma following trauma are outlined in Box 6.1, with the stress hormones (adrenaline, cortisol, glucagon) playing pivotal roles.

Protein metabolism

Amino acids are required for:

- synthesis of proteins necessary for growth, function and structural repair;
- energy substrates for gut, lymphocytes and other rapidly proliferating tissues (mostly glutamine), also as fuel in muscle;
- hepatic gluconeogenesis – glucose is produced from alanine, which itself is produced by transamination reactions from other amino acids;
- maintenance of renal acid–base balance (e.g. arginine);
- production of proteins with specific roles in repair – immunological, endocrine, etc.

In the well-fed state, proteins are synthesised at a rate exceeding breakdown, whereas in the fasting state breakdown predominates. Following prolonged

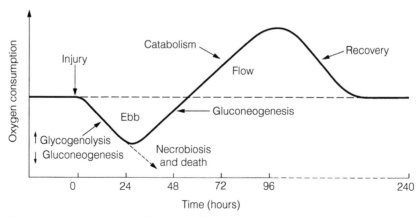

Figure 6.1 • Diagrammatic representation of the ebb and flow phases in the metabolic response to injury. Reproduced from Broom J. Sepsis and trauma. In: Garrow JS, James WPT, editors. Human nutrition and dietetics. 9th ed. Edinburgh: Churchill Livingstone, 1993; p. 456–64. With permission from Elsevier.

Box 6.1 • Changes in hormone concentrations in plasma following trauma

Catecholamines

Rapid increase in concentrations of adrenaline and noradrenaline within a few minutes of injury due to increased sympathetic nervous system activity. Concentrations return to normal within 24 hours

Glucagon

Rises within a few hours; maximal concentration 12–48 hours post-trauma

Insulin

Initially plasma concentration is low following trauma, but rises reaching a maximum several days after the injury

Cortisol

Rapid increase in plasma cortisol concentration, usually returning to normal 24–48 hours later, but may remain elevated for up to several days. Has 'permissive' effects with other hormones such as catecholamines

Growth hormone

Concentration increased following trauma; usually returns to normal within 24 hours

Thyroid hormones

Following trauma, the biochemical features of 'sick euthyroid syndrome' may be present: thyroid-stimulating hormone (TSH) concentration normal or low, concentrations of free thyroxine (T_4) and tri-iodothyronine (T_3) normal, whereas the total concentrations are altered because of changes in binding protein concentration. In addition, reverse T_3 is generally high. These effects may be prolonged for some weeks

Other disturbances of thyroid function may, however, be present, including 'transient hyperthyrotropinaemia of illness' – a transiently raised TSH, not to be confused with hypothyroidism

Renin, aldosterone

Renin produced in response to reduced renal perfusion after trauma stimulates aldosterone secretion, returning to normal within 12 hours

Testosterone

Plasma concentration falls after trauma and may remain low for up to 7 days

Vasopressin/antidiuretic hormone

Plasma concentration rises following trauma and may remain elevated for several days

Prolactin

Plasma concentration increased very rapidly (minutes) following any stress (may even rise during 'stressful' phlebotomy!)

Cytokines

Increased secretion of interleukin (IL)-2, IL-6, tumour necrosis factor, etc.; inter-relationship between these changes leads to differential responses seen in trauma and sepsis

---

fasting for 1–2 weeks, breakdown still predominates but at a lower rate as the metabolism adapts to starvation. Following trauma or sepsis, breakdown exceeds synthesis regardless of whether the patient is fed or fasted; this response is, however, impaired if the metabolism is already adapted to starvation.[2] The magnitude of the nitrogen loss is proportional to the degree of operative trauma or the severity of the sepsis, and the major site of protein breakdown is skeletal muscle (contains 80% of the body's amino acid pool, with 60% being glutamine).

Carbohydrate metabolism

Glucose is the main fuel used by many different tissues, being essential for some. In the well-fed state it is available for absorption from the gastrointestinal tract and, mostly driven by insulin, any excess is converted to glycogen (glycogenesis) in both liver and muscle, and to fatty acids (lipogenesis), the latter predominating when glycogen stores are replete. On fasting, insulin concentrations are lower, peripheral utilisation of glucose is reduced and endogenous production increased – from glycogen (glycogenolysis) or other precursors (gluconeogenesis), e.g. amino acids and fatty acids. Initially, glycogenolysis predominates, but after a number of hours (dependent on demands), gluconeogenesis predominates (colloquially referred to as 'getting your second wind'). Following trauma, there is an increase in hepatic glycogenolysis (caused by increased sympathetic activity), with these stores being substantially depleted within 24 hours. Insulin antagonists are also involved in this metabolic response (see Box 6.1), and the insulin resistance is accompanied by a rise in insulin concentration. The circulating insulin concentration usually reaches a maximum several days after the injury, before returning towards normal concentrations.

In general, the carbohydrate response is to produce hyperglycaemia both in the immediate 'shock' ('ebb' phase) and later 'flow' phase of the metabolic response. The origin of the increased glucose differs between these two phases – while reduced peripheral utilisation of glucose is common to both phases, the glycogenolysis of the ebb phase must be replaced by gluconeogenesis in the flow phase. In the critically ill patient the advent of hypoglycaemia is an indication of major problems – glycogenolysis has slowed with depletion of glycogen stores, but gluconeogenesis is not yet adequate.

Fat metabolism

In the healthy, resting, fed state, triglyceride, being energy-dense, is used to store energy efficiently. When fasting, lipolysis of triglyceride releases free fatty acids, which can be used as respiratory fuel for most cells other than brain and red blood cells, and glycerol that can be converted to glucose by hepatic gluconeogenesis. Fatty acids are also metabolised in the liver to form ketone bodies, which are used as a preferential fuel source by many tissues (humans cannot use fatty acids for gluconeogenesis). Lipolysis is stimulated by glucagon during short-term fasting, by ACTH once the metabolism is adapted to starvation, or by adrenaline during exercise and stress. Following trauma, there is therefore an increase in the turnover of fatty acids and glycerol, although raised concentrations of lactate, for example in hypovolaemic shock, induce re-esterification leading to raised plasma triglyceride concentrations.

Mineral and micronutrient metabolism

Changes in fluid compartments, minerals and micronutrients (micronutrients are broadly defined as substances required in amounts of <1 g daily) are beyond the scope of this chapter, but it is worth re-emphasising that measured serum concentrations rarely reflect body status, and this is even more pronounced in starvation and illness; for example, hyponatraemia is more often associated with an excess of water than with a deficiency of sodium; hypocalcaemia rarely indicates calcium deficiency, but can suggest magnesium deficiency. It is therefore essential to consider the effect of illness before trying to interpret laboratory results.[3]

Sepsis

The metabolic response to sepsis is also characterised by alterations in protein, carbohydrate and fat metabolism, but the following are key differences:[4]

- The breakdown of skeletal muscle and nitrogen losses can be substantial (more than 15–20 g per day);
- There is increased production of glucose by the liver (both gluconeogenesis and glycogenolysis), resulting in an elevated plasma glucose;
- In contrast to the situation following trauma, there is an increased rate of glucose uptake and oxidation by peripheral tissues;
- Decrease in the peripheral uptake of triglyceride and defective ketogenesis in the presence of sepsis leads to hypertriglyceridaemia (in contrast to the situation occurring after trauma).

A significant abnormality in the patient with sepsis is the disruption of the microstructure of the hepatocyte mitochondria, particularly of the inner membrane. There is a block in energy transduction pathways, with consequent reduction in the aerobic metabolism of both glucose and fatty acids. The body therefore depends on *anaerobic* metabolism of glucose, which results in lactate production. An adequate supply of glucose is therefore essential. If gluconeogenesis is impaired or inadequate, then hypoglycaemia may ensue. Hypoglycaemia during sepsis indicates an extremely poor prognosis and is usually associated with mortality.

Nutritional requirements

Proteins and amino acids

Protein is required for the maintenance of normal health and cellular function. Proteins have many functions, including being essential components of cellular structure. They are required for the synthesis of a variety of secretory proteins produced by many organs. The average daily intake of protein is approximately 80 g in the UK, with a recommended daily intake of 0.8 g/kg body weight and with nitrogen comprising approximately 16% of its weight. However, more than 50% of the world's population exist on less!

Conventionally, amino acids have been classified as either 'essential' or 'non-essential'. The 'essential' amino acids cannot be synthesised endogenously and are required in the diet. Paradoxically, the so-called 'non-essential' amino acids are actually so metabolically important that humans have retained the ability to synthesise them. Both groups of amino acids are necessary for normal tissue growth and metabolism.

Dietary intake and endogenous synthesis of amino acids in the body maintain the relevant pool of amino acids, replacing those that have been lost by excretion in the urine, losses from the skin and gastrointestinal tract, utilisation as precursors for non-protein synthetic pathways, irreversible modification and irreducible oxidation.

Under certain circumstances (e.g. sepsis, trauma, growth) endogenous synthesis of some 'non-essential' amino acids may be inadequate; therefore, these amino acids are described as 'conditionally essential': L-alanine, L-glutamate and L-aspartate, produced by a simple transamination reaction, are the three most important amino acids in times of starvation:

- alanine for hepatic gluconeogenesis;
- glutamate as a fuel source for liver, enterocytes and white blood cells;
- aspartate for maintaining renal acid–base balance.

Energy requirements

Energy transduction is accomplished by the breakdown of carbohydrate, fat and proteins. The energy available from various common nutrients is:

- fat 9.3 kcal/g (38.9 kJ/g);
- glucose 4.1 kcal/g (17.1 kJ/g);
- protein 4.1 kcal/g (17.1 kJ/g);
- alcohol 7.1 kcal/g (29.7 kJ/g).

The principal carbohydrates in the diet are polysaccharides (starch and dietary fibre), dextrins and free sugars (monosaccharides), disaccharides, oligosaccharides and sugar alcohols. Dietary fat includes cholesterol and triglyceride, containing long-chain (C_{16}–C_{18}) and medium-chain (C_6–C_{12}) fatty acids.

If the energy intake of an individual is greater than energy expenditure, extra carbohydrate intake, on reaching the liver via the portal vein, will be channelled into synthesis of glycogen or fat. Glycogenesis dominates until hepatic glycogen stores are replete; thereafter, fat synthesis dominates. Additional fat intake will be stored in adipose tissue as triglyceride. In contrast, if there is a negative energy balance, then glycogenolysis dominates until glycogen stores are depleted, then fat and protein will be broken down to provide energy.

Total daily energy expenditure comprises the following:

- resting metabolic expenditure (RME), which is energy required for cardiorespiratory function and synthesis and maintenance of electrochemical gradients across cell membranes;
- activity energy expenditure (depends on type of physical work undertaken);
- diet-induced energy expenditure.

Normally, approximately 25–30 kcal/kg (105–125 kJ/g) are required daily; the magnitudes of changes in requirements in some common conditions are given in Box 6.2.

Box 6.2 • Additional energy requirements in disease states

Trauma: 0.3 × RME
Elective surgery: 0.1 × RME
Sepsis: up to 0.5 × RME
Severe sepsis: up to 0.6 × RME
Massive burns: 1 × RME

RME, resting metabolic expenditure.

Minerals and micronutrients

A number of specific organic compounds (vitamins) and inorganic elements are essential for tissue growth and repair, and for maintenance of body function, playing key roles in metabolism, including the processing of macronutrients (protein, carbohydrate and fat). For many micronutrients, specific deficiency diseases have been described. Details of individual substances are beyond the scope of this chapter and can be found elsewhere,[5] but some examples are given in Box 6.3.

In general, micronutrients are classified into:

- fat-soluble vitamins (A, D, E and K);
- water-soluble vitamins (C and the B vitamins – folic acid, B_{12}, B_1, B_2, B_3, pantothenic acid, biotin and B_6);
- trace elements (iron, zinc, copper, selenium, etc.).

Box 6.3 • Functions of some micronutrients important in surgical practice

Vitamin A
Stabilises epithelial cell membranes; necessary for fibroblast differentiation and collagen deposition

Vitamin D
Role in calcium and phosphate regulation

Vitamin E
Immunostimulant and free radical scavenger

Vitamin K
Required for liver synthesis of clotting factors

Vitamin B_{12}
Important in synthesis of proteins and nucleic acids

Ascorbic acid
Important in hydroxylation (e.g. collagen synthesis) and energy transduction

Thiamine
Necessary for carbohydrate metabolism and ATP synthesis

Iron
Energy transfer

Copper
Collagen synthesis

Selenium
Antioxidant; protection against peroxidation processes occurring in tissue damage and repair

Zinc
Cofactor in numerous enzymes; necessary for wound healing

The exact requirement for micronutrients during trauma and sepsis is unclear and may alter depending on the type of metabolic support provided.

It should be remembered that micronutrients, if given at high doses, can have toxic effects on tissues. In particular, toxicity can be a problem with excesses of vitamin A, iron, selenium, zinc and copper; vitamin D toxicity is no longer thought to be a common problem. Care must be taken when these micronutrients are provided for a prolonged period to ensure that toxicity does not occur. It is also unusual to find isolated deficiencies, so identification of one micronutrient deficiency should stimulate consideration of other deficiencies.

Identification of patients who are malnourished

It is important to assess the nutritional status in all patients undergoing surgery and identify those who are malnourished, or who are at risk of becoming so. Measurements used previously in clinical practice include:

- anthropometric – body structure and composition;
- biochemical;
- functional – muscle (skeletal and respiratory) and immunological responses.

Anthropometric measures

Height and weight

Height and weight are two commonly used indices of nutritional status. Body weight on its own takes no account of frame size but body mass index (BMI; weight divided by the square of the height) is a good anthropometric indicator of total body fat in adults.

Loss of body weight is an indicator of nutritional risk, and is incorporated into the MUST score (see below). Loss of more than 10% of body weight is associated with a significant increase in postoperative mortality. The shorter the period of weight loss, the more significant this is in predicting increased postoperative complications.

Body composition

Various techniques for assessing the body's different compartments (e.g. fat, fat-free mass, total body nitrogen and total body mineral contents) have become available but many require specialised equipment and may not be readily applicable to clinical practice. Relatively simple techniques, such as skinfold thickness and bioelectrical impedance, can be used clinically, although even these tend to be limited to research or clinical audits of nutrition and nutritional support.

Subcutaneous fat thickness

Skinfold thickness has been used as an index of total body fat (50% of total body fat is subcutaneous, depending on age, sex and fat pad). Triceps skinfold thickness is most commonly measured but assessment of skinfolds at multiple sites correlates better with total body fat. Skinfold thickness measurements are however susceptible to intra- and inter-observer variability, limiting clinical use.

Bioelectrical impedance

This entails applying an alternating voltage between electrodes attached to the hand and foot. At low frequencies, current passes through the water and electrolyte compartment of lean tissues, thus total body resistance depends principally on lean body mass. Adipose tissue acts as an insulator at low frequencies, but at high frequencies it acts as a capacitor, thus comparison of current at low vs high frequency can indicate relative body fat. This can give a reasonable estimate of body composition in stable subjects and is frequently used in gymnasia and weight-reduction clinics, but it becomes less reliable in patients with oedema and electrolyte shifts, and so the value of bioelectrical impedance in critically ill patients remains unclear.

Biochemical measures

Serum proteins

Albumin is the major protein in serum and low concentrations are associated with increased risk of complications in surgical patients In starvation, however, serum albumin, which has a relatively long half-life of approximately 21 days, may not fall for several weeks. Conversely, serum albumin acts as a negative marker of the acute-phase response, and so is lowered in malignancy, trauma and sepsis, even in the presence of an adequate intake. Serum albumin should therefore *not* be used as an assessment of nutritional *state*, although low concentrations point to the increased nutritional *risk* associated with underlying disease, and indeed the implied reduction of gut absorption may indicate that the parenteral route may be preferred for provision of nutrition.

Alternatives to using albumin as a marker of nutritional status by measuring other serum protein concentrations, including transferrin (half-life 7 days), retinol-binding protein (half-life 1–2 hours) and pre-albumin (half-life 2 days), had been considered but the serum concentrations of these proteins are also altered in stress, sepsis and cancer, and so, as for albumin, they are not useful for assessing nutritional status in routine clinical practice.

Nitrogen balance

Most of the nitrogen lost from the body is excreted in urine, mainly as urea (approximately 80% of total urinary nitrogen). Urea alone may be measured as an approximate indicator of losses, or total urinary nitrogen may be measured, although this latter technique is not widely available. In addition, there are also losses of nitrogen from the skin and in stool of approximately 2–4 g per day.

Nitrogen balance has not been shown to be a prognostic indicator, but can help assess nutritional requirements or the response to provision of nutritional support.

Tests of function

Immune competence

In malnutrition there is a reduction in total circulating lymphocyte count and impairment in immune functions.

Depression of total circulating lymphocyte count is associated with a poorer prognosis in surgical patients; however, these alterations in immune function are non-specific and affected by trauma, surgery, anaesthetic and sedative drugs, pain and psychological stress, and so are not generally applicable to clinical practice.

Muscle function

Skeletal muscle

Various aspects of skeletal muscle structure and function are deranged in malnutrition. In patients undergoing surgery, handgrip strength (cheap and easy to perform) may predict patients who develop postoperative complications (sensitivity >90%). However, grip strength is influenced by factors such as patients' motivation and cooperation. Furthermore, such tests may be difficult to apply to critically ill patients. Alternatively, stimulation of the ulnar nerve at the wrist with a variable electrical stimulus results in contraction of the adductor pollicis muscle, the force of which reflects nutritional intake.[6]

Respiratory muscle

The function of the respiratory muscles is impaired by malnutrition and can be detected by deterioration in respiratory function tests, in particular vital capacity.[7] Measurements of inspiratory muscle strength have the advantage that they can be performed in patients who are intubated.

How should nutritional status be assessed in clinical practice?

Although the various techniques outlined above can help to predict the risks of complications, there is at present no reliable technique for assessing nutritional status. There is, however, increasing support for using the following techniques, which are applicable to clinical practice.

The Malnutrition Universal Screening Tool (MUST)

This simple, yet effective, tool was developed by the British Association for Parenteral and Enteral Nutrition (BAPEN). Details are available from the website (www.BAPEN.org.uk). This tool has been endorsed by external organisations and its routine use is recommended for all hospital admissions in the UK. It consists of a series of five steps:

1. Measure height and weight to obtain BMI (in kg/m^2) – this is then given a numerical score (>20 = 0; 18.5–20 = 1; >18.5 = 2).
2. Note percentage unplanned weight loss in the previous 3–6 months – then give this a numerical score (<5% = 0; 5–10% = 1; >10% = 2).
3. Establish the 'acute disease effect' and also give this a numerical score (if patient is acutely ill and there is, or will be, no nutritional intake for more than 5 days = 2).
4. Add scores from steps 1, 2 and 3 together to obtain the 'overall risk of malnutrition'.
5. A decision is taken as to what to do depending on the resultant score.

Significance of the resultant score and clinical management

- **Score 0 (low risk)** – repeat the screening process at a future time.
- **Score 1 (medium risk)** – observe by noting the patient's dietary intake for the next 3 days. If this improves then there is little concern. However, if there is no improvement, this is of clinical concern and one should follow the local policies for what to do next, for example referral to nutrition support team/dietician.
- **Score 2 or more (high risk)** – these patients should be referred to the nutrition support team/dietician to try to increase their nutritional intake and there should be policies in place for the nutritional support given to these patients.

✅ The MUST tool should be used routinely to assess nutritional risk for all hospital admissions (www.BAPEN.org.uk).

Re-feeding syndrome

Once a patient's need for nutritional support has been identified, it is important to consider whether the patient is at risk of re-feeding syndrome. This is described in detail elsewhere, but in essence it is the inability of a patient's metabolism to handle macronutrients. After approximately 10 days without nutritional intake, the metabolism adapts to the state of starvation. Re-feeding with full 'normal' required amounts of macronutrients will induce a sudden reversal of this adaptation, with an anabolic drive that may result in catastrophic depletion of available potassium, phosphate and magnesium. Before re-feeding, the serum biochemistry may appear 'normal', and so the possibility of re-feeding must be anticipated on history alone. The other essential nutrient liable to become depleted in this situation is thiamine, a cofactor of pyruvate kinase, which is required for glucose to undergo oxidative phosphorylation, and without which glucose is metabolised to lactic acid. Thiamine must therefore be replenished before feeding is commenced in the starved patient to prevent development of Wernicke–Korsakoff syndrome. The potential for this is considerably higher in patients with a history of chronic excessive ethanol intake, and so even greater caution is required.

✅ Thiamine deficiency must always be considered in patients who have had no nutritional intake for more than 1 week, who have a history of excessive alcohol intake, or in the presence of an unexplained metabolic acidosis.

Nutritional support in surgical practice

Route of nutritional support

The preferred route of administration of nutritional support is through the gastrointestinal tract (enteral), with intravenous (parenteral) nutrient delivery reserved for patients with intestinal failure.

Detailed guidance for enteral nutrition (EN) and parenteral nutrition (PN) in patients is published by the European and American Societies for Parenteral and Enteral Nutrition (ESPEN and ASPEN). Current guidelines are available on their websites (www.espen.org and www.nutritioncare.org).

Enteral nutritional support

If there is an intact and functioning gastrointestinal tract, enteral feeding should be used if oral intake is insufficient. Enteral feeding is contraindicated to various degrees in patients with intestinal obstruction, paralytic ileus, vomiting and diarrhoea, high-output intestinal fistulas or in the presence of major intra-abdominal sepsis.

The importance of enteral nutrition

Studies in animals have shown that in the absence of nutrients into the intestinal lumen, changes occur in the intestinal mucosa. There is loss of height of villi, reduction in cellular proliferation and the mucosa becomes atrophic. Activities of enzymes found in association with the mucosa are reduced and permeability of the mucosa to macromolecules increased. Stimulation of the intestinal tract by nutrients is important for release of many gut-related hormones, including those responsible for gut motility and stimulation of secretions necessary for normal maintenance of the mucosa. The gut acts as a barrier to bacteria, both physically and by release of chemical and immunological substances. Atrophy of the intestinal mucosa is associated with increased translocation of bacteria and endotoxin from the gut lumen into portal venous and lymphatic systems, and loss of gut integrity may account for a substantial proportion of septicaemic events in severely ill patients. However, the extent to which it contributes to sepsis in patients is not fully understood.

Routes of access for enteral nutritional support

Nasoenteric tubes

Nasogastric feeding via fine-bore tubes (polyvinyl chloride or polyurethane) may be used in patients who require nutritional support for a short period of time. The fine-bore tube can be manipulated through the pylorus into the duodenum, reducing the risk of gastric aspiration. In patients with delayed gastric emptying, double-lumen tubes may be used – one lumen resides in the stomach and is used to aspirate gastric contents, while the distal lumen is placed in the jejunum for feeding, thus reducing risks of aspiration. Regardless of initial position, it is common for tubes to become misplaced, with a potential for pulmonary aspiration. In the UK, the National Patient Safety Agency produces reports on incidents (including a number of fatal incidents) related to nasogastric feeding tubes, and advice on reducing potential harm.[8]

Other complications associated with the use of nasoenteric tubes include:

- pulmonary atelectasis;
- oesophageal necrosis, stricture formation;
- tracheo-oesophageal fistulas;
- sinusitis, postcricoid ulceration.

Gastrostomy tubes

A gastrostomy tube can be placed into the stomach at laparotomy, although percutaneous endoscopic or percutaneous fluoroscopic techniques are preferred. Details of how these are performed can be found in standard texts.

The establishment and use of a gastrostomy has certain disadvantages and there is a recognised morbidity:

- infection of the skin at the puncture site;
- necrotising fasciitis or deeper-sited sepsis;
- damage to adjacent intra-abdominal viscera;
- leakage of gastric contents into the peritoneal cavity;
- haemorrhage from the stomach;
- persistent gastrocutaneous fistula following removal of the feeding tube.

The overall mortality rate for a gastrostomy is 1–2%, with major and minor complications occurring in up to 15% of patients. Mechanical complications associated with the tube include blockage, fracture and displacement. Dumping syndrome may occur when the tip of the tube lies beyond the pylorus.

Jejunostomy tubes

A feeding jejunostomy is usually carried out at the time of laparotomy if it is envisaged that a patient will need nutritional support for a longer period. Details of the operative technique are also in standard operative texts and the smaller needle-catheter tubes are to be preferred. Advantages of a feeding jejunostomy compared with a gastrostomy are:

- less stomal leakage;
- gastric and pancreatic secretions are reduced because the stomach is bypassed;
- less nausea, vomiting or bloating;
- reduced risk of pulmonary aspiration.

Nutrient solutions available for enteral nutrition

A range of nutrient solutions are available for use in enteral nutritional support and examples can be found in specialised texts. However, there are four main categories of enteral diet.

Polymeric diets

Polymeric diets are 'nutritionally complete' diets and provided to patients with inadequate oral intake, but whose intestinal function is good. They contain whole protein as the source of nitrogen, and energy is provided as complex carbohydrates and fat. They also contain vitamins, trace elements and electrolytes in standard amounts.

Elemental diets

Elemental diets are required if the patient is unable to produce an adequate amount of digestive enzymes or has a reduced area for absorption (e.g. severe pancreatic insufficiency or short-bowel syndrome). Elemental diets contain nitrogen as oligopeptides (free amino acids are not as easily absorbed as dipeptide and tripeptide mixtures). The energy source is provided as glucose polymers and medium-chain triglycerides. Each oligopeptide molecule contributes as much to the osmolarity of the solution as one molecule of intact protein, and it can be difficult to provide complete requirements without producing side-effects associated with an osmotic load, for example 'dumping' and diarrhoea.

Special formulations

Special formulations have been developed for patients with particular diseases. Examples of such diets include: (i) those with increased concentrations of branched-chain amino acids and low in aromatic amino acids for patients with hepatic encephalopathy; (ii) those with a higher fat but lower glucose energy content for patients who are artificially ventilated; and (iii) diets containing key nutrients that modulate the immune response (see later).

Modular diets

Modular diets are not commonly used but allow provision of a diet rich in a particular nutrient for specific patients. For example, the diet may be enriched in protein if the patient is protein-deficient or in sodium if sodium-deficient. These modular diets can be used to supplement other enteral regimens or oral intake.

Enteral nutrition delivery and complications

Previously, when starting an enteral nutrition feeding regimen, patients received either a reduced rate of infusion or a lower strength formula for the first 2 or 3 days to reduce gastrointestinal complications. Recent studies have demonstrated this is not required and nutritional support can commence using full-strength feeds at the desired rate in those not at risk of developing 're-feeding syndrome'. Feeding may be cyclical (e.g. 16 hours feeding with a post-absorptive period of 8 hours) or continuous.

Enteral nutrition should be administered through a volumetric pump. If not available, then it is possible to use a gravity drip flow but care should be taken to reduce the risk of a large bolus being administered. In patients whose conscious level

Box 6.4 • Complications of enteral nutrition

Gastrointestinal

Diarrhoea, nausea, vomiting, abdominal discomfort and bloating, regurgitation and aspiration of feed/stomach contents

Mechanical

Dislodgement of the feeding tube, blockage of the tube, leakage of stomach/small intestine contents onto the skin with the use of jejunostomies or gastrostomies

Metabolic

Excess or deficiency of glucose, electrolytes, minerals or trace elements. Some of these will be noted through routine testing protocols, e.g. hyperkalaemia, but others such as hypophosphataemia may be missed if not specifically anticipated

Infective

Local effects (e.g. diarrhoea, vomiting) or systemic effects (e.g. pyrexia, malaise)

is impaired or confined to bed, the head of the bed should be elevated by 25° to reduce risks of pulmonary aspiration. Some clinicians prefer patients to be sitting upright when receiving enteral nutrition. The stomach contents should be aspirated every 4 hours during feeding and if a residual volume of more than 100 mL is found, enteral nutrition is temporarily discontinued.

The aspirate is checked again after 2 hours, and when satisfactory volumes are aspirated (<100 mL) feeding is re-instituted. If more than 400 mL per 24 hours is aspirated, then feeding is discontinued. Gastric emptying may be improved by the administration of cisapride or erythromycin, which may allow feeding to be continued.

Metabolic disturbances are less likely with enteral feeding. The other complications of enteral nutrition are those associated with the route of access to the gastrointestinal tract (Box 6.4).

Parenteral nutritional support

Patients who require nutritional support but with enteral feeding contraindicated will require parenteral nutrition. These include:

- patients with a non-functioning or inaccessible gastrointestinal tract;
- those with high-output enteric fistulas (enteral nutrition may stimulate gastrointestinal secretion – discussed further later);
- those for whom it is not possible to provide sufficient intake of nutrients enterally (e.g. because of a short segment of residual bowel or malabsorption, severe burns, major trauma).

Parenteral routes of access

Central venous access

Central venous access is obtained by positioning a catheter into the superior vena cava through subclavian or internal jugular veins. The catheter either emerges through the skin (usually after being tunnelled in the subcutaneous fat) or is connected to a port placed in the subcutaneous fat of the anterior chest wall. A variety of techniques for insertion of central venous lines are used. For example, catheters may be introduced into the internal jugular or subclavian vein directly by 'blind' percutaneous puncture, using small hand-held ultrasound imaging, by 'cut-down' techniques utilising the cephalic vein to access the subclavian vein, or under fluoroscopic control. Details of these techniques, their advantages and disadvantages can be found elsewhere; however, it is important that whoever inserts a central venous line is expert, well practised and carries out the procedure under full aseptic techniques.

Technical aspects of feeding lines

Central lines are manufactured from polyurethane or silicone. Both these materials are tolerated well, with low thrombogenic potential. However, polyurethane does have advantages:

- it is stiffer than silicone at room temperature, but at body temperature is pliable;
- it has a higher tensile strength than silicone and is less likely to fracture;
- polyurethane catheters have smaller outside diameters, making cannulation easier, as well as a greater resistance to thrombus development on their surfaces.

Catheter manufacturers have attempted to reduce risks of bacterial colonisation of the line by bonding antiseptics (e.g. chlorhexidine) and antibiotics (e.g. silver sulphadiazine) into the catheter's fabric. Some catheters have an antimicrobial cuff, usually made of Dacron, around their external surface. This acts as a barrier to micro-organisms, which may migrate from subcutaneous tissues along the external aspect of the catheter to its tip. Although studies have suggested that risks of septicaemia are reduced by using a cuff around the catheter, this makes positioning of the catheter more difficult technically. Complications of central venous catheters are shown in Box 6.5.

Catheter care

Appropriate dressings of the catheter are essential. The dressing should be changed weekly with strict aseptic technique, and the skin exit site cleaned with chlorhexidine. A variety of dressings have been used at the skin exit, but a transparent adherent type of

Catheter-related sepsis: variable, but reported in up to 40% of catheters

Thrombosis of central vein: variable, but reported in up to 20% of catheters

Pleural space damage: pneumothorax (5–10%), haemothorax (2%)

Major arterial damage: subclavian artery (1–2%)

Catheter problems: thrombosis (1–2%), embolism (<1%), air embolism (<1%)

Miscellaneous problems: brachial plexus (<1%), thoracic duct damage (<1%)

dressing has the advantage of allowing a visible check on the puncture site for inflammation or pus.

Infection of the catheter tip is the most serious type of infection. The patient may have systemic signs of sepsis and is usually pyrexial with spiking temperature, often most prominent just after each PN bag is connected. Blood should be taken for cultures, both peripheral and through the catheter. Antibiotic therapy may result in recovery, but in some the feeding line has to be removed to eradicate the infection. However, less serious infection may occur in the skin at the exit site of the catheter. This is recognised by skin erythema, possibly associated with fluid exudate and pus.

Peripheral venous access

Peripheral venous cannulation, using a sterile technique, may be used to supply nutrients intravenously, avoiding complications associated with central venous catheters. Peripheral intravenous nutrition is likely to be used in patients who do not require nutritional support for long enough to justify risks of central vein cannulation or in whom central vein cannulation is contraindicated (e.g. central line insertion sites are traumatised, increased risks of infective complications, thrombosis of the central veins or significant clotting defects).

Problems associated with the delivery of intravenous nutrition using the peripheral route include:

- a limit to nutrient quantity deliverable – this is not the route of choice in those with high requirements for protein or energy;
- a high incidence of complications, particularly phlebitis (occurs in up to 45% of patients), and it is essential to ensure good peripheral venous access.

The lifespan of a peripheral intravenous cannula can be prolonged by treating it as if it is a central line with regard to aseptic care, and by using a narrow-gauge cannula giving better mixing and flow characteristics of the nutrient solution. Risks of phlebitis can be reduced by frequent changes of infusion site, ultrafine-bore catheters or using a vasodilator patch over the cannulation site (e.g. transdermal glyceryl trinitrate). Furthermore, peripheral intravenous nutrition can only be used where fat emulsion is part of the single-phase administration of nutrients to avoid thrombophlebitis.

Nutrients used in parenteral feeding solutions

Various nutrient solutions (amino acids, glucose and fat) are available and a complete list is given in the *British National Formulary* (www.bnf.org/bnf). There are also available a variety of pre-mixed bags containing various concentrations of amino acids and glucose, with or without fat, which are suitable for different clinical situations. These mixtures do not usually contain vitamins or trace elements, which must be given in addition to avoid development of metabolic complications. Care should be taken that patients receive sufficient electrolytes and minerals to satisfy requirements.

Nitrogen sources

Nitrogen sources are solutions of crystalline L-amino acids containing all essential and a balanced mixture of the non-essential amino acids required. Amino acids that are relatively insoluble (e.g. L-glutamine, L-arginine, L-taurine, L-tyrosine, L-methionine) may be absent or present in inadequate amounts.

Attention has focused on the provision of L-glutamine because of its key roles in metabolism. Despite being one of the most abundant amino acids, its use is limited by instability. It is not contained in routine PN fluids but can be added as N-acetylglutamine (hydrolysed in the renal tubule to free L-glutamine) or as L-glutamine dipeptides such as alanylglutamine (broken down to release free L-glutamine). Trial evidence has not however shown improved mortality or morbidity in surgical patients.[9]

Energy sources

Energy is supplied as a balanced combination of dextrose and fat. Glucose is the primary carbohydrate source and the main form of energy supply to the majority of tissues. During critical illness the body's preferred calorie source is fat (fasted or fed states).

Glucose utilisation may be impaired in certain patients and glucose is then metabolised through other pathways. This results in increased production and oxidation of fatty acids, resulting in increased carbon dioxide (excreted through the lungs). In addition, if glucose is the only energy source, patients may develop essential fatty acid (linolenic, linoleic) deficiency.

Fat (e.g. soyabean oil emulsions) provides a more concentrated energy source. Usually, approximately

30–50% of the total calories are given as fat, with non-protein calorie to nitrogen ratio varying from 150:1 to 200:1 (lower in hypercatabolic conditions). The provision of exogenous lipids has also been associated with problems. Intravenous fat emulsions can impair lung function, inhibit the reticuloendothelial system and modulate neutrophil function; recent interest has also focused on the use of fish oils as a source of fat rich in omega-3 polyunsaturated fatty acids, as this appears to be associated with reduced incidence of hepatic dysfunction.[10]

Other nutrients

Commercially available preparations of trace elements (e.g. Additrace®) and vitamins, water-soluble (e.g. Solivito®) and fat-soluble (e.g. Vitlipid®), supply daily requirements. Larger amounts, particularly of the water-soluble vitamins, may be required initially if recent nutritional intake has been inadequate. Additionally, total fluid volume and amounts of electrolytes can be modified daily to meet particular requirements.

Delivery and administration of PN

It is possible to give individual components, but in practice it is safer and more convenient to use compounded bags. Compatibility between different prescribed constituents must be ensured then the parenteral infusion is compounded under sterile conditions in laminar flow facilities. No additions of drugs should be made as this could make the emulsion unstable, affect the bioavailability of the drug or compromise sterility.

Advantages of pre-mixed bags include:

- cost-effectiveness;
- reduced infective risks;
- more uniform administration of a balanced solution over a prolonged period;
- decreased lipid toxicity as a result of the greater dilution of the lipid emulsion and longer duration of infusion;
- ease of delivery and storage and reduced long-term accumulation of triglycerides (occurs with glucose-based PN).

Pre-compounded bags, including micronutrients, are now available covering a range of nutritional requirements, obviating the need for laminar flow facilities. A bag is chosen which approximates to anticipated nitrogen and calorie requirements; nothing should be added to these bags – extra fluid, electrolyte and minerals are given by separate infusion if required.

Complications of parenteral nutritional support

Instant availability of nutrients provided by the intravenous route can lead to metabolic complications if the composition or flow rate is inappropriate. Rapid infusion of high concentrations of glucose can precipitate hyperglycaemia, which may be further complicated by lactic acidosis. Electrolyte disturbances may present problems, not least because the intravenous feeding regimen is usually prescribed in advance for 24 hours. Prediction of the patient's nutrient requirements must be complemented by frequent monitoring. The provision of nutrients may lead to further electrolyte abnormalities when potassium, magnesium and phosphate enter the intracellular compartment. This is particularly noticeable in patients whose previous nutrient intake was especially poor, as highlighted previously. Other complications of PN are shown in Box 6.6.

Monitoring patients receiving nutritional support

Patients receiving nutritional support should be monitored by accurate recording of fluid balance and regular weighing. Daily intake of calories and nitrogen should be documented. Biochemical assessments include daily measurements of renal and liver function, with twice-weekly checks of phosphate, calcium, magnesium, albumin and protein concentrations, and haematological indices (haemoglobin, white blood cell count, haematocrit), until the patient is stabilised. Then, weekly or fortnightly measurements are necessary. Patients receiving PN require urinalysis daily initially in case glycosuria occurs, as this induces further fluid and electrolyte losses. If glycosuria occurs, it may be necessary to commence intravenous insulin on a sliding scale with blood glucose monitoring. It is important to note that if the PN fluid is stopped, insulin requirements will reduce immediately; it is safest to discontinue the insulin at the same time as the PN, reviewing the sliding scale with a view to giving intravenous glucose if required.

Routes of access should be regularly examined to ensure that the catheter remains correctly positioned and mechanically satisfactory.

When feeding is prolonged, other assessments, for example muscle function, nitrogen balance, measurement of trace elements and vitamins, may be performed regularly to ascertain patient progress (see nutritional assessment section above).

Glucose disturbances

Hyperglycaemia: excessive administration of glucose with inadequate insulin response, e.g. sepsis

Hypoglycaemia: rebound hypoglycaemia occurs if glucose is stopped abruptly but insulin concentrations remain high

Lipid disturbances

Hyperlipidaemia: directly through excess administration of lipid, or indirectly through excess calories that will be converted to fat or reduced metabolism (e.g. renal failure, liver failure)

Fatty acid deficiency: essential fatty acid deficiency leads to hair loss, dry skin, impaired wound healing

Nitrogen disturbances

Hyperammonaemia: occurs if deficiency of L-arginine, L-ornithine, L-aspartate or L-glutamate in infusion. Also occurs in liver diseases

Metabolic acidosis: caused by excessive amounts of chloride and monochloride amino acids

Electrolyte disturbances

Hyperkalaemia: excessive potassium administration or reduced losses

Hypokalaemia: inadequate potassium administration or excessive loss

Hypocalcaemia: inadequate calcium replacement, losses in pancreatitis, hypoalbuminaemia

Hypophosphataemia: inadequate phosphorus supplementation, also tissue compartment fluxes

Liver disturbances

Elevations in aspartate and alanine aminotransferases, alkaline phosphatase and γ-glutamyltransferase may occur because of enzyme induction secondary to amino acid imbalances or fatty liver from excess calories

Ventilatory problems

If excessive amounts of glucose are given, the increased production of CO_2 may precipitate ventilatory failure in non-ventilated patients

Nutritional support teams

It is clear that for optimal provision of nutritional support, a multidisciplinary nutritional support team is required. This may comprise a clinician with a special interest in nutritional support and

The provision of nutritional support by such a team results in the most cost-effective use of nutritional support and the least risk of infective, metabolic and feeding-line complications.[11]

understanding of metabolic pathways, a biochemist, a pharmacist, a dietician and a nursing specialist.

Nutritional support in defined clinical situations

Nutritional support in the perioperative period

Parenteral nutrition

Debate continues as to which patients require preoperative and/or postoperative nutritional support. Many studies have evaluated the effects of nutritional support in the perioperative period; clinical benefit with supplemental nutrition has not been a consistent finding. This may be because the studies were small, with many different end-points (e.g. morbidity, mortality), frequently without proper randomisation or allowance for malnutrition prior to the study commencing. It is clear however that benefit is dependent on the nature of surgery required; ESPEN guidance is available for a number of specific situations.

In general, however, the enteral route is the preferred route except in specific circumstances where not possible (e.g. intestinal obstruction, ileus, intestinal ischaemia, etc.) or used in combination with PN if the nutritional requirements cannot be provided by the enteral route alone.

The ESPEN guidance is summarised as follows.[12]

Patients who should receive perioperative nutritional support:

- Those expected not to eat for >7 days perioperatively.
- Those unable to have an oral intake >60% of their recommended intake for >10 days.

Patients who should receive preoperative enteral nutritional support:

- Preoperative nutritional support should be considered in specific situations.

Patients who should receive postoperative nutritional support:

- Early enteral nutritional feeding (i.e. <24 hours after surgery) is recommended for patients who have undergone upper gastrointestinal anastomosis with the tip of a feeding tube placed distal to the anastomosis.

Enteral nutrition given to patients in the perioperative period has been reviewed and published as European Society of Parenteral and Enteral Nutrition (ESPEN) guidelines12 (www.espen.org).

Nutritional support in patients with acute pancreatitis (see also Chapter 14)

Severe pancreatitis produces a major catabolic stress with rapid loss of muscle proteins. The daily nitrogen requirements of such patients are high, reaching 1.2–2.0 g protein/kg body weight (0.2–0.3 g of nitrogen/kg). Daily energy requirements also increase with disease severity to be 28–35 kcal/kg. Previously, patients with pancreatitis were fasted in order to avoid pancreatic stimulation. However, a Cochrane review has shown that for patients with acute severe pancreatitis, early enteral support results in better outcomes, including mortality.[13]

✓✓ Patients with severe acute pancreatitis should commence early enteral nutritional support as this is associated with a better outcome.[13]

Nutritional supplementation in inflammatory bowel disease

A significant number of patients with Crohn's disease and ulcerative colitis become malnourished. The reasons for this include decreased nutrient intake, malabsorption by the small intestine (decreased length, bacterial overgrowth, protein-losing enteropathy) and increased calorie/nitrogen requirements in those with coexistent sepsis. There may be deficiencies of specific vitamins and trace elements.

Nutritional support, therefore, may be required empirically, with some suggestion that relapse rate in Crohn's may be reduced, but to date there are insufficient trial data to confirm specific outcome benefit from either enteral or parenteral nutrition.[14,15]

✓ While systematic reviews have shown some potential for enteral nutrition to maintain remission in Crohn's disease, further studies are required to clarify the use of nutrition in this way.[14,15]

Nutritional support in enterocutaneous fistulas

Nutritional support has an important role to play in management of patients with enterocutaneous fistulas as up to 50% are malnourished. The importance of adequate nutritional support is well established, but whether PN or enteral nutrition is more effective is unknown. Other techniques for providing nutritional support have included collecting the intestinal output from the proximal end of the fistula and re-infusing it into the distal part of the small intestine or by giving enteral nutrition via the fistula. If the fistula output is low, enteral nutritional support should be considered because of the benefits.[16]

✓ Enteral nutrition has theoretical benefits due to its effects on gut mucosa, and case series have suggested that healing rates with enteral nutrition are comparable to those of parenteral nutrition.[16]

Nutritional support in patients with burns

Major burns induce severe hypermetabolic and hypercatabolic states. There is increased skeletal muscle breakdown, nitrogen losses of 15 g daily or more, and up to a doubling of metabolic rate. In patients with burns of greater than 20% of their body surface area, nutritional support is required, orally or by nasoenteric feeding. Feeding early, with glutamine supplementation, is recommended by the ESPEN guidelines.[17]

✓ Glutamine supplementation should be given to patients with substantial burns to reduce their complications and improve healing.[17]

Nutritional supplementation with key nutrients: application to clinical practice

Certain nutrients can have effects on cellular and tissue function. Some of these nutrients modulate immune and inflammatory responses if given in excess of normal intake or requirements. The use of nutrients ('nutriceuticals') in this way has been termed 'nutritional pharmacology'. Examples and specific effects include:

- L-arginine – stimulates aspects of immune function, improves nitrogen retention after surgery, enhances wound healing;[18,19]
- L-glutamine – stimulates immune function, reduces nitrogen loss postoperatively, may be important in maintaining gut-barrier function;[20]
- branched-chain amino acids – may control protein synthesis in muscle and stimulate whole-body protein synthesis, especially in severely traumatised patients;[21]
- essential fatty acids – stimulation or inhibition of immune function, anti-inflammatory effects;[22,23]

- polyribonucleotides and ribonucleic acid – stimulate immune function;
- vitamins, trace elements – stimulation of immune function, antioxidant effects, wound healing;
- selenium – stimulation of immune function, prevention of tissue damage, anti-inflammatory effects;[24]
- omega-3 fatty acids – immunomodulatory effect and avoidance of hepatic dysfunction.[25]

The clinical benefits of supplementation with key nutrients have, however, been difficult to demonstrate.

Combinations of these nutrients and their place in practice

Several studies have evaluated the use of combinations of key nutrients in clinical practice in patients with critical illnesses (trauma, surgery for malignant disease, burns), but particularly in upper gastrointestinal cancer. A combination of L-arginine, n-3 essential fatty acids and ribonucleic acid is commercially available (Impact; Sandoz Nutrition, Minneapolis, MN, USA) and has been

used in many trials. The supplemented nutrition has been given in the postoperative period (nasoenteric tube or feeding jejunostomy), starting within 12–48 hours of the critical events and continued for several days.

The first meta-analysis of the studies that have compared supplemented nutritional versus standard nutritional diets (**Figs 6.2** and **6.3**) showed that supplemented nutrition had clinical benefits:[26]

- reduction in infectious complications (wound infections, intra-abdominal abscesses, septicaemia), with an odds ratio of 0.47 (95% CI 0.32–0.70);
- reduction in length of hospital stay, with a weighted mean difference of −2.4 days (95% CI −4 to −1).

However, there was no significant difference in mortality. A subsequent meta-analysis of 17 trials has confirmed this benefit.[27]

Many of these studies had methodological limitations but, nevertheless, the role of immunonutrition in critically ill patients was further investigated by ESPEN.[17] The conclusion drawn

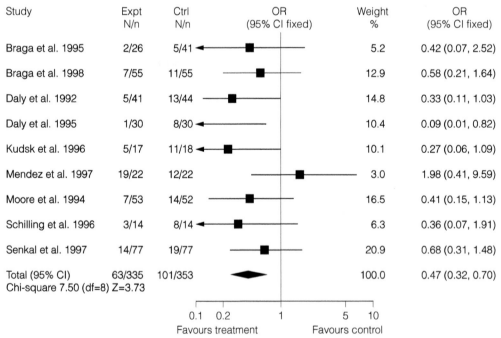

Study	Expt N/n	Ctrl N/n	OR (95% CI fixed)	Weight %	OR (95% CI fixed)
Braga et al. 1995	2/26	5/41		5.2	0.42 (0.07, 2.52)
Braga et al. 1998	7/55	11/55		12.9	0.58 (0.21, 1.64)
Daly et al. 1992	5/41	13/44		14.8	0.33 (0.11, 1.03)
Daly et al. 1995	1/30	8/30		10.4	0.09 (0.01, 0.82)
Kudsk et al. 1996	5/17	11/18		10.1	0.27 (0.06, 1.09)
Mendez et al. 1997	19/22	12/22		3.0	1.98 (0.41, 9.59)
Moore et al. 1994	7/53	14/52		16.5	0.41 (0.15, 1.13)
Schilling et al. 1996	3/14	8/14		6.3	0.36 (0.07, 1.91)
Senkal et al. 1997	14/77	19/77		20.9	0.68 (0.31, 1.48)
Total (95% CI) Chi-square 7.50 (df=8) Z=3.73	63/335	101/353		100.0	0.47 (0.32, 0.70)

0.1   0.2   1   5   10
Favours treatment   Favours control

Figure 6.2 • Effect of immune-enhancing diets on the incidence of major infective complications (wound infections, intra-abdominal abscesses, pneumonia, septicaemia). Expt, patients receiving immune-enhancing diets; Ctrl, patients receiving standard nutrition; n, number of events; N, number of patients in each group on an intention-to-treat basis; OR, odds ratio; CI, confidence interval. (Study sources are given in Heys et al.[20])
Reproduced from Heys SD, Walker LG, Smith IC, et al. Enteral nutritional supplementation with key nutrients in patients with critical illness and cancer. A meta-analysis of randomised controlled clinical trials. Ann Surg 1999; 229:467–77. With permission from Wolter Kluwer Health.

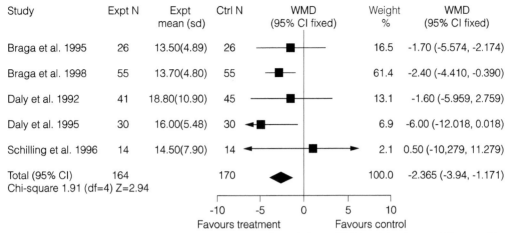

Study	Expt N	Expt mean (sd)	Ctrl N	WMD (95% CI fixed)	Weight %	WMD (95% CI fixed)
Braga et al. 1995	26	13.50(4.89)	26		16.5	-1.70 (-5.574, -2.174)
Braga et al. 1998	55	13.70(4.80)	55		61.4	-2.40 (-4.410, -0.390)
Daly et al. 1992	41	18.80(10.90)	45		13.1	-1.60 (-5.959, 2.759)
Daly et al. 1995	30	16.00(5.48)	30		6.9	-6.00 (-12.018, 0.018)
Schilling et al. 1996	14	14.50(7.90)	14		2.1	0.50 (-10,279, 11.279)
Total (95% CI)	164		170		100.0	-2.365 (-3.94, -1.171)

Chi-square 1.91 (df=4) Z=2.94

-10   -5   0   5   10
Favours treatment   Favours control

Figure 6.3 • Effect of immune-enhancing diets on the length of hospital stay. WMD, weighted mean difference; CI, confidence interval. (Study sources are given in Heys et al.[26])
Reproduced from Heys SD, Walker LG, Smith IC, et al. Enteral nutritional supplementation with key nutrients in patients with critical illness and cancer. A meta-analysis of randomised controlled clinical trials. Ann Surg 1999; 229:467–77. With permission from Wolter Kluwer Health.

from the consensus based on the available evidence was that an immune-modulating nutrition (enriched with arginine, nucleotides and omega-3 fatty acids) was beneficial and recommended for the following:

- patients with mild sepsis (APACHE II score <15);
- patients undergoing elective major intra-abdominal surgery for cancer to receive 5–7 days of immune-enhancing nutrition (arginine, omega-3 fatty acids and polyribonucleotides);
- patients with acute respiratory distress syndrome (ARDS) should receive enteral nutrition supplemented with omega-3 fatty acids and antioxidants.

In addition, there were situations identified where immunonutrition should not be given due to potentially adverse effects:

- patients with severe sepsis;
- patients unable to tolerate more than 700 mL/day of immunonutrition.

✓✓ Immune-modulating nutrition is associated with a reduction in septic complications and a reduced hospital stay. It should be considered in patients with mild sepsis (APACHE II score <15), patients undergoing elective major intra-abdominal surgery for cancer and in patients with ARDS.[17,26,27]

Key points

- Malnutrition is associated with loss of body weight and impairments in organ function.
- The metabolic changes that occur in patients undergoing surgery or in those who have experienced trauma and sepsis can be compounded by inadequate nutritional support.
- Nutritional requirements must take into consideration the underlying pathophysiological changes.
- An assessment of nutritional status should be made in all patients.
- If nutritional support is considered necessary, the route and composition of this support should be considered carefully.
- Remember re-feeding syndrome and possible thiamine deficiency.
- The role of certain key nutrients and their effects, either individually or in combination, on aspects of organ and immune function should be taken into consideration when planning nutritional interventions.
- There is now emerging evidence to indicate that manipulating the composition of nutritional support can affect patient outcome.
- Careful monitoring of patients receiving nutritional support and the role of the multidisciplinary team is essential for all patients.

⊕ Full references available at **http://expertconsult. inkling.com**

Key references

11. National Institute for Health and Care Excellence. www.nice.org.uk/CG32.

NICE guidance on nutrition support in adults: oral nutrition support, enteral tube feeding and parenteral nutrition, including guidelines for the role and function of multidisciplinary nutritional support teams.

12. Weimann A, Braga M, Harsanyi L, et al. ESPEN guidelines on enteral nutrition: surgery – including organ transplantation. Clin Nutr 2006;25(2):224–44. PMID: 16698152.

Evidence-based guidelines summarising the current evidence and making recommendations for clinical practice in patients during the perioperative period.

13. Al-Omran M, AlBalawi ZH, Tashkandi MF, et al. Enteral versus parenteral nutrition for acute pancreatitis. Cochrane Database Syst Rev 2010;CD002837. PMID: 20091534.

17. Kreymann KG, Berger MM, Deutz NEP, et al. ESPEN guidelines on enteral nutrition: intensive care. Clin Nutr 2006;25:210–23. PMID: 16697087.

Evidence-based guidelines summarising the current evidence and making recommendations for clinical practice.

26. Heys SD, Walker LG, Smith IC, et al. Enteral nutritional supplementation with key nutrients in patients with critical illness and cancer. A meta-analysis of randomised controlled clinical trials. Ann Surg 1999;229:467–77. PMID: 10203078.

This is the first meta-analysis that indicated that immunonutrition could result in clinically important benefits for patients in terms of reduction in infectious complications postoperatively.

27. Heyland DK, Novak F, Drover JW, et al. Should immunonutrition become routine in critically ill patients? JAMA 2001;286:944–53. PMID: 11509059.

This is an updated meta-analysis of randomised controlled trials that confirms the previous meta-analysis and extends it further by examining different subgroups of patients in an attempt to try to understand further which patients are the most likely to benefit from immunonutrition.

7

Abdominal hernias

Andrew C. de Beaux

Introduction

A hernia is defined as an abnormal protrusion of a cavity's contents through a weakness in the wall of the cavity, taking with it all the linings of the cavity, although these may be markedly attenuated. They can be described as reducible, incarcerated or strangulated. A reducible hernia is one in which the contents of the hernial sac can be manually introduced back into the abdomen while, conversely, an irreducible or incarcerated hernia cannot be manipulated back into the abdomen. A strangulated hernia occurs when the vascular supply to the contents contained within the hernia is compromised, resulting in ischaemic and gangrenous tissue.

Aetiology

Multiple factors contribute to the development of hernias. Hernias are associated with a number of medical conditions, including connective tissue disorders such as Ehlers–Danlos syndrome, as well as a number of abnormal collagen-related disorders such as varicose veins and arterial aneurysm. In essence, hernias can be considered design faults, either anatomical or through inherited collagen disorders, although these two aetiological factors probably work together in the majority of patients. Anatomical design faults can be considered at any site where structures within the cavity exit through an opening in the wall of the cavity, such as blood vessels, bowel or the spermatic cord. This is typical, for example around the oesophagus and in the groin. However, not everyone develops a groin hernia so other factors must be important in its aetiology. The fascia and surrounding tissues that

cover muscle, acting to hold the muscle bundles together, may appear relatively avascular, but it remains a complex and living structure. The genetic code for fascia is coded on DNA, and within fibroblasts the sequence is messenger RNA, transfer RNA, peptide formation, with fusion of peptides into approximately 1000-amino-acid polypeptides called alpha chains. The endoplasmic reticulum converts these to procollagen. Procollagen is the large building block of collagen, comprising triple-helix strands, stabilised by hydroxylation of proline and lysine, which is vitamin C-dependent. These triple-helix strands form microfibrils, then fibrils, then fibres and finally bundles. These collagen bundles surrounded by extracellular matrix comprise fascia. The control of this process is mediated through matrix metalloproteinases, which in turn are controlled by tissue inhibitory metalloproteinases. If this is not complex enough, there is also control by collagen-interacting proteins and receptors such as fibronectin, tenasin and collagen receptor discoidin domain receptor 2. Fascia and tendon are made up of type I and type III collagen (type II is found in cartilage and type IV in the basement membrane of cells). In cross-section, there is a bimodal distribution of bundle size with the fibres orientated in the line of pull. The larger bundles are type I collagen, imparting the strength to the fascia or tendon. The type III collagen bundles are smaller and are thought to provide elastic recoil following stretch when the tissues have been loaded. The type I to III collagen ratio varies between individuals but is constant in all the fascia of a particular individual.

A clinical observation was made by surgeons in the late 1960s that the anterior rectus sheath some distance from the hernial defect was thinner than normal, especially in those patients with direct hernias.[1] Since then, research has demonstrated a variety of defects in collagen synthesis in such patients.[2] The current notion is that the majority of hernias are a disease of collagen metabolism. One of the key factors in this is the type I to III collagen ratio. The lower this ratio, from an average of around 5, the more likely the individual is to develop a hernia. Currently, collagen typing is not used in clinical practice to help decide perhaps which patients merit a mesh as opposed to a suture repair, but this may well be a development in the near future.

✔ Hernias are a collagen disease, with reduced collagen type I to III ratio.[2]

Classification of hernias

A number of hernia classifications exist, both for the description of hernia characteristics such as size and location and also hernia surgery-related complications. The use of such classifications aids the reporting of hernia series, reducing the risk of comparing 'apples with oranges'. For example, the use of mesh in the repair of small hernias in general, does not have such a marked benefit in terms of reducing hernia recurrence compared to larger hernia defects. Classifications based on size and location allow the surgeon to think more about tailored surgery, as one operation technique does not always fit all. The European Hernia Society inguinal hernia classification[3] and the EuraHS ventral hernia classification[4] are two such useful pragmatic classifications.

Mesh

Much will be mentioned about mesh repairs of hernias in the remainder of this chapter, but this section gives a brief overview of mesh and its science. Many companies produce a variety of mesh for hernia repair. These are either synthetic (man-made) or biological (preparations from animal or human tissue). The majority of synthetic meshes are woven from either polypropylene (monofilament) or polyester (multi- and monofilament), but new polymers continue to be developed. Biological meshes are typically animal collagen, either from skin or bowel, but there are also human preparations. Biological meshes tend to be much more expensive and should be reserved for specialist use.

It goes without saying that any mesh should have the usual properties of any implant, including being non-allergenic, non-carcinogenic, have good incorporation into tissue and mimic the tissue it is replacing or reinforcing. The abdominal wall is not a rigid structure, but regularly copes with increases in abdominal pressure on coughing and sneezing, etc. of up to 200 mmHg. The abdominal wall elasticity is greater in women than in men and is greater in the cranio-caudal direction than transversely or obliquely. The traditional standard weight polypropylene mesh, of around $100 \, g/m^2$, is significantly over-engineered, with a burst strength at least an order of magnitude greater than the anterior abdominal wall and an elasticity of much less. As a result there are now many polypropylene meshes on the market of lighter weight. However, 'lightweight' is a misnomer. Some heavyweight meshes behave in a 'lightweight' fashion and vice versa, as it is not just the weight of the mesh that imparts mesh elasticity and flexibility. The weave of the strands in the mesh may impart varying flexibility or elasticity to the mesh in different directions of pull, so-called anisotropy. Pore size or the size of the large holes in the mesh is also important. Mesh has a volume with length, breadth and thickness. The amount of empty space within the 'volume' of the mesh is the porosity and the effective porosity is the amount of empty space within the volume of the mesh made up of holes that are bigger than 1 mm diameter. It has recently been proposed that an effective porosity of a mesh for hernia repair should be at least 60%.[5] Fibrosis will occur around each strand of the mesh. If the strands are close together, the fibrosis around each strand will coalesce, forming a solid scar plate. As the scar plate matures it will shrink, reducing the overall size of the mesh. The minimum pore size should be about $1 \, mm^2$ but many meshes have pore sizes around 3–5 mm. Increasing the macroporosity of the mesh produces a scar net, rather than a scar plate, with normal tissue in between the fibre/scar complex, reducing mesh/scar shrinkage and improving flexibility (**Fig. 7.1**). Furthermore, increasing the macropore size reduces the bulk of the foreign body implant, and their use in contaminated fields, due to reduced bacterial adherence and increased bacterial clearance, is becoming acceptable practice. In addition to the macropore size, mesh also has micropores within the mesh material itself. These should be at least $10 \, \mu m$ in size. If the micropore size is smaller, bacteria can harbour in the pores out of reach of the larger inflammatory cells.

The majority of synthetic meshes in the UK are polypropylene. Gore-Tex and other poly-tetrafluoroethylene (PTFE)-based meshes also have some popularity. PTFE has no macropores so will be encapsulated by fibrous tissue with minimal tissue ingrowth. Polyester-based meshes are gaining popularity and have some advantages over polyproplyene but are mostly multifilament rather than monofilament. The multifilament arrangement increases the developed surface of the mesh (around 10-fold) and thus improves tissue incorporation.

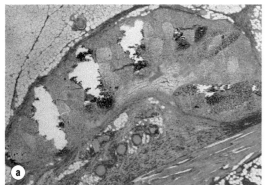
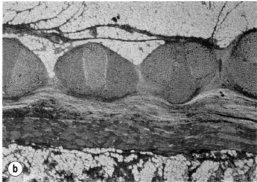
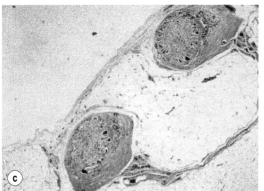

Figure 7.1 • (a) Micrograph of a macropore mesh of <0.5 mm pore size showing scar plate formation and contraction/distortion of the mesh. (b) Micrograph of a macropore mesh of 0.8 mm pore size showing minimal scar bridging and no distortion of the mesh. (c) Micrograph of a macropore mesh of 3 mm pore size showing scar net formation and no contraction/distortion of the mesh.
Micrographs used by permission of Medtronic.

As a result, the peel strength (the effort required to separate the mesh from the tissues once it is incorporated) is greater (**Fig. 7.2**).

The latest mesh category is slowly resorbable synthetic mesh, with resorption taking many months to years. It is hoped that such meshes will reduce the sensation of mesh, or the risk of problems from mesh infection, but there are no long-term data available to comment on hernia recurrence risk, for example.

✔ Preferred mesh should be 'lightweight' (<80 g/m^2), large pore (>1 mm) and macroporous (>10 μm).

Traditional meshes placed within the abdominal cavity have a high rate of adhesions of the omentum and bowel to the mesh. This can result in bowel fistulation or make subsequent laparotomy more difficult, with increased risk of bowel perforation and thus the need for bowel resection during the process of re-entering the abdominal cavity.[6] A number of tissue-separating meshes are available, where the intra-abdominal side of the mesh is coated with a product to minimise adhesion formation. It would be fair to say that while such coatings do reduce adhesion formation, in the majority of patients significant adhesion to such coatings still occurs. The main points of adhesion appear to be the edge of the mesh and to the points of fixation, either

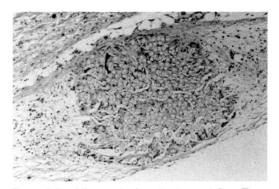

Figure 7.2 • Micrograph of a polyester mesh fibre. There is evidence of fibrosis around the fibre bundle as well as fibrous ingrowth around each strand.
Micrograph used by permission of Covidien UK.

sutures, tacks or staples. Nevertheless, it is likely that these products will improve in the future, as meshes become more physiological, perhaps impregnated with growth hormones and other biologically active molecules to improve the mesh/tissue integration.

Biological mesh (a slight misnomer as most biological meshes are really sheets of collagen) has gained popularity in hernia repair. It is, however, disappointing that, from the thousands of biological meshes that have been implanted worldwide (often at great expense as biological mesh is 10–100 times more expensive than polypropylene mesh), follow-up data on only a few hundred patients have been published. What is becoming evident, though, is that biological meshes are not all the same. The major difference, in addition to the animal and anatomical source of the mesh, is the degree of chemical processing, or cross-linking, of the biological product. The more the collagen is cross-linked, the more resistant it is to bacterial collagenase breakdown in the presence of infection. The downside to cross-linking is that the more the collagen is cross-linked, the less tissue in-growth and integration occurs, with reduction in potential strength to the repair. It is becoming evident that most biological meshes have no role in dirty wounds, acting as little more than a very expensive dressing. They are too expensive for use in clean wounds as any benefit is not worth the huge price difference, and using them for bridging (mesh spanning the fascial gap as opposed to augmentation, where the mesh reinforces or augments the fascial closure) also results in a high percentage of failure. The author's opinion is that there is no good evidence available to suggest that biological mesh is superior or even as good as polypropylene in clean/contaminated operations, or in patients with significant medical comorbidity. Similarly, there is a lack of comparative evidence in contaminated operations, although fortunately this is a very small part of hernia surgery.

Epigastric hernia

An epigastric hernia is defined as a fascial defect in the linea alba between the xiphoid process and the umbilicus.

Aetiology

The aetiology is related to the functional anatomy of the abdominal wall. The anterior abdominal wall aponeurosis consists of tendinous fibres that lie obliquely in aponeurotic sheets, allowing for changes in the shape of the abdominal wall, for example during respiration, or distension. Such abdominal wall movement/change may result in tearing of fibres leading to the development of an epigastric hernia.

Clinical presentation

The majority of epigastric hernias (probably 75%) are asymptomatic. Typical symptoms, if present, include vague upper abdominal pain and nausea associated with epigastric tenderness. The symptoms can be more severe when the patient is lying down (usually the opposite if the pain is caused by a hernia), attributed to traction on the hernial contents. Pain on exertion localised to the epigastrium is also

a common symptom. Incarceration is frequent, and strangulation of pre-peritoneal fat or omentum results in localised pain and tenderness. Incarceration or strangulation of intra-abdominal viscera is rare, the symptoms obviously depending on the incarcerated organ.

The presence of a midline mass on physical examination usually confirms the diagnosis. In obese patients, palpation of the mass may be difficult and confirmation of the diagnosis by ultrasound (US) or computed tomography (CT) may be helpful.

Management

Epigastric hernias are rare in infants and children, and asymptomatic hernias in children under the age of 10 years may resolve spontaneously. The decision for surgical intervention depends on the presence and severity of symptoms.

Operative details

Small solitary defects may be approached with either a vertical or transverse incision in the midline, centred over the hernia. For larger hernias, if the defects are multiple or in the emergency setting when a strangulated viscus is suspected, a vertical incision is preferred. The hernia and its contents are dissected free of the surrounding tissues and, if present, the hernial contents examined and dealt with appropriately. If the defect is small (<2 cm), repair by primary suture closure using non-absorbable material may be sufficient. The orientation of the suture closure remains controversial, some surgeons preferring a vertical closure and others a horizontal orientation. There are few data to support one technique over the other and probably the direction resulting in the least tension is the most appropriate. If the defect is large (>2 cm), or occurs within a divarification of the recti, the hernia should be repaired with prosthetic mesh. This technique is described later in the chapter when considering incisional hernias. The technique applied to intermediate-sized hernias is controversial and suture or mesh techniques are both currently deemed acceptable. Laparoscopic repair of epigastric hernias has grown in popularity. The author prefers an open technique under local anaesthetic whenever possible for smaller hernias (defect < 2 cm), suture or mesh depending on the quality of the tissues, and the laparoscopic approach for larger, multiple, recurrent hernias, or hernias in the obese. At laparoscopic repair, it is important to take down the falciform ligament and remove any pre-peritoneal fat above the linea alba, otherwise the 'hernia' may still be palpable following the alleged repair.

Complications

Complication rates are low and most are the usual complications associated with abdominal wall incisions (haematoma, infection). There are few data on recurrence rates, but a recent study supports mesh repair for even small hernias.[7] In a number of patients, however, the recurrence probably represents the persistence of a second hernia or area of weakness overlooked at the initial procedure, or a new hernia nearby. The laparoscopic technique avoids this problem because all fascial defects are visible laparoscopically if adequate dissection is carried out, and the mesh will re-enforce a large part of the midline at risk of hernia formation.

Umbilical and para-umbilical hernias

There are several distinct types of hernia that occur around the umbilicus: congenital (omphalocele), infantile, para-umbilical and adult umbilical hernias.

Congenital umbilical hernias

A congenital umbilical hernia occurs when the abdominal viscera herniate into the tissue of the umbilical cord. Normally, the gut returns to the abdominal cavity at 10 weeks of gestation. If this fails to occur, normal rotation and fixation of the intestine are prevented, the umbilicus is absent and a funnel-shaped defect in the abdominal wall is present through which viscera protrude into the umbilical cord. The abdominal wall defect may vary in size from no larger than an umbilical stump to a defect that appears to involve the entire abdominal wall. Congenital umbilical hernia occurs in 1 in 5000 births and is associated with other serious congenital anomalies. Congenital and infantile umbilical hernias are discussed in more detail in Chapter 18 and will not be dealt with further here. While some infantile umbilical hernias will persist into adulthood, their management can be considered together with para-umbilical hernias even if their aetiology is different.

Para-umbilical hernias

Para-umbilical hernias are acquired hernias and occur in all age groups. They occur secondary to disruption of the linea alba and generally occur above the umbilical cicatrix. Aetiological factors include stretching of the abdominal wall by obesity, multiple pregnancy and ascites. Para-umbilical hernias are more common in patients over the age of 35 years and are five times more common in females.

Clinical presentation

Clinically, para-umbilical hernias are frequently symptomatic. Patients complain of intermittent abdominal pain (possibly caused by dragging on the fat and peritoneum of the falciform ligament) and, when the hernial sac contains bowel, colic resulting from intermittent intestinal obstruction. The hernia tends to progress over time and both intertrigo and necrosis of the skin may occur in patients with large dependent hernias. Such symptoms are a good indication for surgery.

Management

It is important to distinguish para-umbilical hernias from true umbilical defects as the latter may resolve spontaneously in the young, whereas the former require surgical correction. Umbilical hernias classically produce a symmetrical bulge with the protrusion directly under the umbilicus. This is in contrast to para-umbilical hernias, where about half the fundus of the sac is covered by the umbilicus and the remainder is covered by the skin of the abdomen directly above or below the umbilicus(**Fig. 7.3**). Para-umbilical hernias do not resolve spontaneously and have a high incidence of incarceration and strangulation; therefore surgical repair is nearly always indicated.

Operative details

For solitary hernias separated from the umbilicus, a transverse incision over the hernia produces the best exposure. In patients with a para-umbilical and umbilical hernia, a midline incision may provide

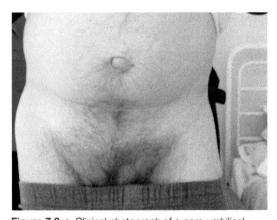

Figure 7.3 • Clinical photograph of a para-umbilical hernia. Note the swelling of the right groin of an associated right inguinal hernia – a common finding consistent with a generalised collagen disorder.

better access. Similarly, if multiple fascial defects are present or there is concern about the integrity of visceral contents of the sac, a vertical incision may be better employed. If the defect simply contains pre-peritoneal fat, this may be reduced. In patients with strangulated or ischaemic pre-peritoneal fat, it is best excised. If there is a sac present, it should be dissected free from the fascial edges, opened and the contents examined. Once the contents have been dealt with appropriately, they may be reduced and redundant sac excised. Repair is performed by fascial apposition either transversely or longitudinally, depending on the defect and the direction of least tension. As this is an acquired defect, non-absorbable sutures are recommended. Indeed, the author usually creates a pre-peritoneal pocket, inserting a 5 cm × 5 cm square (minimum size – bigger if necessary) mesh and closing the fascia over this. Again, the higher recurrence rate for suture repair over mesh repair for small hernias is noted.[7] For larger para-umbilical hernias, with a neck size >2 cm (or smaller hernias in an obese patient), it is the author's preference to repair these laparoscopically and very large hernias with a neck size >7 cm by an open sublay technique (described later).

The overlying umbilical skin need not be excised unless it is macerated or infected, although the cosmetic appearance is often enhanced by judicious removal of excess skin and subcutaneous fat. Patients should be warned that it might be necessary to excise the umbilicus.

Complications

Complications include the development of seromas, haematomas and infection. Sealed suction drains may be employed in the retromuscular and subcutaneous planes to help avoid the development of large seromas. In addition to local problems, these patients may have respiratory and cardiovascular complications.

Adult umbilical hernias

Umbilical hernias in adults represent a spectrum of conditions from the partially unfolded cicatrix to huge dependent sacs. The umbilicus may become partially unfolded in patients with acute abdominal distension. Persistent elevation of intra-abdominal pressure eventually results in the umbilical cicatrix giving way and the development of an umbilical hernia. Although uncommon, causes include ascites from cirrhosis or congestive cardiac failure and patients undergoing peritoneal dialysis. Management should be non-operative where possible, as the majority of these patients have serious underlying comorbidity. Operative repair is not indicated unless the hernia incarcerates or

becomes extremely large and the overlying skin is thinned down to such an extent that spontaneous rupture is possible.

Umbilical hernias in adults do not represent persistence of infantile hernias but are indirect herniations through an umbilical canal, which is bordered by umbilical fascia posteriorly, the linea alba anteriorly and the medial edges of the two rectus sheaths on each side. They have a tendency to incarcerate and strangulate and do not resolve spontaneously. The clinical presentation, management and complications of adult umbilical hernia are very similar to those of para-umbilical hernia, as described above.

Spigelian, lumbar and other primary ventral hernias

Away from the midline, there are a number of anatomical sites where abdominal wall hernia is possible. Sometimes the hernia that develops is called an interstitial hernia – when the hernia protrudes through transversus abdomina and internal oblique, but external oblique remains intact although it may become stretched over the hernia. This can lead to intraoperative uncertainty when, at open surgery, the external oblique is exposed but no hernia is found. Careful marking of the bulge pre-operation, and then incising external oblique at this site will uncover the underlying interstitial hernia. The occasional misdiagnosis of a subcutaneous lipoma as a Spigelian hernia is recognised but is usually obvious at the time of surgery.

As for midline ventral hernias, there are various open and laparoscopic operations for repair, with the type of operation chosen following discussion with the patient taking into account surgeon and patient factors.

Inguinal hernias

Anatomy

The inguinal canal is approximately 4 cm in length and is located just above the inguinal ligament between the internal and external rings. The inguinal canal allows passage of the spermatic cord into the scrotum, along with the testicular, deferential and cremasteric vessels. The superficial ring is a triangular aperture in the aponeurosis of the external oblique and lies about 1 cm above the pubic tubercle. Normally, the ring will not admit the tip of the little finger. The deep ring is a U-shaped condensation of the transversalis fascia and it lies about 1–2 cm above the inguinal ligament, midway between the pubic tubercle and the anterior superior iliac spine.

The transversalis fascia is the fascial envelope of the abdomen and the competency of the deep inguinal ring depends on the integrity of this fascia.

The anterior boundary of the inguinal canal comprises mainly the external oblique aponeurosis with the conjoined muscle laterally. The posterior boundary is formed by the fascia transversalis and the conjoined tendon (internal oblique and transversus abdominus medially). The inferior epigastric vessels lie posteriorly and medially to the deep inguinal ring. The superior boundary is formed by the conjoined muscles (internal oblique and transversus) and the inferior boundary by the inguinal ligament.

Definition

An indirect hernia travels down the canal on the outer (lateral and anterior) side of the spermatic cord. A direct inguinal hernia comes out directly forwards through the posterior wall of the inguinal canal. While the neck of an indirect hernia is lateral to the epigastric vessels, the direct hernia usually emerges medial to these vessels, except in the saddle-bag or pantaloon type, which has both a lateral and a medial component (**Fig. 7.4**).

Inguinal hernia in infants and children (see also Chapter 18)

Repair of congenital inguinal hernia is the most frequently performed operation in the paediatric age group. Although inguinal hernias can present

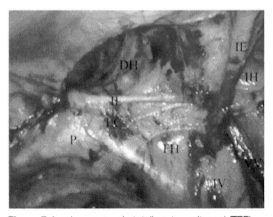

Figure 7.4 • Laparoscopic totally extraperitoneal (TEP) view of the right groin with a direct inguinal hernia (*DH*) lying medial to the inferior epigastric vessels (*IE*), above the inguinal (*IL*) and lacunar (*LC*) ligaments. The pubic bone (*P*), iliac vessels (*IV*), vas and vessels (*VV*) are also seen. The positions of a femoral hernia (*FH*) and indirect inguinal hernia (*IH*) are also marked.

at any age, the peak incidence is during infancy and childhood. About 3–5% of full-term infants may be born with a clinical inguinal hernia, with prematurity increasing the incidence, as does male gender. Congenital inguinal hernias have a 15% bilateral presentation.

Clinical presentation

Examination of the inguinal area for a hernia may show an obvious bulge at the site of the external ring or within the scrotum that can often be gently reduced. However, the bulge may only be seen during severe straining, such as with crying or defaecation. If the infant is old enough to stand, he or she should be examined in both the supine and standing positions. If not, the parent can hold the infant upright so that the surgeon can closely observe the inguinoscrotal area. Sometimes, photographs taken by the parent when a swelling appears can aid in the diagnosis in the difficult case. It is essential to make sure that the testis is within the scrotal sac to avoid mistaking a retractile testis for a hernial bulge. The presence of an empty scrotum should alert the examining surgeon to a possible undescended or ectopic testis, which is associated with an inguinal hernia in more than 90% of patients. Although routine orchidopexy is usually delayed until the child is 1 year of age, a coexisting symptomatic hernia should be promptly repaired and orchidopexy accomplished at the same time.

Inguinal hernias in infants and children are prone to incarcerate, with the overall rate being around 10%. Incarceration is most common in the first 6 months of life, when more than half of all instances are observed. An incarcerated hernia usually presents as an acute tender mass in the inguinal canal. The mass may protrude beyond the external inguinal ring or into the scrotum. The skin over the mass may be discoloured, oedematous, erythematous or blue. Strangulation, characterised by abdominal distension, vomiting, failure to pass faecal material, tachycardia and radiological evidence of small-bowel obstruction, demands emergency operative intervention for relief of obstruction, intestinal salvage and hernia repair. In contrast to the adult with an incarcerated hernia, in children testicular ischaemia is far more common than intestinal ischaemia, and it is therefore appropriate to be aggressive about early reduction and surgery to the hernia (see also Chapter 18).

Management

In general, hernias in children and particularly infants should be managed by experienced paediatric surgeons (see also Chapter 18). However, this is not always possible depending on geography and availability. In these circumstances the general surgeon on call may be required to manage these patients. As most (80%) incarcerated hernias in children may be managed initially by non-operative measures, which include sedation, and then gentle reduction when the baby is quiet, exploration may be safely delayed for about 24–48 hours, allowing, if possible, a more experienced paediatric surgeon to become involved. However, if the hernia remains irreducible at this stage, emergency repair is indicated, accepting that the complications rate of emergency surgery is much greater than that of elective surgery. This is covered in more detail in Chapter 18.

Operative details

Surgical access is achieved through a short (2–3 cm) transverse incision in the lowest inguinal skin crease. The superficial fascia (Scarpa's fascia) is incised and the external oblique fascia identified. The aponeurosis is traced inferiorly and laterally to identify the inguinal ligament and the exact location of the external inguinal ring. The hernial sac is always located in an anteromedial position in relation to the cord and gentle blunt dissection of the cremasteric fibres usually brings the sac into view. The sac is elevated with a haemostat and the cremasteric fibres carefully freed from the anterior and lateral aspects. Retraction of the sac medially allows identification of the spermatic vessels and vas deferens, and these structures may be carefully teased away from the sac in a posterolateral direction. Injection of 1–2 mL of saline into the cord may help to define the planes of separation. The vas itself should not be grasped and the floor of the canal not disturbed. Once the end of the sac has been freed, the dissection of the sac is carried superiorly to the level of the deep inguinal ring. If the sac extends down into the scrotum, it may be divided once the cord structures are identified and protected. The base of the sac may then be gently twisted to reduce any fluid or viscera into the peritoneal cavity. The base of the sac should be suture ligated with an absorbable suture and, once the suture is cut, the peritoneal stump should retract proximally through the deep inguinal ring. Free ties should not be used because of the risk of them becoming dislodged if abdominal distension occurs. Absolute haemostasis is essential to prevent postoperative haematoma formation. The position of the testis within the scrotum should be confirmed to avoid iatrogenic entrapment within the inguinal canal. There is an increasing role for laparoscopic hernia repair in infants and young children.[8] An emergency operation is required for patients with an incarcerated hernia, with toxicity and obvious intestinal obstruction or after failed attempts at reduction. As previously mentioned, a paediatric surgeon should be involved in all cases if possible as this can be a difficult undertaking. After appropriate resuscitation, prophylactic antibiotics and insertion of a nasogastric tube, the operation begins with preparation of the whole abdomen in case laparotomy is required. An inguinal incision is utilised and the incarcerated intestine carefully inspected for viability once the obstruction at the internal ring is relieved. A rapid return of pink colour, sheen, peristalsis and palpable or visible pulsations at the mesenteric border should be observed. If there is any question regarding intestinal viability, resection and anastomosis should be carried out and hernial repair accomplished.

In certain circumstances, the incarcerated intestine may reduce during surgical manipulation, before the intestine has been visualised. However, such spontaneous reduction of infarcted bowel is very rare. Laparoscopy through the hernial sac can be undertaken if there are serious concerns regarding bowel viability. Surgery for incarcerated hernia may be difficult because of oedema, tissue friability and the presence of the mass, which may obscure the anatomy. The gonad should be carefully inspected because it may become infarcted by vascular compression caused by the incarcerated intestine. The undescended testis is more vulnerable to this complication in the presence of incarcerated intestine.

Complications

Complications may be divided into intraoperative and postoperative categories. Intraoperative complications include: division of the ilioinguinal nerve, which can be avoided if the external oblique fascia is elevated before incision; division of the vas deferens, which should be repaired with interrupted 7/0 monofilament sutures; and bleeding, which can usually be controlled with the application of pressure and cautious diathermy.

Postoperative complications include wound infection, scrotal haematoma, postoperative hydroceles and recurrence. The wound infection rate is low (1–2%) and recurrence rates of less than 1% are reported, 80% of recurrences being noted within the first postoperative year. The major causes of recurrence in infants and children include: (i) a missed hernial sac or an unrecognised tear in the peritoneum; (ii) a broken suture ligature at the neck of the sac; (iii) injury to the floor of the inguinal canal, resulting in the development of a direct inguinal hernia; (iv) severe infection in the inguinal canal; and (v) increased intra-abdominal pressure, as is noted in patients with ascites after ventriculoperitoneal shunts, in children with cystic fibrosis, after previous operation for incarceration and in patients with connective tissue disorders. Although failure to repair a large internal inguinal ring is a possible (and very occasional) cause of recurrence, attempts to tighten the internal ring at the time of the first repair by approximating the transversalis fascia medial to the inferior epigastric vessels risk compromising the blood supply to the testicle and should be avoided where possible. Simple excision of the sac is all that is required in most patients. Re-operations for recurrent inguinal hernia may be a technical challenge and a pre-peritoneal approach is a useful alternative for recurrent hernias.

Adult inguinal hernias

Inguinal hernias are more frequent in males (1 in 4 males will develop an inguinal hernia in their lifetime), with a male to female ratio of 12:1. Around two-thirds are indirect, and a right-sided hernia is slightly more common than a left-sided hernia. Bilateral hernias are four times more common in direct than indirect forms (1 in 2 males who develop an inguinal hernia will present with bilateral hernia or develop a contralateral hernia).

Aetiology

The pathogenesis of groin hernias is multifactorial. It was initially believed that persistence of a patent processus vaginalis into adult life was the predisposing factor for indirect inguinal hernia formation. However, post-mortem studies have shown that up to a third of adult males without a clinically apparent inguinal hernia have a patent processus vaginalis. Similarly, review of the contralateral side in infantile inguinal hernias reveals a patent processus vaginalis in 60% of neonates and a contralateral hernia in 10–20%. During 20 years of follow-up after infantile hernia repair, only 20% of men will develop a contralateral hernia.

It is therefore apparent that the problem of indirect inguinal hernia is not simply one of a congenital defect. The high frequency of indirect inguinal hernia in middle-aged and older people suggests a pathological change in connective tissue of the abdominal wall to be a contributory factor, as discussed earlier.

Diagnosis

The diagnosis of an inguinal hernia is usually straightforward. The patient presents with a swelling in their groin, which is often associated with discomfort on activity, coughing and sneezing. On lying down, the swelling often disappears. On examination, asymmetry between the two groins is often obvious (**Fig. 7.5**), even with bilateral presentation. Where there is diagnostic doubt, a dynamic ultrasound scan may help, but a word of warning: a small hernia evident on ultrasound which is not clinically detectable is rarely the cause of the patient's symptoms! Many clinical tests have been described to determine between a direct and indirect hernia and indeed a femoral hernia, but in practice, they perform no better than tossing a coin!

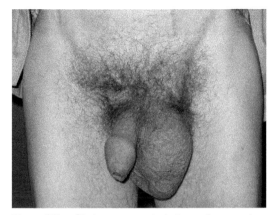

Figure 7.5 • Obvious asymmetry between the normal right side and small inguinoscrotal hernia on the left side.

Management

The goal of hernia repair is to restore the functional integrity of the groin. It is beyond the scope of this chapter to review the history of the various repair techniques that have been previously employed and are now mainly historical. Only the latest techniques (i.e. prosthetic repairs) will be considered here.

'Tension-free' open mesh repair

Lichtenstein first described the technique of tension-free repair of groin hernia, which now bears his name.[9] 'Tension-free' repair of primary groin hernias may be performed as an outpatient procedure under local anaesthesia, although in the UK open mesh repair is still more commonly performed under general anaesthetic.

Once the local anaesthesia has been administered (typically a mixture of 0.5% bupivacaine and 1% lignocaine) along the line of the proposed incision, an incision is made in the groin-crease through the skin and subcutaneous tissues including Scarpa's fascia exposing the external oblique aponeurosis (from just lateral to the deep ring to close to the midline). Additional anaesthetic is then injected under the external oblique aponeurosis, following which a small incision is made in the external oblique along the line of the fibres, to the superficial ring. The edges are lifted with haemostatic forceps avoiding damage to the ilioinguinal nerve. After the contents of the inguinal canal have been gently separated from the external oblique aponeurosis, a self-retaining retractor is inserted under its edges. The spermatic cord is then mobilised utilising the avascular space between the pubic tubercle and the cord itself to avoid damage to the floor of the canal, injury to the testicular blood flow and crushing of the genital nerve, which always lies in juxtaposition to the external spermatic vessels (**Fig. 7.6**).

In order to thin out the spermatic cord and remove any lipoma present, the cremaster fibres are incised longitudinally at the level of the mid-canal.

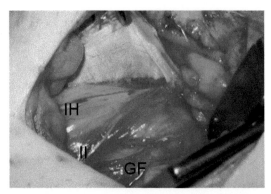

Figure 7.6 • Open right inguinal hernia repair. External oblique has been opened. Medial is to the right of the picture with superior at the top. Note the iliohypogastric (*IH*), ilioinguinal (*II*) that splits into two branches, and the small genitofemoral nerve (*GF*) lying inferiorly.
Clinical photograph used with permission of Mr Martin Kurzer, London, UK.

Complete excision of the cremaster fibres from the spermatic cord is unnecessary and may result in damage to the vas deferens, increasing the likelihood of postoperative neuralgia and ischaemic orchitis. Indirect hernial sacs are opened and digital exploration performed to detect any other defects or the presence of a femoral hernia. The sac can be suture-ligated at the deep ring, but Lichtenstein states that the sac may be simply inverted into the abdomen without excision, suture or ligation, which he feels is unnecessary and may contribute to postoperative discomfort.[9] To minimise trauma to the cord structures and prevent postoperative hydrocele formation, inguino-scrotal sacs are transected at the midpoint of the canal, with the distal section left open and in situ. If performing the procedure under local anaesthetic, handling of the sac at this stage can cause pain and often further local anaesthetic to the sac area in the region of the deep ring is required.

In the event of a large direct hernia, the sac (transversalis fascia) is invaginated with an imbricating suture to achieve a flat surface over which to lay the prosthetic mesh. The external oblique aponeurosis is separated from the underlying internal oblique muscle at a point high enough to accommodate a mesh measuring around 12 cm × 7 cm. This size will vary depending on the size of the patient and the size of the hernial defect.

The mesh is trimmed as appropriate so that the patch overlaps the internal oblique muscle and aponeurosis by at least 2 cm above the border of the Hesselbach triangle. The medial portion of the mesh is rounded to the shape of the medial corner of the inguinal canal. The mesh is sutured to the aponeurotic tissue over the pubic bone, overlapping the bone to prevent any tension or weakness at this critical point, but ensuring the periosteum is not caught in the suture as this is believed to be a source of chronic pain. The medial part of the mesh should extend at least 2 cm medial to the pubic tubercle to reduce the risk of medial recurrence. The same suture is continued along the lower edge, attaching the mesh to the shelving portion of the inguinal ligament to a point just lateral to the deep ring.

A slit is made at the lateral end of the mesh, creating a wider tail above the cord and a narrower one below the cord. This manoeuvre positions the cord between the two tails of the mesh and avoids the keyhole opening, which is less effective at preventing recurrence. The upper edge of the patch is sutured to the internal oblique aponeurosis using a few interrupted sutures or widely spaced continuous suture. Retraction of the upper leaf of the external oblique aponeurosis from the internal oblique muscle is important because it provides the appropriate amount of laxity for the patch. When the retraction is released, a 'tension-free' repair is taken up when the patient strains on command during the operation (if under local anaesthetic) or resumes an upright position afterwards. Using a single non-absorbable monofilament suture, the edges of the two tails are re-approximated snugly around the cord structures creating a new deep ring of mesh (**Fig. 7.7**).

The excess patch is trimmed on the lateral side, leaving 3–4 cm beyond the deep ring. This is tucked underneath the external oblique aponeurosis and the external oblique aponeurosis closed with a continuous suture. Unrestricted activity is

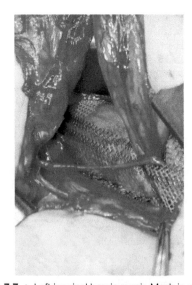

Figure 7.7 • Left inguinal hernia repair. Mesh in place. Note continuous suture attaching inferior edge of mesh to inguinal ligament and mesh fish-tailed laterally to create a new deep ring. Cord structures and ilioinguinal nerve are intact. The mesh is lying flat and 'tension' free.

encouraged and patients are expected to return to their normal activity 2–7 days after surgery.

In the past few years, there has been an explosion in different mesh types for the open repair of inguinal hernias. The plug and patch utilises a cone-shaped mass of mesh that can be inserted, tip side inwards, into either the deep or superficial rings, depending on the type of hernia. A flat mesh is then placed over the plug akin to the Lichtenstein technique. The prolene hernia system is two flat meshes secured together by a small cylinder of mesh. The aim is to insert one mesh into the pre-peritoneal space and the other is secured akin to the Lichtenstein technique. There is also the open pre-peritoneal approach. All these alternatives report good results in the hands of experts, but the open flat mesh technique in its various forms, akin to the Lichtenstein technique, remains the commonest technique in Western countries to date. It is also the author's prejudice that if a mesh is to be inserted into the pre-peritoneal space, it makes sense to do this under direct vision using a laparoscope rather than using a largely blind, blunt finger dissection technique.

Laparoscopic repair

The alternative to an open operation is a laparoscopic approach. Since the early 1990s, laparoscopic hernia repair has evolved from simple closure of a small indirect hernia, through the placement of mesh plugs and a small mesh patch over the internal ring, to the current use of large pieces of prosthetic mesh to reinforce the lower abdominal wall. Although a variety of laparoscopic repairs have been described, they can be categorised in general according to the approach used to expose the defect. Three exposures are used: the intraperitoneal approach, in which the prosthesis is placed as an onlay graft over the peritoneum; the transabdominal pre-peritoneal (TAPP) repair; and the totally extraperitoneal (TEP) repair.

Intraperitoneal prosthetic repair

In the intraperitoneal repair with an onlay graft, the prosthesis is placed within the peritoneal cavity. Compared to the TAPP and TEP approaches, it has the advantages of being less time-consuming to perform and requires no dissection of the pre-peritoneal space. It has the disadvantage of leaving the prosthetic material exposed within the peritoneal cavity and has a higher recurrence rate. It is the author's view that this operation is very much an operation of last resort, when other open or laparoscopic techniques have failed.

Transabdominal pre-peritoneal prosthetic (TAPP) repair

TAPP repair is one of the most popular approaches used for laparoscopic herniorrhaphy, particularly in Europe. The abdomen is insufflated with carbon dioxide and the laparoscope introduced through an umbilical incision. Two accessory trocars, placed above and slightly medial to the anterior superior iliac spines, are used to provide access for the dissecting instruments. After both groins have been inspected, an incision is made in the pelvic peritoneum several centimetres above the hernia defect and the peritoneum then peeled away to expose the hernia defect. The peritoneum is dissected (with a combination of blunt and scissor dissection) away from the abdominal wall, allowing the hernia sac to be inverted and dissected free of adherent tissue, with sufficient mobilisation to create a large enough pocket for the mesh. A mesh of approximately $10\,cm \times 15\,cm$ is inserted and manipulated into position so that it covers the entire myopectineal orifice. Some surgeons fix the mesh in place with staples, sutures or glue, although there is little evidence to support such practices (except in larger direct hernias).[10] The peritoneum is closed over the mesh with staples/ sutures/glue. This approach has the advantage of permitting inspection of the abdominal cavity in general, and of the opposite side in particular, enabling bilateral repairs to be performed if necessary. In addition, exposure is usually excellent. The disadvantage is that the intra-abdominal instruments present the possibility of injury to intraperitoneal structures and the peritoneal incision in the groin increases the potential for adhesion formation and late bowel obstruction. Furthermore, port site hernia at the umbilicus is recognised.

Totally extraperitoneal prosthetic (TEP) repair

TEP repair is a laparoscopic adaptation of the open posterior pre-peritoneal approach first described by Annandale.[11] The laparoscope is introduced into the pre-peritoneal space through an infra-umbilical incision. The pre-peritoneal space is dissected towards the symphysis pubis, Cooper's ligament and the iliac vessels with a blunt instrument or space-making balloon. Carbon dioxide is insufflated into the pre-peritoneal space to maintain exposure. Care must be taken to avoid entering the peritoneum; if this occurs, loss of pressure in the pre-peritoneal space can result, making exposure more difficult. A venting Verres needle in the right iliac fossa will usually resolve this problem, or alternatively a structural balloon attached to the umbilical port will help to keep the pre-peritoneal space open. Two additional 5-mm ports are inserted, either in the right and left iliac fossa, after extending the dissection laterally or in the midline below the umbilicus. Direct hernial sacs usually reduce with ease, but an indirect hernial sac may need more work. The key landmark here is the vas. The indirect hernial sac lies above and lateral to the vas, taking the dissection away from the iliac vessels, preventing their inadvertent injury. A mesh of minimum size

$10 \, cm \times 15 \, cm$ is used to cover all the inguinal and femoral myopectineal orifices, ensuring good cover laterally and superiomedially. As with TAPP repairs, there is now good evidence that suturing, tacking or stapling of mesh does not reduce the risk of hernia recurrence but is a cause of postoperative chronic pain.[10] The author does occasionally tack the mesh, confined mainly to the patient with a very large direct hernial defect or when there has been more bleeding than usual, especially patients on aspirin. In all circumstances tacks are placed medial to the inferior epigastric vessels and superior to the pubic bone only. More recently, the author has attempted laparoscopic suture closure of large direct inguinal hernias with a non-absorbable suture rather than using tacks. The TEP approach avoids the risks of entering the peritoneal cavity and subsequent intraperitoneal adhesion formation as well as minimising port site hernias.

There is little evidence to support TEP versus TAPP and the technique used is largely down to the individual surgeon.[10]

Single incision laparoscopic surgery (SILS) and robotic surgery

Single port hernia surgery for both the TEP and TAPP approach is described. There is also increasing use of robots in laparoscopic hernia surgery. At present, these should be considered an alternative surgical approach, with little proven benefit – and in the case of the robot, a significant increase in both cost and time of the surgery.

✓✓ Laparoscopic repair of inguinal hernias causes less acute and chronic pain, thus earlier return to work, less wound and mesh infection, fewer wound complications and less numbness than the open operation. Where expertise in laparoscopic inguinal hernia surgery is present, it is now the preferred technique suggested for primary unilateral inguinal hernia and recommended for recurrent inguinal hernias after anterior open repair, bilateral primary inguinal hernias, and groin hernia in women.[10]

Complications

Complications of herniorrhaphy include recurrence, urinary retention, ischaemic orchitis and testicular atrophy, wound infection and nerve injuries. A wide variation in recurrence rates is reported in the literature, depending on both the surgical technique employed and the method and length of follow-up (questionnaire, physical examination, etc.). In general, studies comparing mesh to suture repair note lower recurrence rates in the mesh group.[10] Furthermore, direct inguinal hernias are more likely to recur than indirect inguinal hernias.[12] Nevertheless, the percentage of recurrent to primary

hernia repair has remained largely constant in industrialised countries over the past 30 years at around 10%. Perhaps the only role for suture repair remains in the adolescent age group, where perhaps a herniotomy alone is insufficient and the risks of mesh insertion not merited.[10] There has been a suggestion that mesh repairs in the groin can affect fertility in males. This is a very controversial area, as the occurrence of a hernia per se in the young is associated with reduced fertility. There is no convincing evidence to support the view that a mesh repair affects fertility except when there is obviously direct trauma to the vas or vessels to the testicle.[10]

The complication that is becoming the benchmark for comparing hernia repairs is the incidence of chronic pain, rather than recurrence rate. Risk factors for chronic pain include nerve damage, preoperative pain in the hernia, young age, male sex, chronic pain syndromes at other sites of the body, postoperative complications and psychosocial features.[10] Pain response to a standardised heat stimulus appears to be a useful tool in assessing risk of postoperative chronic pain.[13]

Open suture, open mesh or laparoscopic repair?

Which technique is performed on a particular inguinal hernia will depend on a number of factors, and it is true that no one technique fits all. The concept of 'tailoring' surgery to the patient is important.[10] The skills and resources of the local surgical team, applied to the variation in hernia size and type as well the comorbidity and previous abdominal surgery present in the patient will all play a part in the decision for which operation for a particular patient. The process of informed consent with the patient will also help decide the operative technique. In general, there are few patients with a hernia that are not suitable for a general anaesthetic, which would exclude the laparoscopic approach. (There are reports of laparoscopic repairs undertaken under local anesthetic with sedation but these are on ASA 1 and 2 patients with no generalisability to the comorbid patient.) The laparoscopic repair, as opposed to the open repair, is associated with less acute pain and thus a quicker return to daily activities and work, fewer wound complications such as haematoma, seroma and infection, and less risk of chronic pain. There is a similar recurrence rate (in experienced hands accepting a longer learning curve), and a similar risk of major vessel, bowel or bladder injury. The disadvantage of a laparoscopic approach has traditionally been along the lines that surgery takes longer and is more expensive. Current studies would now support the laparoscopic repair being just as quick if not quicker, especially with bilateral hernia repair.[10] Costs can be minimised by avoiding disposable equipment and unnecessary fixation devices, and the use of standard synthetic flat mesh. The cost of open surgery has to be set against the price of open surgery for the patient and society, namely more acute and chronic pain, more time off work and more wound complications. Indeed, for laparoscopic surgery, current guidelines propose that patients can return to all activities as soon as they want, within their level of discomfort, without any increased risk of hernia recurrence.[14] Nevertheless, a caution about widespread laparoscopic repair is the increased complication rate over open surgery in national registry studies.[15]

Contralateral repair

Inguinal hernia arises as a design fault, both anatomically and at the level of collagen metabolism, so there is every reason why it should be a bilateral disease. Furthermore, clinical assessment of bilateral or unilateral hernia has a false positive and negative rate of around 10%. The rate of development of a contralateral inguinal hernia following open repair is around 25% at 10 years,[16] with up to a 50% life-time risk. Bilateral repair as a routine is not recommended, but in skilled laparoscopic hands, bilateral exploration at TEP with prophylactic mesh inserted even if no contralateral hernia is found is suggested.[10] At TAPP, the contralateral side is more easily examined, but will miss cases of lipoma of the cord. Again, bilateral repair is suggested with appropriate informed consent, especially when the finding is of a direct hernia in a younger patient.

Recurrent inguinal hernias

The repair of recurrent inguinal hernia remains a common operation and there is now some evidence to suggest that the increasing use of mesh may be having a small effect in reducing the number of recurrent hernia repairs[17] (see section on prophylactic hernia repair at the end of this chapter). As a result there is little role now for suture repair of recurrent inguinal hernias, except in centres where mesh is unavailable or too expensive for routine use. As a general rule, the anterior approach should be used for recurrent posterior/laparoscopic repairs, and a laparoscopic repair for previous anterior repairs.[10] Thus repair techniques that involve both the anterior and posterior planes at the first operation, are to be avoided as they make revisional surgery much more difficult.[10] However, redo laparoscopic surgery is possible in experienced hands, and allows assessment as to why the first laparoscopic repair failed. The TAPP approach is likely safer than redo TEP surgery, and the dissection plane is to take down the peritoneum along with the original mesh.

Open mesh repair of recurrent inguinal hernias

The Lichtenstein repair remains the commonest open operation for recurrent inguinal hernias. Rate of re-recurrence depends to an extent on the length of follow-up, but is typically around 10%. When a Lichtenstein repair is performed for a recurrent hernia after a previous laparoscopic repair, the complication rate is similar to that of a primary repair. However, when a redo Lichtenstein is performed, the risk of testicular ischaemia rises dramatically from around 0.1% to as high as 5%.

Laparoscopic repair of recurrent inguinal hernias

The advantages of the laparoscopic approach include: elimination of one of the commonest causes of recurrence – the missed hernia (hernia present but not detected by the operating surgeon). In addition, the laparoscopic approach allows the surgeon to identify those patients with complex hernias (inguinal and femoral/obturator); and to cover the entire myopectineal orifice with mesh, buttressing the intrinsic collagen deficit, thereby overcoming one of the causes of late recurrence. The complication rate is low, and the majority of such repairs are as easy as primary laparoscopic repair. The data from the Swedish Hernia Registry would support the benefit of a pre-peritoneal repair (open or laparoscopic) for recurrent inguinal hernia following a previous open non-peritoneal repair.[18]

The asymptomatic hernia

Traditional teaching used to suggest that once an inguinal hernia was detected, it merited repair to prevent hernia-related complications unless the patient was not fit for such surgery. However, increasing awareness of complications following hernia repair, particularly chronic pain, has questioned this approach. Two randomised trials have reported similar results but come to different conclusions.[19,20] In essence, chronic pain on follow-up is similar between the operation group and the watchful waiting group, but the watchful waiting group have not had their operation with its attendant chronic pain risk. Furthermore, significant numbers in the watchful waiting group crossed over to the surgery arm because of increasing symptoms (at a rate of around 10% a year).[21] These trials also noted that the risk of incarceration or strangulation is much lower than previously thought. Thus, following informed consent, surgery or watchful waiting for an asymptomatic hernia is an acceptable management strategy. The younger the patient, or less fit the patient on presentation, then perhaps the earlier surgery should be offered, with suitable informed consent of the risks, benefits and alternatives to the proposed surgery.

✅✅ Repair of an asymptomatic hernia does not increase the incidence of chronic pain as compared to a wait-and-see policy. Either treatment option is acceptable with appropriate informed consent.[19,20] The majority of wait-and-see patients will cross over to surgery with time as their hernia increases in size and/or becomes more symptomatic.

Femoral hernia

Femoral hernia represents the third commonest type of primary hernia. It accounts for approximately 20% of hernias in women and 5% in men, strangulation being the initial presentation in 40%. Its incidence increases with age.

Anatomy

The femoral canal occupies the most medial compartment of the femoral sheath, extending from the femoral ring above to the saphenous opening below. It contains fat, lymphatic vessels and the lymph node of Cloquet. The femoral ring is bounded anteriorly by the inguinal ligament and posteriorly by the iliopectineal (Cooper) ligament, the pubic bone and the fascia over the pectineus muscle. Medially, the boundary is the edge of the lacunar ligament, while laterally it is separated from the femoral vein by a thin septum (see Fig. 7.4).

Aetiology

Femoral hernias are likely to have an aetiology similar to inguinal hernias. The multifactorial factors will include a significant component related to an underlying collagen disorder.

Management

The treatment of femoral hernia is surgical repair due to the high risk of incarceration and the associated risk of strangulation. Several operative approaches have been described: the low approach, the high approach and the inguinal approach. To these can now be added the laparoscopic approach.

Operative details

The low approach (Lockwood)

The low approach is based on a groin-crease incision and dissection of the femoral hernia sac below the inguinal ligament. The anatomical layers covering the sac should be peeled away and the sac opened to inspect its contents. Once empty, the neck of the sac is pulled down, suture-ligated as high as possible and redundant sac excised. The neck then retracts through the femoral canal and the canal is closed with a plug or cylinder of polypropylene mesh, anchored to the inguinal ligament and iliopectineal ligament with non-absorbable sutures.[22] Suturing of the iliopectineal ligament to the inguinal ligament may result in tension due to the rigidity of these structures and may predispose to recurrence.

Transinguinal approach (Lothiessen)

Techniques of femoral hernia repair that open the posterior inguinal wall for exposure and repair should rarely be used, except at open inguinal hernia surgery when no inguinal hernia is found (and a missed femoral hernia is suspected). This technique usually involves ligation and division of the inferior epigastric vessels at the medial border of the internal inguinal ring followed by incision of the transversalis fascia to expose the extraperitoneal space and the femoral hernia sac. This is reduced and the defect closed by either suture (as in the original description) or, increasingly, with mesh. However, the need to incise the natural fascial barrier in Hasselbach's triangle for exposure results in this technique being inferior to either the low or high approach, both of which leave the inguinal floor intact.

High approach (McEvedy)

The high approach was classically based on a vertical incision made over the femoral canal and continued upwards above the inguinal ligament. This has now been replaced with a lateral transverse incision on the affected side. The dissection is continued through the subcutaneous tissue to the anterior rectus sheath, which is divided transversely. The rectus muscle is retracted laterally and the pre-peritoneal space entered (or sometimes with a low arcuate line, anterior to the posterior rectus sheath). The femoral hernia sac is identified medial to the iliac vessels and reduced by traction. If the hernia is incarcerated, the sac may be released by incising the insertion of the iliopubic tract into Cooper's ligament at the medial margin of the femoral ring. The sac is then opened, the contents dealt with appropriately and the sac ligated at its neck. The hernioplasty may then be completed by either suturing the iliopubic tract to the posterior margin of Cooper's ligament or by insertion of a flat mesh, covering the whole of the myopectineal openings. The wound is closed in layers. This technique is particularly useful in the presence of a strangulated femoral hernia as it is easy to convert to laparotomy for bowel resection.

Laparoscopic approach

The laparoscopic approach is the same as for inguinal hernias and may employ the TAPP or TEP technique. The femoral ring is easily seen during either of these approaches and, indeed, visualisation of the whole of the myopectineal opening is frequently quoted as one of the advantages of laparoscopic herniorrhaphy. Furthermore, the laparoscopic repair appears to reduce the risk of re-operation for recurrence.[23] However, there appears to be little difference in short-term quality of life between open and laparoscopic surgical approaches for femoral hernia.[24]

Incisional hernia

Aetiology

Incisional hernias are unique in that they are the only hernia to be considered iatrogenic and constitute the commonest complication of a laparotomy. The cause of wound complications after laparotomy is multifactorial, influenced by local and systemic factors and by preoperative, perioperative and postoperative factors. Again, inherited collagen-type abnormalities have a significant role to play.[25] In addition, several factors including smoking, advanced age, pulmonary disease, morbid obesity, malignancy and intra-abdominal infection are associated with impaired wound healing and predispose patients to serious wound complications such as wound dehiscence, wound infection and incisional herniation. It is always easy to blame the patient for complications but surgeon or technical factors influencing wound complications include surgical technique and suture material choices.

What is the best way to close the abdominal wall? It is amazing that today we still do not know for sure. A recent review[26] proposed mass closure (as compared to layered closure), continuous (as compared to interrupted sutures), slowly absorbable monofilament (as compared to non-absorbable monofilament and absorbable multifilament), with a suture length to wound length ratio of at least 4:1. Controversy over the 4:1 ratio also exists. This ratio can be achieved by big bites far apart or small bites close together. The first small-bite small-stitch randomised controlled trial (RCT)[27] reported a 50% reduction in wound infection and a 67% reduction in incisional hernia rates in the 2/0 polydioxanone 20-mm-needle small-bite arm compared to more conventional closure techniques. Using such a suture technique, suture-to-wound length ratios greater than 4:1 were not associated with increasing wound complications.[28] A further RCT[29] of small-bite small-stitch midline closure recently reported a reduction in incisional hernia rate from 21%

to 13% at 1-year follow-up, although in this trial there was no significant difference in wound infection or burst abdomen (sometimes called an acute hernia or deep wound dehiscence). However, patients who were obese and undergoing emergency laparotomy were excluded from these trials, so the generalisability of the small-bite small-stitch closure to all laparotomy wounds is not known. Nevertheless, the development of an incisional hernia is inevitable if there is separation of the fascia by 12 mm at 12 weeks, so it is not difficult to see that the events that lead to an incisional hernia are determined early in the healing phase, and technical issues are likely to have a significant part to play.

✓✓ Closure of a laparotomy wound to minimise incisional hernia formation includes:[26]
avoid the midline;
mass closure;
simple running technique;
absorbable monofilament;
suture length to wound length ratio of at least 4:1;
small-stitch small-bite technique.[27,29]

Management

The diagnosis of an incisional hernia is usually easy except in the very obese. However, CT is helpful to identify the size of the defect and the state of the abdominal wall muscles (**Fig. 7.8**). Part of the CT assessment is considering the degree of 'loss of domain' – the percentage of the abdominal cavity contents that lie within the hernia sac. When these contents are returned within the confines of the abdominal wall, they will increase the dimensions of the hernial defect. Restoring integrity of the abdominal wall with significant loss of domain will require a variety of ways to elongate the abdominal wall musculature, such as Botox injections into the

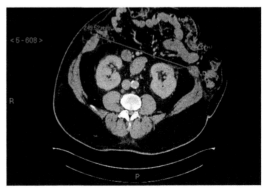

Figure 7.8 • CT scan of a large incisional hernia demonstrating loss of domain. The gap between the medial ends of the left and right recti muscles on this slice is 25 cm.

lateral muscles 1 month prior to surgery,[30] progressive pneumoperitoneum[31] or component separation techniques (described below). Sometimes excision of abdominal cavity contents such as omentectomy or right hemicolectomy may be necessary. Occasionally, bridging the gap in the abdominal wall muscles (as opposed to mesh augmentation of the primary closure) with mesh is necessary. Weight loss prior to surgery is to be encouraged, especially for larger hernias. As a rough rule of thumb, for every 3 kg of weight loss, about 1 litre of abdominal volume is gained, which is very helpful when there is loss of domain.

The large number of surgical procedures described in the literature to repair incisional hernias illustrates that no single technique has stood out as being effective. While 50% of incisional hernias occur within 1 year after the primary operation, 20% are diagnosed more than 5 years later. Any study reporting re-recurrence rates following incisional hernia repair should therefore ideally have at least 5 years of follow-up data for analysis. Unfortunately, prospective randomised trials comparing different types of incisional hernia repair are lacking and the majority of studies are retrospective.

As a consequence of the disappointing data on mesh-free repair of incisional hernias, including the Mayo ('vest-over-pants') procedure, meshes were introduced to strengthen the abdominal wall repair. Several different techniques were developed: inlay, onlay and sublay (**Fig. 7.9**). Mesh implantation as an inlay does not achieve any strengthening of the abdominal wall and is essentially a suture repair at the muscle/fascia mesh interface. It has the highest recurrence rate of the three techniques. The results of randomised trials comparing mesh to suture repair demonstrate a clear advantage for mesh repair, even for small hernias.[32] However, incisional hernia should be considered an incurable disease, mesh just increasing the time from repair to recurrence. Although suture repair is now rarely indicated, it might still have a role in young women who wish repair of an incisional hernia but are also contemplating further pregnancy.

✔✔ Mesh repair of incisional hernia reduces the recurrence rate, even for small hernias.[32,]

Mesh repair

The onlay technique remains the commonest technique in industrialised countries, largely because it is relatively easy to perform. The technique is dependent on closure of the anterior abdominal wall and adequate fixation of the mesh to the fascia, and a minimum overlap of 5–8 cm is recommended. If the connection between the mesh and the fascia is lost, a buttonhole hernia develops at the edge of the mesh. Good results

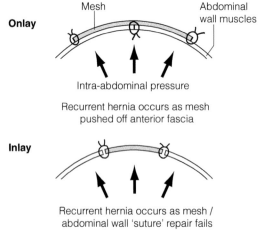

Onlay

Mesh   Abdominal wall muscles

Intra-abdominal pressure

Recurrent hernia occurs as mesh pushed off anterior fascia

Inlay

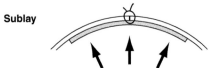

Recurrent hernia occurs as mesh / abdominal wall 'suture' repair fails

Sublay

Recurrent hernia minimised as intra-abdominal pressure pins the mesh against the abdominal wall

Figure 7.9 • Cross-sectional appearance of mesh position in incisional hernia repair.
Reproduced from Schumpelick V, Klinge V. Immediate follow-up results of sublay polypropylene repair in primary or recurrent incisional hernias. In: Schumpelick V, Kingsnorth AN, editors. Incisional hernia. Berlin: Springer-Verlag; 1999. p. 312–26. With kind permission of Springer Science + Business Media.

can be reported with attention to detail, namely wide overlap of the mesh and obliteration of large skin flaps with fibrin glue.[33] However, for many surgeons the relatively high rate of hernia recurrence, seroma formation, mesh infection and skin flap complications make this operation a poor option for the patient.

The sublay technique is the procedure favoured by the author. A mesh in the sublay position is not only sutured into position but is also held in place by the intra-abdominal pressure. Mesh in this position is therefore able to strengthen the abdominal wall both by mechanical sealing and by the induction of strong scar tissue. The sublay operation is effective for both midline and transverse wounds. A number of studies have compared the recurrence rate in a single institution where all three techniques have been used,[34] demonstrating the superior results achieved by the sublay technique.

Open, intraperitoneal onlay mesh is also described. It is a useful technique when the abdominal wall is very scarred from previous surgery or when the abdominal wall is very attenuated. However, placing a large mesh in the abdominal cavity has a significant adhesion risk, and the open technique is still associated with significant wound complications, in effect combining the worst of the open and laparoscopic techniques.

Open sublay repair

The sublay operation begins by excising the old scar in the skin and performing a laparotomy. Adhesions tend to be maximal at the neck of the sac, so entering the abdominal cavity through the hernia sac is usually straightforward. It is helpful to mobilise adhesions off the underside of the anterior abdominal wall. It is not the author's routine practice to mobilise all the bowel adhesions unless there is a good history of recurrent episodes of bowel obstruction. The sublay space is then developed, which is the space anterior to the posterior rectus sheath, although this becomes pre-peritoneal below the semi-arcuate line. Care should be taken to mobilise the inferior epigastric vessels up with the belly of the rectus muscle to minimise bleeding. It is also important to preserve as many of the intercostal nerves as possible to minimise muscle denervation (**Fig. 7.10**). The pre-peritoneal space can be developed behind the pelvis, akin to a TEP repair, especially if the hernia arises in a Pfannensteil incision. Superiorly, the sublay space can be developed behind the xiphisternum if necessary. The posterior rectus sheath is divided on either side close to the linea alba to expose the area known as the fatty triangle (**Fig. 7.11**). The posterior rectus sheath is approximated with an absorbable suture. The mesh is cut to size, aiming to have at least a 6-cm overlap in all directions. This mesh is sutured to the posterior rectus sheath with interrupted absorbable sutures, avoiding any obvious nerves. These sutures are purely to hold the mesh flat until it is encased in fibrous tissue. A suction drain is often left anterior to the mesh. Any further redundant skin and hernial sac is excised and the anterior rectus sheath

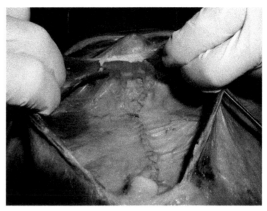

Figure 7.11 • Fresh cadaveric dissection demonstrating the fatty triangle by division of the posterior rectus sheath as it attaches to the linea alba. This allows development of the sublay space behind the xiphisternum. Courtesy of Dr J Conze, Berlin, Germany.

closed with an absorbable suture, as is the skin, minimising any subcutaneous dead space. The cross-sectional appearance is illustrated in **Fig. 7.12**. If an abdominoplasty is performed at the same time, then further drains are placed to the subcutaneous space. In larger incisional hernias, the peritoneal flaps can be used to aid anterior and posterior fascial closure.[35]

Component separation techniques to allow midline closure for large ventral hernias are described. The anterior technique involves dividing the tendon of the external oblique as it attaches to the anterior rectus sheath from above the costal margin to close to the inguinal ligament, followed by mobilisation of this muscle off the internal oblique. The posterior approach involves mobilising the transversus muscle in a similar manner but from the inside, avoiding the larger skin flaps created by the open anterior approach and the risk of seroma, skin necrosis and wound breakdown. (The anterior release can also be undertaken using endoscopic techniques.) Both these techniques rob Peter to pay Paul and weaken the abdominal wall at these sites, which in some cases results in lateral bulging in the longer term. Use of the peritoneal flap technique[35] avoids the need for component separation in the majority of cases.

✓ The open sublay technique for incisional hernia repair has a lower recurrence rate and wound complication rate compared to onlay or inlay repair techniques.[34] Randomised trials comparing the three mesh position techniques are lacking.

Laparoscopic repair

The laparoscopic (intraperitoneal) approach has also been applied to incisional hernias. The laparoscopic approach has the advantages of shorter hospital stay, lower analgesic requirements, fewer wound

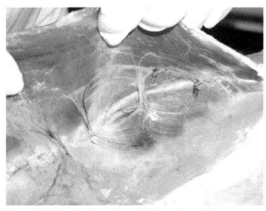

Figure 7.10 • Fresh cadaveric dissection of the retromuscular space for sublay incisional hernia. Courtesy of Dr J Conze, Berlin, Germany.

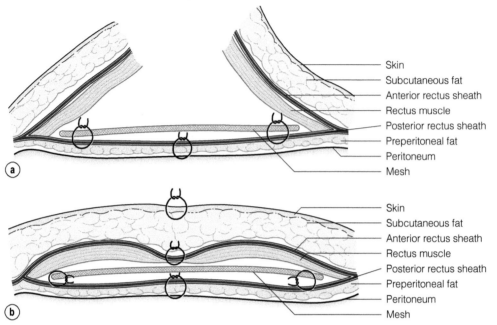

Figure 7.12 • **(a)** Cross-sectional appearance of posterior fascia/peritoneum closure showing the sublay position of the mesh, which is fixed to the posterior sheath of the rectus muscle with an interrupted absorbable suture. **(b)** The anterior and posterior rectus sheath is closed continuously.

complications and an earlier return to normal activities over open surgery. However, while the complication rate is lower overall when compared to open surgery, there is concern that when complications do arise with the laparoscopic approach, they are more likely to be life-threatening or require further surgery to deal with compared to open surgery.[36] Furthermore, the cosmetic result for larger hernias may not be as good, as there is no abdominoplasty component to the laparoscopic approach. Remember, the majority of patients wish surgery for their incisional hernia because of the cosmetic deformity rather than symptoms related to the hernia. The laparoscopic approach works well for smaller incisional hernias, with a hernia neck size less than 7 cm and when cosmesis is not a significant concern. A number of controversies exist in the technique, related to (i) the method of fixation of the mesh, (ii) whether the hernia defect should be closed or not and (iii) the size of the mesh overlap. The method of mesh fixation divides surgeons between those who believe transfascial sutures to be essential to prevent hernia recurrence and those who believe such sutures cause chronic pain post-surgery and their use should be avoided. The author prefers a double-crown tack technique (two rings of tacks around the hernia defect), although there is a lack of quality studies to make this an evidence-based decision. The recent introduction of absorbable tacks may reduce the risk of chronic pain and bowel adhesion to the tacks. Centring the mesh over the hernial defect is important to minimise

hernia recurrence. The mesh can be centred with a central stitch, although two or four corner sutures are probably more accurate.

What about closure of the defect? Bridging of the defect is recognised to be a problem at open surgery, so why bridge with laparoscopic surgery? It is clear that once adhesions to the abdominal wall are taken down, inserting a mesh and tacking it in place is usually quick and easy. Closing the defect is thus not attractive to the majority of laparoscopic surgeons, introducing tension and perhaps increasing postoperative pain. However, many groups are talking about pseudo-recurrence[37] – the redevelopment of a bulge at the hernia site several years after laparoscopic repair as the mesh slides into the hernia sac. Whether closing (either completely or partially) will reduce recurrence and pseudo-recurrence is still unknown but would seem likely.[38] The size of the mesh overlap in a bridged repair, and the mesh size when the defect is closed are still controversial.

One of the main long-term risks of the laparoscopic repair of incisional hernias is the placement of the mesh in direct contact with the intra-abdominal structures. As mentioned earlier, the use of meshes that have one side coated with a relatively non-adhesive material will help reduce (but not abolish) adhesion formation to the mesh. The other main risk is infection of the mesh, which is nearly always due to contamination from a bowel injury. Care should be taken with any adhesiolysis to minimise bowel injury, with thermal sources such as diathermy dissection kept to a minimum. The current consensus is that if the colon is injured, then it should be repaired, laparoscopically or open, according to the skills of the surgeon and no mesh inserted at this time. The patient can return in a number of months for a further attempt at repair. If the small bowel is injured with minimal contamination, then laparoscopic repair of the injury, washout and mesh insertion, is acceptable. If there is significant small-bowel injury and risk of failure of the bowel repair, then no mesh should be inserted. The patient should be observed in hospital and if they remain well 4–5 days later, then it is appropriate to re-laparoscope the patient and if no continuing contamination/infection is observed, the laparoscopic mesh repair can be completed. The use of antibiotic-impregnated mesh may allow a change to this policy with placement of such a mesh at the same time as bowel injury and repair.

Parastomal hernia

Parastomal hernias occur at the site of an abdominal wall stoma. Indeed, the majority of patients with a stoma will develop such a hernia. Techniques to fashion a stoma to minimise parastomal hernia are outwith the scope of this chapter. However, many patients with a parastomal hernia will seek repair because of pain, cosmetic deformity and poor-fitting stoma appliances. Localised suture repair always fails. Moving the stoma to another location will have short-term benefit until a new hernia develops, and perhaps a hernia at the original site! Mesh can be inserted in the onlay, sublay and intraperitoneal positions. Traditionally this mesh is key-holed around the stoma, not too tight to cause ischaemia and not too loose for early failure. In practice, this is easier said than done. More durable results are being reported for the laparoscopic Sugerbaker technique, especially if performed with a keyhole mesh at the same time. However, lateralisation of the colon is usually straightforward, but for small-bowel stomas this is often more difficult, and can result in kinking of the bowel as it passes over the mesh, with resultant bowel obstruction.

Emergency hernia surgery

Much of what has been mentioned above is applicable to hernia repair in the emergency situation. However, there are a few dilemmas that occur more frequently in the emergency setting. Patients who present as an emergency but have no bowel compromise can be treated as per elective hernia surgery. When bowel is compromised, especially when there has been significant contamination, current opinion is that synthetic mesh should not be used. However, there is little in the way of evidence apart from anecdote to support such a view and this view has been challenged.[39] The case for biological mesh in such scenarios is also lacking in evidence.[40] For those who support the laparoscopic approach, it is not unreasonable to offer this in the emergency setting and laparoscope the patient with an irreducible groin hernia. If the bowel can be reduced and is viable, then convert the operation to a TEP/TAPP and place mesh as usual. If the bowel is compromised, then resect the bowel through a small incision and return 6 weeks later for a TEP. In the emergency incisional/ventral hernia setting, if the hernia is large, then proceed directly to open sublay mesh repair. If the hernia is smaller, then laparoscopy and intra-abdominal mesh are appropriate if there is no bowel compromise. If there is bowel ischaemia, then convert to the open sublay repair. The use of mesh in the sublay space in the emergency setting should not be associated with an increase in mesh infection as it lies external to the peritoneal cavity, but clearly each case will need to be assessed individually.

Emergency hernia surgery remains a high-risk surgical procedure, with the main risk factor for postoperative mortality being infarcted bowel.[41,42] Such operations should not be left to junior members of the surgical and anaesthetic teams. Appropriate resuscitation, followed by timely and appropriate surgery, may save lives. Occasionally, the techniques of damage limitation surgery (see Chapter 19) may be appropriate.

> ✓ Bowel infarction is the main risk factor for mortality in emergency hernia surgery.[40,41]

Port-site hernia

This is a hernia with an increasing incidence associated with the increase in laparoscopic surgery. Insertion of larger ports through the midline as opposed to more laterally appears to be a significant risk factor.[26] This is especially true in the presence of a divarification of the recti or an unrecognised umbilical hernia. There is little evidence to support closure of the fascia except when a cut-down is performed for the first port. The use of dilating rather than cutting trocar tips may reduce the incidence of port-site hernia formation. However, the risk of port-site hernia at the umbilicus with larger ports such as the SILS technique, is associated with an increased port-site hernia risk.

Antibiotic prophylaxis in hernia surgery

In general, elective hernia surgery to the groin and ventral regions does not require antibiotic prophylaxis.[10,43] However, as the risk of bowel injury is always present in incisional hernia surgery, it would be reasonable to give routine antibiotic prophylaxis for such surgery. Patients at increased risk of infection, including the immunocompromised, skin conditions with higher bacterial carriage such as psoriasis and in the emergency setting, all merit antibiotic prophylaxis.

All theatres have bacteria (called colony-forming units) in the circulating theatre air. It therefore makes sense to open the mesh just before it is required during the operation. Changing to fresh gloves before the handling of the mesh, minimising mesh contact with the skin and inserting the mesh deep to the subcutaneous tissues may all help reduce the risk of mesh contamination. The author uses a gentamicin solution (240 mg gentamicin in 250 mL normal saline) to irrigate larger meshes following insertion, although there is no evidence-based medicine to support this manoeuvre. Methicillin-resistant *Staphylococcus aureus* (MRSA) bacteria have been found on mesh several years after insertion, so prophylaxis to MRSA is appropriate if a previous repair has been complicated by MRSA infection.

✔✔ Antibiotic prophylaxis is unnecessary for uncomplicated elective hernia surgery to the groin and ventral regions.[10,43]

'Prophylactic' hernia surgery

The topic of prophylactic mesh insertion to minimise subsequent incisional hernia formation in high-risk groups of patients remains controversial but is an active area of surgical research. High-risk patients, such as the obese, aneurysm surgery and the creation of a permanent stoma are all under study.[26,44,45] These studies report significantly reduced incisional or parastomal hernia rates at the same time point, with no increase in morbidity related to the prophylactic mesh, even in clean-contaminated situations. It is likely that prophylactic mesh to minimise subsequent hernia formation will become more mainstream practice, but there are many unanswered questions, including mesh type, mesh size and position of the mesh within the abdominal wall. The selective use of prophylactic mesh may be supported by preoperative collagen type I/III ratio typing to identify patients more at risk. This concept of collagen disease is important, and introduces the notion that hernia repair of any type will fail if the patient lives long enough. It is true that some surgeons' repairs last longer than others, so technical factors remain important, and mesh repairs at any time point are more likely to be intact compared to a suture repair. (Re-operation rates are a surrogate for recurrence rates, although re-operation will underestimate the true recurrence rate.) However, a hernia repair at present is a patch-up job, and

will probably fail eventually (if the patient lives long enough). Nevertheless, randomised trials of prophylactic mesh use in patients at high risk of developing incisional hernia are ongoing.

Management of an infected mesh

In general, an infected mesh has to be removed or exposed to the surface. If the mesh is lying in a pool of pus with no adherence to the patient, then the only real option is removal of the mesh. This is the more likely scenario with early infection in the first week or so following repair. If the mesh is partly embedded in tissue, then if there is adequate drainage through an open wound (or a laparoscopically placed drain for meshes in the pre-peritoneal space), many infected meshes will slowly granulate over and remain sound (**Fig. 7.13**). The exposure of the mesh to the skin surface, aided with negative pressure therapy,[46] will salvage the majority of meshes, especially those placed in the sublay position. However, sometimes chronic sinuses will develop and the only option is excision of these along with as much of the visible mesh as possible. Not all patients who require mesh removal will develop a hernia recurrence, although the majority probably will at some stage in the future on longer follow-up.[47] If mesh has to be removed/ excised, it is best to remove as much of the mesh foreign body material as possible, control the sepsis and return at a later date for further hernia repair. The use of biological mesh in such a contaminated field is rarely indicated. The use of vacuum-assisted dressing to control the fluid exudates from the wound may aid wound care in such patients.

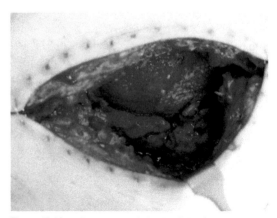

Figure 7.13 • Early wound infection following onlay large pore mesh repair of incisional hernia. There is good granulation tissue through the mesh pores already. Opening the wound, washout and negative-pressure therapy salvaged this mesh repair.

Key points

- Herniorrhaphy is one of the commonest operations performed.
- Techniques advanced considerably during the 1990s.
- The use of prosthetic mesh should now be considered for the repair of all hernias.
- The laparoscopic approach may be more appropriate than a traditional open approach.
- Recurrent hernias may be best managed in specialist centres or by surgeons with a specialist interest in hernia surgery who are technically competent to perform both open and laparoscopic procedures.
- A multidisciplinary approach, including plastic surgeons, may be appropriate for complex, multiply recurrent hernias.

Full references available at **http://expertconsult. inkling.com**

Key references

3. Miserez M, Alexandre JH, Campanelli G, et al. The European Hernia Society groin hernia classification: simple and easy to remember. Hernia 2007;11:113–6. PMID: 17353992
   Pragmatic, easy to remember and use classification.

9. Lichtenstein IL, Shulman AG, Amid PK, et al. The tension-free hernioplasty. Am J Surg 1989;157: 188–93. PMID: 2916733.
   The original description of an operation that has been considered the gold standard repair of inguinal hernia.

10. www.herniasurge.com World inguinal hernia guidelines.
    The first world inguinal hernia guidelines!

13. Aasvang EK, Gmaehle E, Hansen JB, et al. Predictive risk factors for persistent postherniotomy pain. Anaesthesiology 2010;112:957–69. PMID: 20234307.
    Chronic pain can be predicted prior to surgery with simple bedside tests.

19. O'Dwyer PJ, Norrie J, Alani A, et al. Observation or operation for patients with an asymptomatic inguinal hernia: a randomized clinical trial. Ann Surg 2006;244:167–73. PMID: 16858177.
    The first randomised trial on surgery versus no surgery in the asymptomatic hernia.

26. Muysoms FE, Antoniou SA, Bury K, et al. European Hernia Society guidelines on the closure of abdominal wall incisions. Hernia 2015;1–24. PMID: 25618025.
    Excellent review of key step of every laparotomy.

32. Luijendijk RW, Hop WC, van den Tol MP, et al. A comparison of suture repair with mesh repair for incisional hernia. N Engl J Med 2000;343: 392–8. PMID: 10933738.
    The first randomised trial to demonstrate the benefit of mesh in reducing recurrence in incisional hernia repair.

43. Scottish Intercollegiate Guidelines Network (SIGN). Antibiotic prophylaxis in surgery. Guideline 104. 2008. www.sign.ac.uk.
    The SIGN website allows all guidelines produced to date to be downloaded for free. An excellent reference source on current best practice in a variety of medical and surgical conditions.

8

Neck surgery for the general surgeon

Iain J. Nixon

Introduction

A neck mass is a common clinical presentation. Surgeons should be familiar with common causes, red flag symptoms and characteristic examination findings. A wide range of conditions can present with a neck mass and an exhaustive explanation of investigation and management of all such conditions is beyond the scope of this text. Instead, the aim of this chapter is to review the surgical investigation of a neck mass and to outline the surgical approach to managing common conditions which may face general surgeons as well as those with an interest in diseases of the head and neck.

Diagnostic approach to neck masses

Initial assessment (Table 8.1)

A full clinical history is critical and should include not only features relating to the mass (duration, tenderness, growth etc.) but also associated symptoms that may point to the underlying diagnosis, such as fevers, hoarseness, dysphagia and weight loss. Patient features including smoking and drinking habits as well as comorbidities may be critical in overall case management. On occasion, family history may be relevant, particularly in hereditary thyroid and parathyroid conditions such as familial thyroid cancer and multiple endocrine neoplasia (MEN).

The majority of neck masses requiring investigation arise within lymph nodes. However, salivary and thyroid masses are also common. Although

vascular and neurogenic tumours are uncommon, an appreciation of such conditions is useful for forming a differential diagnosis (Table 8.2).

In areas of the world where tuberculosis is endemic, tuberculous cervical lymphadenopathy is common. Patients present with cold collar and stud abscesses and may have systemic features of the infection. An accurate diagnosis may be aided by aspiration of pus in order to target antibiotic therapy. Open incision and drainage should be avoided as this often results in an unsightly chronic sinus.

Malignancy should always be considered when investigating cervical lymphadenopathy presenting as a neck mass. A careful head and neck examination is indicated to look for an upper aerodigestive tract primary lesion. In order to assess all at-risk sites appropriately, visualisation of the mucosal surfaces of the upper aerodigestive tract is required. Although the oral cavity can be adequately assessed using a light, further examination requires mirror (indirect) or endoscopic (direct) assessment.

When considering the high-risk sites for primary disease, an understanding of lymphatic drainage from the head and neck is key. Malignancy from the oral cavity will tend to drain to the submandibular (level I) nodal basin. Lesions more posteriorly in the throat (the oropharynx) commonly metastasise to the jugular nodal chain (level II/III/IV). Laryngeal and thyroid cancers spread first to nodes in the central (level VI) or low lateral (level III/IV) neck. When metastatic nodes are encountered in the posterior triangle (level V), primary disease may be present in the nasopharynx, scalp (skin cancer) or sites below the clavicle (lung, breast or GI metastases to Virchow's node). Lymphoma commonly presents with cervical lymphadenopathy, and can affect any or all lymph node groups.

Table 8.1 • Approach to assessing a neck mass

Modality	Specific technique	Advantages/Disadvantages
Clinical history		
Examination		
Imaging	Chest X-ray	Identification of primary lung disease or metastases
	Ultrasound	Cheap, no ionising radiation
	CT scan	Quick, readily available but exposure to radiation
	MRI scan	Slow, leading to claustrophobia and swallow artefact but no radiation
Biopsy	Fine-needle aspiration	Minimally invasive but small number of cells
	Core	More invasive but provides greater cell number, useful for immunohistochemistry and also provides cellular architecture
	Open (avoid where possible)	Large number of cells but potential for seeding

Table 8.2 • Differential diagnosis of neck mass

Lymphadenopathy	Salivary	Thyroid	Congenital	Vascular	Neurogenic
Infective	Infective (sialadenitis)	Neoplastic (benign goitre or malignant)	Thyroglossal duct cyst	Carotid artery ectasia	Neuroma
Malignant	Neoplastic (benign or malignant)	Inflammatory (Graves' disease)	Branchial arch anomalies	Carotid body tumour	
	Inflammatory (Sjögren syndrome)	Infective (thyroiditis)		Lymphovascular abnormality	

Following a full history and examination, basic investigations including full blood count, ESR, glandular fever screen and chest X-ray, should be considered on a case-by-case basis. Some patients will require further investigation for an overt primary malignancy. However, a large percentage of patients without evidence of primary malignancy will require further investigation of the neck mass itself.

Imaging

Ultrasound scanning (USS) has become widely accepted as a routine investigation in assessment of the neck mass. It is non-invasive, provides an accurate assessment of the tissue characteristics of the mass and allows targeted tissue sampling where appropriate. However, it is not without limitations. The accuracy of findings is operator-dependent and the images produced are less useful for surgical planning than those from cross sectional imaging. Certain areas of the neck, including the parapharyngeal space and the central neck, are poorly visualised on USS. Despite this, the majority of neck masses that require further assessment should be considered for USS in the first instance.

Contrast enhanced computed tomography (CT) scans are the mainstay of assessment of potential malignancy. As well as accurately displaying the relationship of the mass to the great vessels of the neck, CT also provides valuable information about the mucosal surfaces of the head and neck. When extended to the thorax, mediastinal nodes and lungs can be assessed for metastatic disease and possible synchronous primary lesions. However, dental amalgam produces significant artefact which may obscure the structures within the oral cavity and oropharynx.

Magnetic resonance imaging (MRI) has the advantage over CT of avoiding ionising radiation. Excellent soft-tissue definition and increasing availability has led some groups to adopt MRI as the first-choice imaging modality for assessment of the neck. In addition, dental amalgam is less of an issue than for CT. However, images take longer to capture and may be degraded by movement.

Positron emission tomography (PET) scanning involves the use of a radiolabelled tracer (most commonly FDG-18F) to provide functional imaging. In the field of head and neck surgery it tends to be used for identification of unknown primary disease in the setting of squamous cell carcinoma within a neck node, and for detection of recurrence following treatment.

Biopsy

Many neck masses will require a tissue diagnosis in order to plan treatment. In most situations fine-needle aspiration (FNA) is the biopsy of choice. Ideally this can be US-guided in order to sample the area of highest suspicion, but free-hand biopsy is used by many groups who do not have access to USS. The samples obtained by FNA allow cytologists to assess cell groups in order to guide diagnosis. There is minimal bleeding, and seeding (although technically possible) is extremely rare with this technique.

Increased cell yield with sampling to allow analysis of tissue architecture can be achieved by core biopsy. This technique, ideally USS-guided, removes a core of the neck mass for histological analysis. Core biopsy is slightly more invasive than FNA, although complication rates are low.

If a diagnosis cannot be reached using FNA or core techniques, open biopsy may be considered. Although appropriate for certain conditions (salivary tumours and lymphoma, for example), surgeons are warned against this approach if squamous cell carcinoma is in the differential diagnosis. This caution stems from historical evidence that open biopsy is associated with seeding of tumour and recurrence within the skin. However, surgical and radiotherapy techniques have improved significantly and hence open biopsy is increasingly considered outdated. The vast majority of patients can be diagnosed by accurate assessment and appropriate tissue sampling without proceeding to open surgery for diagnosis.

Thyroid mass

Thyroid disease is common, and as increasingly our population is screened with modern imaging techniques, so the number of incidental thyroid nodules referred to surgeons is increasing.[1] For this reason, an appreciation of the investigation and management of thyroid masses is important for the surgeon.

Indications for thyroid surgery include malignancy, pressure symptoms, hyperthyroidism and cosmesis. With this in mind, the approach to a thyroid mass should include a clinical history, examination, basic blood tests, imaging and biopsy as indicated.[2,3] Risks of thyroid surgery include damage to the recurrent laryngeal nerve.[4] As such, all patients considered for surgery should undergo dynamic assessment of the recurrent nerve using direct endoscopic or indirect mirror assessment of the larynx. This is of particular importance in the setting of preoperative voice change, previous surgery or when there is suspicion of thyroid cancer with extra-thyroidal extension, which places the recurrent laryngeal nerve at risk.[2,3]

✅ Where there is suspicion of involvement of the recurrent laryngeal nerve in the setting of thyroid malignancy, the dynamic function of the larynx should be assessed with laryngoscopy.[2,3]

In almost all circumstances, ultrasound will be the first investigation for thyroid masses. Not only does this give information about the size and number of nodules present, but features such as the shape and structure of the nodule allow accurate prediction of the risk of malignancy. These features have been standardised into a 'U' staging system 1–5, which objectively groups nodules in ascending order of risk of malignancy.[2] In those patients with a thyroid that extends behind the sternum, or in the setting of malignant disease with nodal metastases, cross-sectional imaging (normally CT) is a useful adjunct.[5]

Complications from thyroid surgery range from minor to life-threatening (Box 8.1). All patients require an incision and therefore a scar is inevitable. For most, an incision in a skin crease around the level of the cricoid will afford excellent access and minimal cosmetic impact.

In some cultures, however, a neck scar is associated with significant negative connotations. In response, groups in the Far East are using a transaxillary approach to the neck using endoscopes or robotic techniques.[6] Such procedures involve wide-field dissection, high levels of expense and significant operative time. An alternative is the 'minimally invasive' endoscopic technique.[7] With this approach a small (<2-cm) incision is placed in the central neck and with video-endoscopic assistance, adequate exposure can be achieved to allow thyroid surgery.

Such modern techniques of thyroidectomy have significant potential advantages. The cosmetic outcome from surgery is superior due to the absence or reduction of a cervical incision. However, there are significant limitations. Large goitres cannot be removed through small incisions, therefore such 'minimally invasive' approaches are not suitable for the majority of patients who require thyroid surgery for compressive symptoms. In addition, these techniques do not allow lymphadenectomy or wide-field thyroidectomy to address extra-thyroidal extension. In particular, those techniques that approach the thyroid from a lateral position

---

Box 8.1 • Complications of thyroid surgery

- Any thyroid resection
  - Scar
  - Haemorrhage
- Thyroid lobectomy
  - Late hypothyroidism
  - Unilateral nerve injury (recurrent laryngeal and external branch of superior laryngeal)
- Total thyroidectomy
  - Definite hypothyroidism
  - Hypocalcaemia (early and late)
  - Bilateral recurrent laryngeal nerve injury (requires tracheostomy)

(transaxillary approach) prevent access to the contralateral lobe and as such these techniques are not appropriate for total thyroidectomy. Furthermore, the oncological safety of opening a wide field of dissection in the setting of malignancy has been questioned following reports of recurrence.[8] However, as experience is gained in these techniques groups are reporting favourable outcomes and expanded indications.[9,10] One of the significant limitations is cost. The duration of the procedure and the cost of consumables make such procedures extremely expensive and at a time of global healthcare rationing this has prevented widespread adoption of these techniques.[11]

The most serious complication from thyroidectomy is haemorrhage, affecting around 2% of patients.[12] In the UK, all thyroid surgeries are performed with an overnight stay[13] to allow patients to be regularly assessed and dealt with promptly in the event of haemorrhage. Some groups have found that modern electrosurgical devices are associated with lower rates of haemorrhage and recommend these devices to facilitate same day discharge. Despite all efforts, the risk of haemorrhage cannot be completely avoided.[14]

If a postoperative patient develops increasing neck swelling, urgent intervention is required. Arterial bleeding increases the pressure in the central neck compartment until it exceeds venous pressure. This leads to venous oedema of the larynx with progressive stridor and asphyxiation. If there is audible airway compromise (stridor) at the time of presentation, the skin incision and deep fascial (platysma) closure should be opened on the ward to evacuate haematomas and allow a temporary reduction in pressure. Instrumentation to allow suture or clip removal should be available at the bedside for all neck surgery patients. An anaesthetist should be alerted to secure the airway immediately. Ideally, haematoma evacuation and haemorrhage control should be completed under general anaesthesia.

Damage to the nerves that supply the muscles of the larynx is also of concern. The recurrent laryngeal nerve supplies all laryngeal muscles apart from cricothyroid. Injury to this nerve leads to significant voice change. Although reported nerve injury rates depend on when the larynx is examined, permanent damage occurs in around 1–2% of most major series.[4] The precise risk to an individual patient is likely to depend on the nature of the disease and the experience of the surgeon.[15] Previously, surgeons believed that identifying the recurrent laryngeal nerve was not mandatory during thyroid surgery. However, contemporary practice requires the nerve to be visualised in order to minimise the risk of inadvertent injury while mobilising the gland.[16–21] This approach is now endorsed by both American and British guidelines.[2]

Clearly, unilateral thyroid lobectomy places only one nerve at risk; total thyroidectomy places both nerves at risk. In the event of a bilateral injury, laryngeal function is significantly compromised and permanent tracheostomy may be required in order to provide a safe airway. Although this is extremely rare (around 0.02% of all cases), rates are higher in total thyroidectomy versus lobectomy where it is only encountered if a pre-existing contralateral vocal cord palsy is present.[15]

The external branch of the superior laryngeal nerve approaches the larynx from above to innervate the cricothyroid muscle. It has a variable position in relation to the superior thyroid artery and its branches. Most authors do not advocate specific identification during thyroidectomy but recommend taking branches of the artery low in order to minimise the risk of injury.[3] Permanent injury leads to a loss of high-pitch voice which is most evident during singing.

✔✔ The recurrent laryngeal nerve should be identified in all thyroidectomy procedures. Steps should be taken to minimise the risk to the external branch of the superior laryngeal nerve during dissection.[3,16–21]

The parathyroid glands are small organs with a key role in calcium homeostasis and are located on the posterior surface of the thyroid. They should be identified and protected during thyroid surgery. Following thyroid lobectomy, up to 25% of specimens will be found to contain parathyroid tissue on histological analysis.[22] Removal or devascularisation of the glands will interfere with function. Around 20% of patients suffer temporary hypocalcaemia following total thyroidectomy but only 1–2% will have long-term problems.[4] This complication is almost never seen after thyroid lobectomy and is more common when a central neck dissection is performed along with total thyroidectomy.

If half of the thyroid is removed (thyroid lobectomy) less than one-third of patients will become hypothyroid.[23] This is more common if there is a background of Hashimoto's thyroiditis (such patients are at risk of becoming hypothyroid even without surgery). Clearly if the entire gland is removed the patient will require lifelong thyroxine therapy.

Surgery for malignancy

A spectrum of malignancies affects the thyroid gland. However, differentiated thyroid cancer is most common (90%), of which papillary cancer is the most frequent subtype. Medullary[24] and anaplastic[25] thyroid cancers are uncommon, while thyroid lymphoma and metastases to the thyroid are rare.

Most thyroid cancers present either with a palpable mass, or as an incidental finding on imaging.[27] Assessment of the regional nodes with ultrasound scan is critical. Assuming there are suspicious findings on USS, biopsy will be indicated to confirm the diagnosis. For differentiated thyroid cancer (papillary and follicular), FNA is considered the gold standard and ideally should be ultrasound-guided. The results can be stratified by the 'THY' staging system (1–5) in order to allow cytologists to communicate effectively with surgical colleagues.[2]

✅✅ Patients considered at risk of thyroid malignancy should have fine-needle aspiration biopsy.[2,3]

In patients with lesions that are clearly malignant (THY 5), therapeutic surgery is indicated. In those with lesions that are not confirmed as malignant (THY 3f or THY 4), diagnostic surgery is indicated. Generally THY3a lesions will be re-biopsied unless sufficient clinical concern exists to recommend surgery. If investigations suggest benign disease (THY 2), the patient may be suitable for reassurance and discharge.[2]

The details of surgical procedure in each case are beyond the scope of this chapter. However, broadly speaking, for differentiated thyroid cancer with significant extra-thyroidal extension, regional nodal or distant metastases, total thyroidectomy is indicated (Box 8.2). This procedure removes disease and renders the patient suitable for adjuvant radioactive iodine (RAI) therapy, which would otherwise be absorbed by any remnant thyroid lobe. Radioactive iodine is preferentially taken up by native thyroid tissue, which is more iodine-avid than metastatic thyroid cancer. If residual normal thyroid tissue remains present in the neck following surgery, the radiation dose delivered to malignant cells is reduced.

The issue of appropriate oncological management of the thyroid and neck remains highly controversial. In addition to the thyroid gland procedure, resection of any obvious nodal disease should be performed with a 'compartment orientated' neck dissection.[28] For low-risk patients with disease within the thyroid and no evidence of spread beyond the gland, simple thyroid lobectomy should be adequate. In such patients, oncological outcomes are excellent, and the morbidity of thyroid lobectomy is significantly lower than that of total thyroidectomy.[15]

Proponents of both aggressive (total thyroidectomy and prophylactic neck dissection) and conservative (thyroid lobectomy and no regional lymphadenectomy) exist. The reason for the controversy is the excellent outcomes enjoyed by low-risk patients with differentiated thyroid cancer. As outlined above, if an indication for RAI exists, total thyroidectomy is indicated. If there is evidence of nodal disease at the time of presentation, neck dissection is indicated. For most patients, however, disease is limited to the thyroid and 30-year survival in this group is >95%. When the American Thyroid Association performed a feasibility analysis of determining the optimal approach to therapy their power calculation suggested almost 6000 patients would be required in a prospective randomised trial. As such, it is unlikely that a definitive answer will ever be provided.

A more detailed approach to the management of differentiated thyroid cancer is available in British and American Thyroid Association Guideline Documents.[2,3]

Box 8.3 • Choice of primary thyroid procedure for malignancy

- Total thyroidectomy
  - Large primary tumour (>4 cm)
  - Evidence of extra-thyroid extension
  - Nodal or distant metastatic disease
  - Contralateral nodular disease
- Thyroid lobectomy
  - Small primary tumour
  - Intra-thyroid disease only
  - No evidence of contralateral nodules

Box 8.2 • THY cytological grading system

THY category	Clinical meaning
THY1	Non-diagnostic sample
THY2	Benign
THY3a	Atypical cells
THY3f	Follicular neoplasm
THY4	Suspicious for malignancy
THY5	Diagnostic for malignancy

Box 8.4 • Primary neck procedure for malignancy

Evidence of disease in the central neck (cN1a)	Dissection of levels VI and VII
Evidence of disease in lateral neck (cN1b)	Dissection of levels II–V
No evidence of neck disease (cN0)	Controversial – consider prophylactic surgery if high-risk features (extra-thyroidal extension or large primary tumour)

✅ For patients with thyroid cancer and evidence of nodal metastases, compartment-orientated neck dissection is indicated. For those patients without evidence of nodal metastases, elective nodal dissection should only be considered in those at highest risk of harbouring occult disease.[2,3]

Surgery for pressure symptoms

As the thyroid enlarges, it does so within the confines of the neck. Initial growth is asymptomatic. However, as the gland increases in size, and in particular if it encroaches on the thoracic inlet, pressure on surrounding structures, including the oesophagus and trachea, may increase. Such patients initially complain of a vague feeling of something in the throat, progressing to dysphagia and even airway compromise in severe cases. Compression of the great vessels may impede venous return, particularly with the arms raised (Pemberton's sign). Such patients should be considered for surgery.[5] For the vast majority of patients, even those with retrosternal goitre, a cervical approach to surgery is adequate. However, sternotomy may be required for those patients with a goitre exceeding the dimensions of the thoracic inlet or those involving the posterior mediastinum.[29,30]

Preoperative investigation is similar to that for those patients considered at risk of malignancy with USS and FNA as indicated. However, if there is significant retrosternal extension, cross-sectional imaging with CT is preferred as it allows assessment of the relationship of the goitre to mediastinal structures.

It should be remembered that although thyroidectomy does remove the thyroid gland, entering the pretracheal fascia replaces native thyroid tissue with scar. As such, patients with mild throat discomfort and a small thyroid goitre may not notice a significant improvement in symptoms following surgery. Indeed, if there is injury of the recurrent laryngeal nerve intraoperatively, postoperative symptoms may exceed preoperative symptoms. In such patients, a barium swallow may help to identify the extent of impingement caused by the gland, and is useful in counselling the patient in relation to postoperative expectations.

Rates of recurrent laryngeal nerve injury are greater in surgery for large goitres. Not only can the position of the nerve be affected by the unpredictable growth of the gland, but the nerve is in apposition with the gland for a greater distance requiring significant dissection to allow the gland to be mobilised safely. The recurrent laryngeal nerve will tend to lie deep to the thyroid, making visualisation impossible as the gland is mobilised up out of the neck. For this reason the nerve is at risk throughout the surgery and great care should be taken, particularly in bilateral procedures.

Surgery for hyperthyroidism

Patients who present with hyperthyroidism require careful investigation to determine the cause and select the most appropriate treatment. The most common cause of hyperthyroidism is Graves' disease, a diffuse toxic goitre. Functioning nodules can also cause hyperthyroidism as an isolated finding or within a multinodular goitre. Investigation of this patient group will include basic thyroid function tests and serum autoantibodies. USS is also used in conjunction with radioactive iodine scanning in order to identify functioning nodules.

Most patients will not require surgery initially. Medical therapy with antithyroid drugs offers the advantages of avoiding surgery in diffuse toxic goitre, but has a failure rate of up to 50%.[31] Radioactive iodine can be used to destroy thyroid cells and reduce the function of the gland. This may be suitable for diffuse or nodular toxic disease. However, treatment requires quarantine during treatment and pregnancy must be avoided during and for a minimum 6-month period after therapy.

Surgery will be required for patients who have failed medical therapy or for specific subgroups: for example, large toxic nodular goitres tend to respond poorly to radioactive iodine therapy[32] and those patients with significant eye signs related to Graves' disease show better response to surgical than medical therapy.[33]

When the decision is made to proceed with surgery, the extent of the operation will depend on the nature of the disease. Patients with diffuse toxic goitre (Graves' or multinodular) will be candidates for total thyroidectomy and thyroxine replacement therapy. In the setting of a single functioning nodule, lobectomy alone will suffice.[34]

This patient group should be managed by a team that includes an endocrinologist. Not only should non-surgical therapy be managed by a clinical team with endocrine experience, but input to preoperative preparation and postoperative management is invaluable. Prior to surgery, antithyroid drugs should be used to achieve euthyroid status. In those patients who cannot be adequately controlled, beta-blockers may be used to abolish the systemic features of hyperthyroidism in the peri- and postoperative period. Iodine has also been used orally to reduce the vascularity of the thyroid in the run-up to surgery.[35,36]

Surgery for Graves' disease (total or near total thyroidectomy)[34] is challenging due to the firm nature of the gland and the inflammatory response that surrounds it. Careful dissection with prompt control of pin-point haemorrhage is required in order to safely identify nerves and parathyroid glands during the dissection and minimise the risk of postoperative complications. UK data suggest that patients with Graves' disease who opt for surgery are at a significantly increased risk of complications compared with those operated on for other conditions.[4]

Postoperative management following thyroidectomy

Following surgery, patients will require close observation for haemorrhage and airway compromise. Immediately following extubation, stridor should alert the team to the risk of a bilateral nerve injury. In this situation, ideally the larynx is examined with a flexible scope. However, if the patient is clinically unstable (tachypnoeic or significant hypoxaemia), re-intubation may be required. Re-exploration of the recurrent laryngeal nerves at this point is best deferred. Even if divided nerves are identified and repaired, the acute situation will not be affected. The patient will require ventilation and most authors recommend steroids and a trial of extubation in 24–48 hours. There is evidence to suggest that re-exploration can be beneficial in the long term if injured nerves can be identified and repaired.[37] If there is a certainty about bilateral injury, early tracheostomy will be required. This should be an extremely rare event.

Transient hypocalcaemia is a common complication of thyroid surgery. Many units have local policies, and measuring serum levels on the first postoperative day will allow those with hypocalcaemia to be identified. Late hypocalcaemia can occur and patients should be aware of the symptoms so they can seek medical attention if this develops. Some units now prefer to use rapid assessment of parathyroid hormone which can reliably identify those at risk of developing hypocalcaemia. However, this is an expensive resource which is unavailable in many centres.

Those patients undergoing total thyroidectomy should start on replacement therapy (approximately 1.6 µg/kg of thyroxine daily) and this can be fine-tuned in the postoperative period. Those who had thyroid lobectomy should have assessment of thyroid function 4–6 weeks after surgery to determine the need for thyroxine.

Congenital masses

Although many different types of congenital mass may arise in the head and neck region, the most common are branchial cysts and thyroglossal duct cysts.

As the embryo matures, the branchial arches fuse to obliterate the spaces between. If, however, that process is incomplete, communications between the pharynx and skin can persist. A persistent communication between two mucosal surfaces is termed a branchial fistula. These are rare, complex and may be associated with various anatomical structures, including the carotid artery and facial nerves.

More commonly, if the skin surface connections are lost, a branchial cyst forms. These most commonly present in children and young adults, often following an infection that results in swelling and pain. The diagnosis can be made clinically, and imaging will demonstrate an isolated cystic structure, medial to the sternomastoid muscle and lateral to the carotid sheath (**Fig. 8.1**). Classically this is found at the junction of the upper and middle third of sternomastoid.

Treatment is indicated to prevent further infections and confirm the diagnosis.[38] The main risk of surgery is damage to the marginal mandibular branch of the facial nerve. In order to prevent permanent damage, a skin crease incision is placed a minimum of 2 finger-breadths below the mandible. Continuing the incision on to the sternomastoid muscle and raising a plane deep to platysma will protect the nerve, which runs immediately deep to platysma, and therefore this approach maintains the nerve within the skin flap. Although temporary injury can occur from excessive retraction, division of the nerve should be prevented with this approach.

The diagnosis of branchial cyst should raise suspicion in an older patient as there is a risk of malignancy. Previously, 'malignant degeneration of branchial cysts' was thought to be the cause of such cases. However, squamous cell carcinoma from the tonsillar area typically presents with cystic masses in the lateral neck and the primary lesion can be

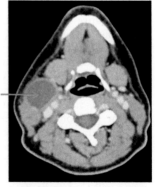

Smooth encapsulated cyst medial to sternomastoid muscle and lateral to carotid sheath

Figure 8.1 • CT scan showing branchial cyst deep to sternomastoid and lateral to the carotid sheath.

small. It is likely that these are the main cause of such cystic metastases rather than a squamous cyst lining undergoing dysplastic change. As endoscopic and imaging techniques have improved, previously occult head and neck primary tumours can be identified and treated appropriately. As outlined above, diagnosis should be made without open biopsy and therefore all such patients should undergo a full head and neck examination, cross-sectional imaging and FNA biopsy prior to considering surgical excision in those with negative results.

As the thyroid gland descends from its initial position at the junction of the anterior two-thirds and posterior one-third of the tongue (foramen caecum) to its adult position anterior to the 2nd and 3rd tracheal rings, it does so along the thyroglossal duct. If the duct fails to regress, a thyroglossal tract may remain and cells within the tract can present later as cystic inclusions. Most lie inferior to the hyoid, although they can present anywhere along the route of descent (**Fig. 8.2**).

The classic clinical finding is of a midline mass which moves both on swallowing (adherence to the pre-tracheal fascia) and on tongue protrusion (adherence to the base of the tongue). This is in contrast to thyroid masses which move only on swallowing.

Again, ultrasound and fine-needle aspiration are useful investigations to confirm the diagnosis. The majority of patients will be candidates for surgical excision to prevent recurrent infections. Ultrasound scan and thyroid function tests are helpful to confirm the presence of a normal thyroid prior to surgery. However, it is extremely rare to find a patient with

no functioning thyroid tissue in the normal position and if a sole site of ectopic thyroid was identified most clinicians would consider surgical excision in this unusual setting.

Initial attempts at thyroglossal cystectomy resulted in high rates of recurrence. These observations led to the Cistrunk procedure, where the entire tract, including the central portion of the hyoid bone, are excised. This more radical approach has reduced recurrence rates to <5%. More recently, histological analysis of excised thyroglossal tracts has demonstrated a branching structure.[39] In response, many authors now recommend an en-bloc excision of a medial portion of the strap muscles along with the tract to encompass any branches.[40,41]

Parathyroid disease

Parathyroid surgery is complex, demanding multidisciplinary input and an understanding of the embryological development of the parathyroid glands. The majority of parathyroid surgeons will work closely with an endocrine team with the support of colleagues in diagnostic and interventional radiology, nuclear medicine, pathology and biochemistry.

The parathyroids are small, tan-coloured glands located in the space around the thyroid gland. The inferior parathyroids develop from the dorsal aspect of the third pharyngeal pouch. They descend, along with the thymus, to lie in the inferior neck. The superior glands arise in the dorsal wing of the fourth pharyngeal pouch and descend along with the thyroid. Due to the longer route of descent, the position of the inferior parathyroid glands is more variable. Over 80% of patients have four parathyroids, 13% have more than four and less than 5% have fewer than four glands.

Primary hyperparathyroidism usually presents with hypercalcaemia detected on routine biochemistry. If advanced, it may present with clinical manifestations including fatigue, thirst, dehydration, renal stones, muscle weakness and bony fractures. Diagnosis is secured by demonstrating raised calcium and raised parathyroid hormone levels. Treatment is surgical, as medical therapy to reduce calcium levels does not correct the underlying pathology.

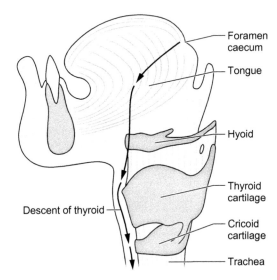

Figure 8.2 • Route of the descent of the thyroid and therefore possible locations of a thyroglossal duct cyst.

Foramen caecum

Tongue

Hyoid

Thyroid cartilage

Descent of thyroid

Cricoid cartilage

Trachea

Box 8.5 • Indications for surgical intervention for primary hyperparathyroidism

Symptoms
Nephrolithiasis
Age <50 years
Serum Ca >1.0 mg/dL above normal limit
Reduced creatinine clearance
Loss of bone mineral density

Having made a diagnosis and decided to pursue surgical treatment, the next issue is whether to perform preoperative localisation. Bilateral neck exploration performed by an experienced surgeon cures primary hyperparathyroidism in 95% of cases. In addition, localisation studies have historically been inaccurate. However, improvements in imaging, in addition to the observation that >90% of patients will have only one parathyroid adenoma, mean that most surgeons now rely on imaging to guide the surgical procedure.

USS is cheap, readily available and non-irradiating. However, it is operator-dependent and poor at visualising areas in the deep central neck. Therefore it has significant limitations and is best used in conjunction with other modalities. Cross-sectional imaging with contrast enhanced CT or MRI is useful for surgical planning, particularly in the re-operative setting. Technetium-99 m sestamibi is concentrated in abnormal parathyroid glands and has revolutionised parathyroid surgery (**Fig. 8.3**). Sestamibi can be combined with CT to produce three-dimensional single-photon emission computed tomography (SPECT) scans to provide further anatomical detail (**Fig. 8.4**).

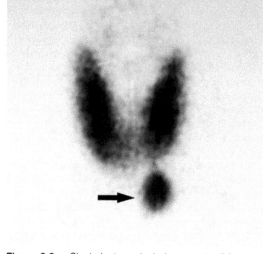

Figure 8.3 • Single-isotope dual-phase sestamibi scan. Sestamibi tracer can be seen concentrating in both the thyroid gland and a left lower pole parathyroid adenoma (*arrow*) in this early-phase image. Delayed-phase images would demonstrate washout of tracer from the thyroid gland but not the parathyroid adenoma.

Figure 8.4 • CT-enhanced SPECT scan. This image shows a mediastinal parathyroid adenoma identified precisely by SPECT enhancement and CT. The top two rows of images mark the parathyroid adenoma on CT scan (crosshair). The bottom row of images marks the parathyroid adenoma on SPECT scan.

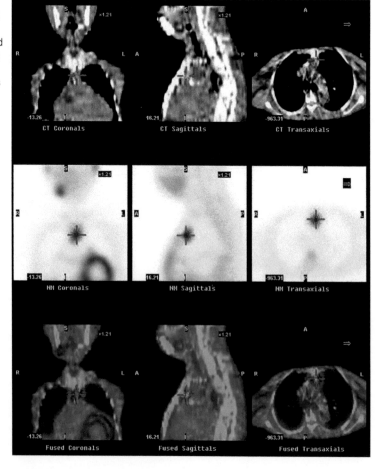

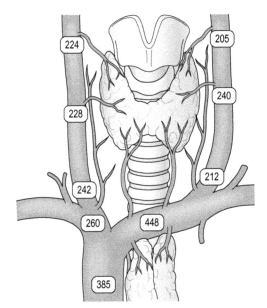

Figure 8.5 • Selective venous sampling data. This image of parathyroid hormone values represents an adenoma in the cervical thymus.

The ability to localise disease to a single gland has made targeted unilateral exploration an alternative to routine bilateral procedures. Interventional radiology can contribute to localisation with targeted angiography (where the parathyroid adenoma is seen as a 'stain') or selective venous sampling (**Fig. 8.5**). Drawbacks of these techniques include need for nephrotoxic contrast and risk of embolic events, meaning most centres reserve these scans for re-operative cases.

Ninety per cent of cases of primary hyperparathyroidism are caused by a single adenoma, 5% multiple adenomas, 5% four-gland hyperplasia and <1% carcinoma.[42] The normal gland weighs approximately 40 mg. Diseased glands weigh upwards of 70 mg. Adenomas are either tan or beefy red in colour. Carcinoma is difficult to diagnose preoperatively and is often a diagnosis based on later metastases. If a parathyroid is palpable this should alert the clinician to the risk of malignancy, as should an extremely high serum calcium. Intraoperative findings may include local invasion which will confirm the diagnosis clinically. If malignancy is suspected, an en-bloc resection including the ipsilateral thyroid gland is recommended. If the capsule of the gland ruptures, recurrent disease presents secondary to seeding and can be impossible to resect.

Having completed investigation of the patient with primary hyperparathyroidism, the surgeon must decide on the most appropriate operation.

For patients with a single adenoma confirmed on preoperative localisation, unilateral open or minimally invasive surgery may be chosen. In those with suspicion of multigland disease (due either to family history or imaging studies), a bilateral exploration will be preferred.[43] This is a controversial subject with conflicting opinions.[44] Improvements in preoperative localisation make the targeted approach attractive. The potential for low morbidity and high success rates has led to an increase in interest in this technique. However, some authors report higher recurrence rates with unilateral than standard bilateral exploration, and low complication rates of bilateral procedures in experienced hands. The approach chosen by the management team will be influenced by factors including preoperative investigations and local complication rates.[45]

Secondary hyperparathyroidism arises when factors other than primary hyperparathyroidism cause overproduction of parathyroid hormone. The most common cause is chronic renal failure, which leads to hypocalcaemia and overproduction of parathyroid hormone. Medical management comprises calcium, vitamin D supplementation and a low phosphate diet. The definitive therapy is renal transplantation. For those who fail medical treatment (5–10%), surgical parathyroidectomy with four-gland excision with or without autotransplantation or three-and-a-half-gland excision is indicated.[46]

Tertiary hyperparathyroidism is a rare condition where patients with chronic renal failure and secondary hyperparathyroidism have resolution of their renal dysfunction (usually after renal transplantation). A small group of these patients will have developed an autonomously functioning parathyroid gland which continues to produce parathyroid hormone without normal feedback inhibition. The majority of these cases resolve spontaneously and surgery is only indicated if the situation persists beyond 12 months.

Conclusion

A wide spectrum of surgical disease presents with head and neck manifestations. These include malignant and benign conditions, including congenital, endocrine and inflammatory processes. The complex neurovascular anatomy in conjunction with the functional aspects of visceral physiology in the neck make surgery in this area particularly demanding. A thorough understanding of embryology and anatomy in conjunction with an appreciation of the underlying pathology will allow the surgeon to investigate the case in the appropriate manner and provide treatment with minimal morbidity.

Key points

- Full head and neck examination is critical in all patients who present with a neck mass.
- Fine-needle aspiration biopsy is preferred to open biopsy to avoid the risk of seeding.
- Patients with thyroid cancer require ultrasound imaging and fine-needle aspiration biopsy.
- In patients requiring thyroidectomy with risk of recurrent laryngeal nerve involvement, preoperative assessment of laryngeal function is advised.
- During thyroidectomy, identification of the recurrent laryngeal nerve is mandatory.
- Older patients presenting with a branchial cyst should be considered at risk of having metastatic squamous cell carcinoma and investigated prior to excision.
- Thyroglossal duct cysts should be excised with a portion of the hyoid bone to minimise recurrence.
- Parathyroid disease is complex and requires multidisciplinary management.
- Surgery for primary hyperparathyroidism can often be targeted with modern preoperative investigations.

Recommended videos:
- Thyroidectomy – https://youtu.be/93xwBssEC2k
- Sistrunk procedure – https://youtu.be/0oxhRpSq850
- Thyroid cancer management – https://youtu.be/VVyuAith2EM
- ENT masterclass – https://tinyurl.com/lxkqu3b

Full references available at **http://expertconsult.inkling.com**

Key references

2. Perros P, Boelaert K, Colley S, et al. Guidelines for the management of thyroid cancer. Clin Endocrinol (Oxf) 2014;81(Suppl 1):1–122. PMID: 24989897.
   This is the UK guideline which outlines a management approach to thyroid cancer. This 2014 update introduces the U staging system for radiological assessment of thyroid nodules. In addition there is a movement away from total thyroidectomy for all thyroid cancers and towards a more conservative approach to managing low risk cases.

3. Haugen BR, Alexander EK, Bible KC, et al. 2015 American Thyroid Association Management guidelines for adult patients with thyroid nodules and differentiated thyroid cancer: The American Thyroid Association Guidelines Task Force on Thyroid Nodules and Differentiated Thyroid Cancer. Thyroid 2016;26(1):1–133. PMID: 26462967.
   This is the US version of the guidelines for managing thyroid nodules and thyroid cancer. This is an exhaustive review and covers many aspects in great detail. In particular this iteration of the guideline refines the approach to risk stratification in terms of recurrence rather than simple survival. Again there is a move away from the aggressive one-size-fits-all approach to management of low-risk cancer.

4. Chadwick D, Kinsman R, Walton P. The British Association of Endocrine and Thyroid Surgeons fourth national audit report. Dendrite Clinical Systems Ltd: The Hub, Station Road, Henley-on-Thames, Oxfordshire RG9 1AY, UK; 2012. http://www.baets.org.uk/wp-content/uploads/2013/05/4th-National-Audit.pdf.
   This is the most recent report of the British Association of Endocrine and Thyroid Surgeons. All UK thyroid surgeons are encouraged to contribute to this prospective database which is then reported in the public domain. Results currently include not only number of cases per surgeon and length of stay but also hypocalcaemia and recurrent nerve injury rates. Individual surgeon level reporting is also available through the website.

13. Doran HE, England J, Palazzo F. Questionable safety of thyroid surgery with same day discharge. Ann R Coll Surg Engl 2012;94(8):543–7. PMID: 23131222.
    This document represents a UK survey of surgeons who were asked to vote on the safety of day case thyroidectomy. It was this vote which led to a move away from day case surgery in the UK, although it is widely practiced elsewhere in the world.

15. Hauch A, Al-Qurayshi Z, Randolph G, et al. Total thyroidectomy is associated with increased risk of complications for low- and high-volume surgeons. Ann Surg Oncol 2014;21(12):3844–52. PMID: 24943236.
    This national database study reports on the increased incidence of complications associated with more aggressive surgery (total thyroidectomy versus lobectomy). Also, it provided further evidence that high-volume surgeons have lower rates of complication than low-volume surgeons.

16. Lahey FH, Hoover WB. Injuries to the recurrent laryngeal nerve in thyroid operations: their management and avoidance. Ann Surg 1938;108(4):545–62. PMID: 17857252.

Landmark paper which led to the modern day opinion that the recurrent laryngeal nerve should be formally identified in all thyroidectomy procedures.

24. Wells Jr. SA, Asa SL, Dralle H, et al. Revised American Thyroid Association guidelines for the management of medullary thyroid carcinoma. Thyroid 2015;25(6):567–610. PMID: 25810047.
An internationally accepted and updated guideline for the management of medullary thyroid cancer. This iteration reflects the understanding that calcitonin may be used in the preoperative staging of medullary thyroid cancer with prophylactic neck dissection considered if calcitonin is high but clinically there is no evidence of metastatic nodes. Also a useful approach to risk stratification based on the genetics of those familial cases of medullary thyroid cancer.

25. Smallridge RC, Ain KB, Asa SL, et al. American Thyroid Association guidelines for management of patients with anaplastic thyroid cancer. Thyroid 2012;22(11):1104–39. PMID: 23130564.
Another American guideline paper which summarises the current state of evidence as it relates to anaplastic thyroid cancer. Although almost always there is no therapeutic option, this introduces the concept of stratifying anaplastic cancer by whether it was identified preoperatively or as part of a resection for a heterogeneous lower risk cancer, in which case outcome may be slightly better.

33. Bahn RS, Burch HB, Cooper DS, et al. Hyperthyroidism and other causes of thyrotoxicosis: management guidelines of the American Thyroid Association and American Association of Clinical Endocrinologists. Endocr Pract 2011;17(3):456–520. PMID: 21700562.
This document discusses the approach to selecting therapy for hyperthyroidism. There is a balanced approach to the pros and cons of antithyroid drugs, radioactive iodine and surgery, including the kinds of patients who may opt for one over the other.

45. Wilhelm SM, Wang TS, Ruan DT, et al. The American Association of Endocrine Surgeons guidelines for definitive management of primary hyperparathyroidism. JAMA Surg 2016; 151(10):959–68. PMID: 27532368.
This review document outlines an approach to the management of primary hyperparathyroidism. The paper explores the pros and cons of targeted versus four-gland exploration and provides a framework for management of these complex cases.

9

Human factors and patient safety in surgery

Craig McIlhenny

The scale of medical error

As surgeons, we are arguably practitioners of one of the most entitled, rewarded and rewarding occupations in the world. We are empowered to the completely legal action of putting a knife to work in a human body. Unfortunately ... our patients are frequently caught in the 'friendly fire' of surgical care – health care providers causing unintentional harm when their only intent was to help.[1]

The practice of healthcare in general, and surgery in particular, is a hazardous business. It was not until the 1990s, however, that the exact nature and scale of that hazard became apparent. In that decade several high profile cases of medical error were reported in the USA and in the UK, such as the enquiry into perioperative deaths from paediatric cardiac surgical care in Bristol Royal Infirmary,[2] which threw the adverse effects of medical intervention into stark relief.

This prompted further investigation into the possible scale of harm perpetrated by modern healthcare. The Harvard Medical Practice Study in 1991[3] demonstrated a major adverse incident rate in 3.7% of all patients treated. Studies conducted in Utah and Colorado,[4] Denmark,[5] New Zealand[6] and Canada[7] reported remarkably similar adverse events rates of between 8% and 12% in all patients admitted to acute hospitals, and this range is now generally accepted as being typical of healthcare systems in developed countries. Crucially, throughout these studies about half of all these adverse events are deemed to be preventable.

Not surprisingly these publications brought about a sharp focus on patient safety, which has now become, quite rightly, a permanent part of healthcare policy. Numerous changes have since been advocated to improve patient safety, including the mandating of minimum nurse-to-patient ratios, reducing working hours of trainee doctors, introduction of 'care bundles', the use of safety checklists and advances in the science of simulation and teamwork training.

Adverse events in surgery

The surgical domain can be seen as more complex and high risk in its delivery of care than other non-interventional specialities. It is therefore not surprising that in the majority of studies of adverse events in healthcare, at least 50% occurred within the surgical domain and the majority of these in the operating theatre. Furthermore, at least half of these adverse events were also deemed preventable.

Just as the multiple studies in the developed world have similar figures for adverse events in hospitalised patients across all specialities, there appears to be a similar rate of harm in surgery. A review of 14 studies, incorporating more than 16000 surgical patients, quoted an adverse event occurring in 14.4% of surgical patients.[8] This was not simply minor harm; a full 3.6% of these adverse events were fatal, 10% severe and 34% moderately harmful.

Gawande, a surgeon from Boston, made one of the first attempts to clarify the source of these adverse events.[9] This paper pioneered the concept that the majority of these adverse events were not due to lack of technical expertise or surgical skill on the part of the surgeon, finding instead that 'systems factors' were the main contributing factor in 86% of adverse events. The most common system factors quoted were related to the people involved and how they were functioning in their environment. Communication breakdown was a factor in 43% of incidents, individual cognitive factors (such as decision-making) were cited in 86%, with excessive workload, fatigue and the design or ergonomics of the environment also contributing. These findings were confirmed in the systematic review of surgical adverse events, where it was found that errors in what were described as 'non-operative management' were implicated in 8.32% of the study population versus only 2.5% contributed to by technical surgical error.[8]

In accordance with other high-risk industries, such as commercial aviation, the majority of these adverse events are therefore not caused by failures of technical skill on the part of the individual surgeon, but rather lie within the wider healthcare team, environment and system. Lapses and errors in communication, teamworking, leadership, situational awareness or decision-making all feature highly in post-hoc analysis of surgical adverse events. This knowledge of error causation has been prominent and acknowledged in most other high-risk industries for many years, but it is only recently that healthcare has appreciated this.

Human factors

Enhancing clinical performance through an understanding of the effects of teamwork, tasks, equipment, workspace, culture and organisation on human behaviour and abilities and application of that knowledge in clinical settings.

Ken Catchpole, http://chfg.org/about-us/
what-is-human-factors/

Human factors encompass all the issues to do with humans working in a system – how we see, hear, think, behave and function physically as individuals and teams – which need to be considered to optimise performance and assure safety[10] (**Fig. 9.1**). This also extends to the design of tools, machines, systems, tasks and environments to ensure safe and effective human use. So a human factors perspective helps highlight why a piece of clinical equipment that has not taken human strengths and limitations into account in its design, or a work environment and shift pattern that is disruptive and stressful, is likely to lead to less-than-optimal human performance and so likely to result in error and compromise patient safety. In surgery these range from the design of surgical instruments or operating theatres, to services and systems, as well as the working

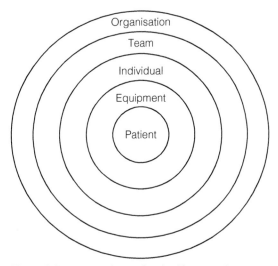

Figure 9.1 • Human factors in a healthcare system.

environment and working practices such as rotas, roles, team behaviours and so on.

Surgical adverse events are almost invariably caused by several factors, often combining unsafe systems and unsafe behaviours.[11] Unsafe systems (such as poorly managed operating lists) produce unsafe behaviours (such as disruption during swab counts). Equally, unsafe behaviours (such as disrespect towards junior staff) undermine safety processes (such as use of the World Health Organisation [WHO] Safer Surgery checklist). Examples of poor systems and practices in the National Health Service (NHS) include: widespread toleration of variation in standard procedures, such as surgical counts; operating lists with multiple changes in list order; failure to adhere to surgical site marking procedures; inadequate staffing; and absent or inadequate training, particularly in team working and human factors. All of which contribute to adverse events.

As evidenced from previous literature, it is apparent that the vast majority of adverse events and errors in surgery occur due to failures in these human factors domains, rather than technical ineptitude on the part of the operating surgeon. Many of these human factors can exist in a latent form within our environment, but they affect those of us working in the operating theatre at the 'sharp end', as it is the surgical teams who are the final common pathway for harm to occur to that patient (**Fig. 9.2**).[11a] While in other high-risk industries considerable work has been done by human factors scientists to engineer out many of these latent threats that lurk in our work systems, in healthcare we are still at a very rudimentary stage in this journey. At present in healthcare we still need to rely on humans to act as our final line of defence to prevent harm coming to our patients, and to optimise our surgical outcomes.

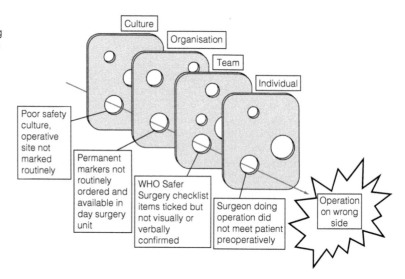

Figure 9.2 • The Swiss cheese model applied to a case of wrong site surgery. The slices of cheese are defensive layers within the healthcare system, the holes are transient or permanent gaps in these defences. When the holes align, a significant adverse event occurs.

While technical skills undoubtedly play a part in this, it is equally important that we are able to deploy good non-technical skills to minimise the risk of harm to our patients.

Non-technical skills in surgery

Although there is undoubtedly a link between technical surgical skill and patient outcomes,[12] it is clear that the majority of error and unintended harm arises from poor non-technical skills on the part of the surgical team,[13] with loss of situation awareness, poor decision-making, compounded by poor leadership, teamwork and suboptimal communication all implicated. Despite this, until recently there was no way of describing, categorising, or rating these non-technical skills, and as a result they were not formally acknowledged, taught or assessed in surgeons.

A collaboration between the University of Aberdeen Industrial Psychology Unit and the Royal College of Surgeons of Edinburgh produced the Non-Technical Skills for Surgeons (NOTSS) taxonomy to describe and assess these non-technical skills in the intraoperative environment.[14] This taxonomy was designed specifically for use in the operating room and is currently the most widely validated tool for rating and classifying surgical non-technical skills.[15]

The NOTSS classification (see **Table 9.1**) describes two cognitive non-technical skill categories – those of situational awareness and decision-making – and two social non-technical skill categories – teamworking and communication, and leadership – Each of the four categories can be subdivided into a further three elements that describe each category in further detail. This taxonomy can be used to rate

and improve the non-technical skills of surgeons in the intraoperative environment – and they will now be considered in turn.

Table 9.1 • NOTSS skills taxonomy v1.2

Category	Elements
Situation awareness	Gathering information
	Projecting information
	Projecting and anticipating future state
Decision-making	Considering options
	Selecting and communicating option
	Implementing and reviewing decisions
Communication and teamworking	Exchanging information
	Establishing a shared understanding
	Coordinating team activities
Leadership	Setting and maintaining standards
	Supporting others
	Coping with pressure

Situation Awareness (SA)

Situation awareness can best be simply described as 'knowing what is going on around you'. To delve a little deeper, situation awareness is the awareness of what is going on around you at any one time, the correct understanding of what is going on and a projection into the future of what that means is likely to happen next (**Fig. 9.3**). This three-level

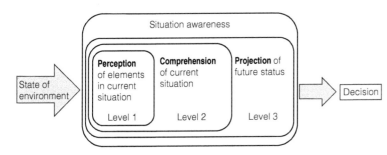

Figure 9.3 • Three-level model of situation awareness. Reproduced with permission from Endsley MR. Theoretical underpinnings of situation awareness: a critical review. In: Endsley MR, Garland DJ, editors. Situation awareness analysis and measurement. Mahwah, NJ: Lawrence Erlbaum Associates; 2000.

model of SA described by Mica Endsley has been well described in aviation and is often referred to as "What?, So What? and Now What?".[16]

The concept of knowing what is going on around you in the operating theatre may seem obvious, but as human beings we think that we notice far more of our environment than we actually do. At any one time there is an overwhelming amount of information available to us, so in order for us to make sense of the world we become very selective in what we consciously attend to, otherwise we would be constantly overwhelmed by masses of competing information. What we focus our attention on depends on the environment (we are easily distracted from a task by loud noises for example), but it also depends on our past experiences – so our knowledge of how the world works will guide us in focusing our attention – for instance looking out for moving cars when we cross a road.

We have a limited capacity for monitoring our current state, interpreting new incoming information, and planning our future actions, and that capacity is easily overwhelmed. This is very powerfully demonstrated in a classic experiment,[17] in which observers were asked to watch a video of a basketball game and count the number of times the ball was passed between team members. In this experiment 60% of observers were so engrossed in the task of counting the passes that they failed to notice a man in a gorilla suit walking across their field of vision. This demonstrated eloquently and powerfully how selective our attention can be, and that concentrating on one task can overwhelm our perception of reality and our ability to process and understand information that was clearly available to our senses at the time. (Watch the video at https://www.youtube.com/watch?v=vJG698U2Mvo.)

Maintaining situation awareness is crucial to patient safety and one does not have to look very far to find accidents where loss of situation awareness was implicated. In aviation, loss of SA has been implicated in 88% of aviation accidents in which human performance was implicated.[18] Likewise, in surgery, good SA within the surgical team has been associated with improved operating times and fewer errors during surgery.[19]

Given the importance of situation awareness and the implications of loss of SA and its connection to accidents and adverse outcomes, we should seek to minimise the risks of reduced or absent situation awareness. A simple way to enhance the SA of the whole team is the use of a robust preoperative briefing. This means that everyone starts the day 'singing from the same hymn sheet'. A good briefing should ensure that the whole team has a correct mental model of the forthcoming task or operating list. In many other high-risk industries, a pre-task briefing is an accepted safety procedure, such as pilots briefing for an aborted take-off before every flight.

Another method to maintain good SA in your operating theatre is to minimise the incidence of interruptions and distractions. Distractions are common in operating theatres, with pagers and phones going off and multiple conversations occurring between different team members at once. An observational study reported an average of 3.5 procedure-irrelevant conversations occurring per surgical case.[20] They also reported that as the number of interruptions in theatre increased, so did the number of team miscommunications, revealing a direct link between team performance and interruptions occurring in theatres.

Distractions are just as deadly to SA, and this includes not concentrating on the job at hand. A well-known aviation case involved a DC-9 in the USA. During the approach to the airport the crew were so busy chatting about matters unrelated to the flight that they failed to notice they were too low, and the aircraft crashed with 74 fatalities. This led to the introduction of the 'sterile cockpit', where the crew are prohibited from performing non-essential duties or conversations during crucial phases of the flight such as take-off and landing. This sterile cockpit rule helps minimise distraction to the flight crew and helps them maintain their SA. In my own hospital, we have implemented a form of sterile cockpit into our operating theatre routine to try to mirror this effect. During these phases, music must be turned off, staff are forbidden to talk about anything not directly related to the current case, staff are not allowed to enter or leave the theatre unless on a task directly related to the case etc. This sterile cockpit state occurs automatically at certain phases of the surgery such as the surgical pause and the postoperative sign out, and during any instrument counts. In addition, any member of the team can call for sterile cockpit during crucial phases of the case – if the anaesthetist is having airway difficulties for instance, or if the surgeon is approaching a technically challenging part of the case. Of course, as well as sterile cockpit drill it is important to take simple steps to minimise other interruptions and distractions such as not having bleeps or mobile phones in theatre.

To help maintain both individual surgeon's and the surgical team's SA it is important to regularly update your mental model and that of the team. Regularly check your current mental model with real-world cues and also with your team's mental model to make sure that they match. And remember that if they do not match, it may not be your mental model that is correct! In this regard it is also important that your team feels empowered to speak up if they see unsafe behaviour, or if their mental model of what is happening does not seem to coincide with either what is going on or what should be going on. Set the tone for this hierarchical challenge culture at your preoperative brief.

Maintaining good time management is also crucial to maintaining good SA. Rushing to get through a procedure, or complete a task, is not conducive to good SA. In a study of aviation accidents the pilots were found to be behind schedule in 55% of them, and were hurrying to get their flight onto the ground on time. This added time pressure serves as a distraction and also utilises precious cognitive capacity; it is a sure recipe for decreased SA and poor decision-making.

Decision-making

Decision-making is intrinsically linked to situation awareness – without the correct mental picture of the situation it is very difficult to make a good decision. As humans we have two main pathways by which we can make decisions – automatic or analytical.[21] The traditional method of decision-making involves critically assessing the situation, then formulating a series of possible options to take, and then carefully weighing up the pros and cons of each before committing to carrying out one of these options. This analytical method of making decisions has long been taught and studied as the classic method of decision-making, and it involves considerable expenditure of mental effort.

Experienced surgeons, on the other hand, spend most of their time using recognition-primed decision-making, which is an almost unconscious, automatic method of decision-making. This relies on 'fast and frugal' pattern matching to recognise familiar situations and apply actions that have been used successfully in previous similar situations. This system of thinking is, however, entirely dependent on previous experience, so is very accurate in experts but highly prone to error in novices. An example of this would be to think about your drive into work – you made thousands of decisions during this drive, but were probably not aware of any of them as you perform this task now on 'automatic pilot' as you are so familiar with it. If you asked a novice to drive you, the result would be very different and you would see them resort to slow effortful analytical decision-making mode – having to consciously think about every junction and road sign along the way.

In crisis situations, or if we stray into unfamiliar surgical territory, we too will resort to a more analytical mode of decision-making because we may not have a pattern to match to. While this still enables us to make decisions it takes much more conscious, cognitive 'thinking power' to do this, and it is a much slower method of decision-making, so we will see ourselves slowing down. We must also be conscious in these situations to try to preserve enough space in our working memory to enable us to make these analytical decisions. If this cognitive capacity is exceeded, then there can be a spiralling deterioration in performance. In these situations, stress can act to reduce cognitive capacity, leading to loss of SA, with concomitant deterioration in decision-making and motor skills that in turn causes more stress. Effective utilisation of leadership and teamwork can help in re-distributing tasks and their associated cognitive load to other team members, thus protecting high performance for successful completion of the surgical task. Effective use of non-technical skills is thus directly related to technical performance of the surgical task.

It is also vital to the rest of the surgical team that they are kept 'up to speed' with the decision-making processes, and the reasoning behind them. Effective teamworking depends on all of the members of the surgical team having the same, accurate SA, or mental model. This is especially important when recognition-primed decision-making is being used, as it can look to the team as if you have just plucked a course of action out of nowhere, so it is vital that the course of action, and its reasoning, are verbalised to the rest of the team so that they can update their mental models and make them congruent with your own. Likewise it is vital for you to review your decision and its consequences – 'have we made this situation better or worse?' 'Do we need to implement another course of action?' etc.

Teamwork and communication

The practice of surgery is not the premise of an individual, but can only be delivered by a surgical team. Teams can only function effectively through good communication – and it is no coincidence that teamwork and communication have been singled out[22] as the 'main contributors to error'.

As surgeons, we tend to think we are better at teamworking than we are – surgeons thinking that they are very good at team working about 85% of the time, whereas only 48% of the nursing staff would agree.[23] It is now well known that teamworking has a real and demonstrable effect on surgical outcomes, with directly observed poor teamworking behaviours in the operating room having worse outcomes for patients than good teamworking, to the extent that teamworking ability was a more powerful predictor of patient outcome than the ASA (American Society of Anesthesiologists) status of the patient.[24] In addition, a team training programme has been shown to significantly improve both morbidity and mortality compared to no training.[25] This has been further emphasised in a randomised trial involving over 182 000 operations and 74 hospitals, which demonstrated an 18% reduction in surgical mortality after initiation of a team training programme.[26]

Teamwork and communication in the NOTSS taxonomy is again divided into the three elements listed above – exchanging information, establishing a shared understanding and coordinating team activities.

The first element emphasises the vital importance of communication within the team. The surgeon should ensure that the entire team feel safe to freely share information within the team. After almost all adverse events someone will say that they thought that something was going to happen but they did not feel empowered to speak up so it is essential that the lead surgeon encourages free flow of information amongst team members, best brought about by consciously trying to 'flatten' the hierarchy between team members. The preoperative briefing is a useful opportunity to set this tone and explicitly encourage team members to speak up if they see something concerning.

This information sharing is used to ensure that all team members have a shared understanding of the current situation. Situation awareness is key to patient safety, and building shared SA among team members is one of the hallmarks of a high-performing surgical team. Again, the preoperative briefing is the first step to establishing this shared understanding, and continuous progress updates from all team members during the course of the procedure ensure that the team hold a shared mental model at all times.

The lead surgeon should also be instrumental in explicitly coordinating team activities, by assessing team members' abilities and then clearly assigning tasks to team members. In the dynamic situation of an operation it may be necessary to re-assign tasks, and to share workload so that any individual team member does not become cognitively overloaded. This explicit assigned role clarity is often taken as read, but clearly defined roles and monitoring of team members' workload is again a mark of excellence in teamwork. Such re-assignment of tasks can of course be coordinated by any member of the team, such as the floor nurse and anaesthetist, especially in times of stress when the surgeons are deeply occupied.

Leadership

In the NOTSS taxonomy the leadership category involves the surgeon leading the operating team and providing a clear direction and goal. It involves demonstrating the highest standards of clinical practice and care, being considerate and supportive of the other members of the operative team, and being able, and seen to be able, to cope with pressure and stressful situations.

Setting and maintaining standards is vital, and being a role model for the rest of the surgical team is crucial. Demonstrating a positive leadership style through modelling positive behaviours has been shown to have a major impact on how patient safety initiatives are viewed and accepted amongst the other members of the medical or surgical team. The surgeon who demonstrates positive attitudes towards protocols and models attention to best surgical practice will be rewarded with a more positive attitude towards safety within the whole team.

The time when modelling good behaviour and being a role model is perhaps most important is during the preoperative briefing. The lead surgeon can set the tone for the entire day with this briefing; simply introducing the briefing with the phrase 'Welcome to today's safety briefing' focuses the entire team onto a safety-oriented footing. Also one can use the introduction to set the tone for the team regarding hierarchy, and encouraging other team members to speak out if they see or think they see unsafe or potentially unsafe events or behaviours.

In addition to setting and maintaining standards within the operating team, it is a vital aspect of leadership that the lead surgeon supports others within the team. Effective leadership means not just focusing on completing the task; truly effective leadership means that the leader must also demonstrate behaviours to improve and enhance team functioning and performance.

The third element in this category is coping with pressure. Demonstration of an outwardly calm demeanour when under increased stress is essential in emphasising to the rest of the team that you have this high-pressure situation under control. This can also mean adopting a forceful manner if such is appropriate in urgent or emergency situations, but without undermining the role of the other team members. This last part is vital as the surgeon who remains completely laid back and laconic even during an emergency situation and who does not convey the urgency or seriousness of the situation is not demonstrating a positive behaviour in this situation.

Conclusion

Our next challenge in improving surgical practice is how to make it safer for our patients who are subject to preventable adverse events. The majority of these unintended outcomes are not due to a lack of technical surgical skill, but are down to poor systems and lack of non-technical skills within the surgical team. The NOTSS taxonomy allows us all to classify, rate and improve non-technical skills, both in ourselves and others. This in turn will permit all surgeons to optimise their performance and make surgery safer for our patients.

Key points

- The incidence of adverse events in surgical patients worldwide is around 10%.
- Human factors play a major role in adverse events.
- Better non-technical skills and team training reduce surgical errors and improve outcomes.

▶ **Selective attention test**

Recommended video:
- The original awareness test from Daniel Simons and Christopher Chabris – goo.gl/TO804q

---

🌐 Full references available at **http://expertconsult. inkling.com**

Key references

3. Brennan TA, Leape LL, Laird NM, et al. Incidence of adverse events and negligence in hospitalized patients. Results of the Harvard Medical Practice Study I. N Engl J Med 1991;324(6):370–6. PMID: 1987460.
   This large review of over 30 000 case records was one of the first studies into iatrogenic harm and reported an adverse event rate of 3.9% in hospitalised patients in the USA. It concluded that many of these adverse events were 'the result of substandard care'.

4. Gawande AA, Thomas EJ, Zinner MJ, et al. The incidence and nature of surgical adverse events in Colorado and Utah in 1992. Surgery 1999;126(1):66–75. PMID: 10418594.
   This retrospective case review was the first study to specifically look at the incidence of adverse events in surgery. It concluded that of all hospital-related adverse events, 66% occurred within the surgical domain, and crucially, that at least 50% of these were preventable.

8. Anderson O, Davis R, Hanna GB, et al. Surgical adverse events: a systematic review. AJS 2013;206(2):253–62. PMID: 23642651.
   This systematic review incorporated over 16 000 surgical patients and found an overall adverse event rate of 14.4%, with preventable adverse events occurring in 5.2%. The review also concluded that errors in 'non-operative management' caused more frequent adverse events than errors in surgical technique.

9. Gawande AA, Zinner MJ, Studdert DM, et al. Analysis of errors reported by surgeons at three teaching hospitals. Surgery 2003;133(6):614–21. PMID: 12796727.
   This study was the first to attempt to classify the cause of surgical adverse events by interviewing surgeons about past adverse outcomes. It highlighted that the majority of surgical adverse events occur during the intraoperative phase of care and that most were due to 'system errors' such as poor leadership or communication rather than errors in surgical technique.

12. Birkmeyer JD, Finks JF, O'Reilly A, et al. Surgical skill and complication rates after bariatric surgery. N Engl J Med 2013;369(15):1434–42. PMID: 24106936.
    In this study surgical skill was assessed by blinded review of surgeons' videos of laparoscopic bariatric surgery. Technical skill as measured using OSATS correlated directly with outcomes.

13. Yule S, Flin R, Paterson-Brown S, et al. Non-technical skills for surgeons in the operating room: a review of the literature. Surgery 2006;139(2):140–9. PMID: 16455321.
    This paper reviewed the literature on non-technical skills in surgery and was the first to identify 'core categories' of non-technical skills in surgery, namely communication, teamwork, leadership and decision-making.

14. Yule SS, Flin RR, Paterson-Brown SS, et al. Development of a rating system for surgeons' non-technical skills. Med Educ 2006;40(11):1098–104. PMID: 17054619.

This paper analyses the identification of crucial non-technical skills for surgeons through a combination of critical incident analysis, direct observation and interviews. It details how these data were then used to develop the NOTSS skills taxonomy and behavioural ratings system to structure observation and feedback in surgical training.

24. Mazzocco K, Petitti DB, Fong KT, et al. Surgical team behaviors and patient outcomes. AJS 2009;197(5):678–85. PMID: 18789425.

Direct observation of surgical teams was used in this study to ascertain a behaviour marker score that reflected how good surgical teams were at teamworking. Teams with good teamworking had better patient outcomes compared to those with poor teamworking. The quality of surgical teamworking was a more powerful predictor of patient outcome than the patient's ASA score.

25. Armour Forse R, Bramble JD, McQuillan R. Team training can improve operating room performance. Surgery 2011;150(4):771–8. PMID: 22000190.

This cohort study demonstrated that a surgical team training programme improved the teamworking in surgical teams, and led to a fall in both morbidity and mortality for surgical patients.

26. Neily J, Mills PD, Young-Xu Y, et al. Association between implementation of a medical team training program and surgical mortality. JAMA 2010;304(15):1693–700. PMID: 20959579.

This randomised trial involving over 182 000 procedures demonstrated an 18% reduction in annual surgical mortality in institutions where a team training programme was implemented for their surgical teams.

10

Principles of organ donation and general surgery in the transplant patient

Diana A. Wu
Gabriel C. Oniscu

Introduction

In just 50 years, organ transplantation has revolutionised the treatment of end-stage organ failure. Innovations in surgical technique, immunosuppression and organ preservation have propelled transplantation to the forefront of pioneering medicine. What was once an experimental procedure is now a highly successful treatment with excellent survival rates (Table 10.1). Consequently, it is increasingly common for general surgeons to encounter transplant patients presenting with a general surgical problem unrelated to the transplant procedure. It is essential for general surgeons to be aware of the particular issues associated with the management of transplant patients in the context of elective or emergency general surgery. Likewise, general surgeons may be involved in the care of patients who become potential organ donors, and as such require an adequate understanding of the principles of organ donation.

This chapter summarises the key issues related to organ donation as well as the management of transplant recipients requiring general surgery.

Principles of organ donation

Organs for transplantation may be donated from living donors, donors after brain death (DBD) or donors after circulatory death (DCD). Worldwide, the number of donors falls drastically short of the number of patients in need of a transplant, and this is arguably the greatest challenge currently faced by the transplant community.

Ethical and legal aspects of organ donation

Consent is the cornerstone of ethical organ donation. The process of consent for organ donation varies according to medical, ethical, societal and legal factors in each country. For deceased organ donation, the legislative framework for consent may be an 'opt-out' system (consent for organ donation is presumed unless the person has specifically registered to opt out) or an 'opt-in' system (explicit consent for organ donation is required). Both systems can be implemented on either a 'hard' basis, where primacy is given to the donor's wishes, or a 'soft' basis, where family members' views are considered (Table 10.2).[1] There is no international consensus on the best system of consent for deceased organ donation (Table 10.3).[2] At the time of writing, England, Northern Ireland and Scotland operate under a soft opt-in system,[3,4] with consent given verbally, in writing, by ownership of a donor card or by registration on the NHS Organ Donor Register (ODR). If neither consent nor refusal to organ donation was specified by the deceased during life, the decision can be made by a person who was in a 'qualifying relationship' (e.g. spouse, parent, child, etc.). In December 2015, Wales introduced an opt-out system for deceased organ donation.[5] This legislation is applied 'softly'; thus if objection from family members exists, organ donation will not proceed.

Living organ donation is a unique clinical situation, whereby a healthy individual undergoes a major surgical procedure that entails a risk of harm, but no physical benefit. As such, the consent process is governed by strict legislation in most countries. It is crucial to ensure that consent for living organ

Table 10.1 • National 1-year and 5-year adult patient survival rates for abdominal organ transplantation in the UK

	1-year patient survival (%)*	5-year patient survival (%)†
Kidney		
Living donor	99	95
Deceased donor	96	88
Pancreas	98	78
Simultaneous kidney–pancreas	97	88
Liver		
Elective	93	81
Super-urgent	89	79

*Includes transplants performed between 1 April 2011 and 31 March 2015.
†Includes transplants performed between 1 April 2007 and 31 March 2011.
Sources: NHS Blood and Transplant. Annual Report on Kidney Transplantation 2015/16, Pancreas and Islet Transplantation 2015/16 and Liver Transplantation 2015/16. https://nhsbtdbe.blob.core.windows.net/umbraco-assets-corp/1313/organ_specific_report_kidney_2016.pdf
https://nhsbtdbe.blob.core.windows.net/umbraco-assets-corp/1316/organ_specific_report_pancreas_2016.pdf
https://nhsbtdbe.blob.core.windows.net/umbraco-assets-corp/1314/organ_specific_report_liver_2016.pdf

donation is given voluntarily, without coercion, without any form of reward and from a person who has full capacity to make informed decisions.

The global shortage of organ donors has led to the emergence of unethical practices in transplantation. Organ trafficking, transplant commercialism and transplant tourism (Box 10.1) exploit vulnerable and impoverished populations through the removal and sale of organs, most commonly to patients travelling from more economically developed countries. These practices are prohibited by the World Health Organisation (WHO) Guiding Principles on Human Cell, Tissue and Organ Transplantation[6] and the Declaration of Istanbul,[7] which provide international ethical standards for organ transplantation.

Table 10.3 • Consent systems for deceased organ donation in different countries

Opt-out	Opt-in
Argentina	Australia
Austria	Brazil
Belarus	Canada
Belgium	Cuba
Bulgaria	Denmark
Columbia	England
Costa Rica	Germany
Croatia	Guatemala
Czech Republic	Hong Kong
Ecuador	Republic of Ireland
Finland	Israel
France	Japan
Greece	Lebanon
Hungary	Lithuania
Italy	Malaysia
Latvia	Mexico
Panama	The Netherlands
Poland	New Zealand
Portugal	Northern Ireland
Russia	Puerto Rico
Singapore	Romania
Slovak Republic	Scotland
Spain	Taiwan
Sweden	United States
Tunisia	Venezuela
Wales	

Source: Shepherd L, O'Carroll RE, Ferguson E. An international comparison of deceased and living organ donation/transplant rates in opt-in and opt-out systems: a panel study. BMC Med 2014;12(1):131.

Types of organ donation

Living donation

The limited availability of deceased donor organs has led to a rise in living donor transplantation. Besides expanding the donor pool, living donor transplantation provides additional advantages. Firstly, living donor

Table 10.2 • Different consent systems for deceased organ donation

	Opt-out	Opt-in
Hard	Consent for deceased organ donation is presumed, unless a person has registered to opt out. If a person has not registered to opt out, organ donation can proceed even if family members object	Consent for deceased organ donation is based on whether a person has registered to opt in. If a person has registered to opt in, organ donation can proceed even if family members object
Soft	Consent for deceased organ donation is presumed, unless a person has registered to opt out. If a person has not registered to opt out, organ donation does not proceed if family members object	Consent for deceased organ donation is based on whether a person has registered to opt in. If a person has registered to opt in, organ donation does not proceed if family members object

Box 10.1 • Definitions of unethical practices in organ transplantation as set out by the Declaration of Istanbul

Organ trafficking is the recruitment, transport, transfer, harbouring or receipt of living or deceased persons or their organs by means of threat or use of force or other forms of coercion, of abduction, of fraud, of deception, of the abuse of power or of a position of vulnerability, or of the giving to, or the receiving by, a third party of payments or benefits to achieve the transfer of control over the potential donor, for the purpose of exploitation by the removal of organs for transplantation.

Transplant commercialism is a policy or practice in which an organ is treated as a commodity, including by being bought or sold or used for material gain.

Travel for transplantation is the movement of organs, donors, recipients or transplant professionals across jurisdictional borders for transplantation purposes. Travel for transplantation becomes **transplant tourism** if it involves organ trafficking and/ or transplant commercialism or if the resources (organs, professionals and transplant centres) devoted to providing transplants to patients from outside a country undermine the country's ability to provide transplant services for its own population.

Reprinted from The Lancet, Vol. 372, Steering Committee of the Istanbul Summit, Organ trafficking and transplant tourism and commercialism: the Declaration of Istanbul, (9632):pages 5-6, Copyright (2008) with permission from Elsevier.

organs have not been exposed to the detrimental effects of the dying process or prolonged periods of ischaemia, thus leading to optimal post-transplant organ function. Secondly, the transplant procedure can be scheduled electively, at a time when both donor and recipient health are optimal, enabling recipients to avoid long waiting times and the associated risk of waiting-list morbidity and mortality. Nevertheless, the benefits of living donor transplantation must be carefully weighed against the small but not insignificant risks to the donor.[8–11] The safety and welfare of the potential living donor always take precedence over the needs of the potential transplant recipient.[12]

Currently, kidney and liver transplantation from living donors is common practice in many countries, while lung and pancreas living donation have been reported in smaller series.[13–15] In the UK, living donation accounts for 33% of kidney transplants and 4% of liver transplants,[16,17] and this is fairly representative of most Western countries. In contrast, in many Asian and Middle Eastern countries such as Japan, South Korea and Turkey the vast majority of transplants are from living donors, due to the lack of cultural acceptance of deceased organ donation.[18,19]

Living donation may be *'directed'* to a specific identified recipient, or *'non-directed'* to an unknown recipient. Altruistic donation, i.e. where the donor does not have a genetic or pre-existing emotional relationship with the recipient, accounts for an increasing number of transplants.

The assessment of all potential living donors is a multistep, multidisciplinary process. A comprehensive medical and psychosocial assessment is required to minimise risk and ensure suitability for donation. Assessment must include function and anatomy of the donor organ, general medical health, risk of transmissible disease and psychiatric morbidity.

Living kidney donation

Living donor kidney transplantation is associated with significantly better graft and recipient survival compared with deceased donor kidney transplantation, and is therefore the treatment of choice for patients with end-stage renal disease (ESRD).[20] Sharing schemes have been developed to enable blood or human leukocyte antigen (HLA) incompatible donor-recipient pairs to be matched with other incompatible pairs, in order to achieve compatible transplants. Paired donation includes two pairs, while pooled donation includes at least three pairs (**Fig. 10.1**). When a non-directed altruistic donor donates their organ into the paired/pooled scheme, a chain of transplants can be created, with the remaining organ at the end of the chain offered to the best matched recipient on the national transplant waiting list (**Fig. 10.2**).

Living donor nephrectomy may be performed using a variety of open, laparoscopic and hand-assisted techniques via a trans- or retroperitoneal approach (Box 10.2). The laparoscopic approaches are now standard in most centres. Several randomised controlled trials have demonstrated shorter hospital stay, less pain, quicker recovery and quicker return to normal activities for laparoscopic versus open techniques, with equivalent complication rates and graft outcomes.[21,22] Generally, there is a preference for left kidney donation due to the longer left renal vein; however, there is no difference in outcomes using either kidney.[23] Computerised tomography (CT) angiogram assessment of renal anatomy should guide the decision as to which kidney is most suitable. Assessment of donor renal function (overall and split function) is required to ensure sufficient residual renal function post-donation and adequate recipient graft function. Direct measurement of radioisotope (e.g. ^{51}Cr-EDTA, ^{125}Iothalamate) clearance allows accurate evaluation of the glomerular filtration rate (GFR). A GFR <80 mL/min/1.73 m^2 generally precludes kidney donation.[24,25] However, since GFR declines with increasing age, lower thresholds may be accepted for older donors.[26]

Since age alone is not associated with increased surgical mortality or complications,[8,27,28] there is no specific age cut-off for kidney donation. Individual risk should be considered within the context of renal function, comorbidities and overall health. Hypertension ($>140/90$ mmHg) with evidence of

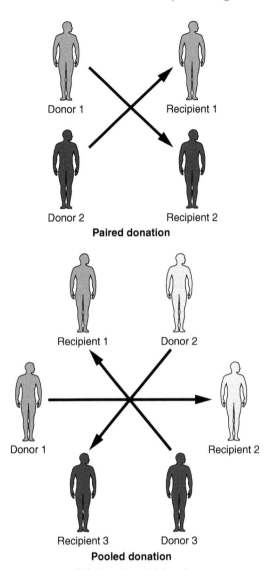

Paired donation

Pooled donation

Figure 10.1 • Paired and pooled donation.

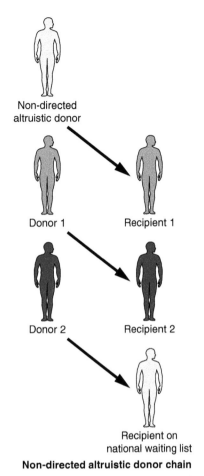

Non-directed altruistic donor chain

Figure 10.2 • Non-directed altruistic donor chains.

Box 10.2 • Surgical approaches to living donor nephrectomy

Open
Mini-incision
Laparoscopic
   Transperitoneal
   Retroperitoneal
   Anterior
   Lumbar
Hand-assisted
   Transperitoneal
   Retroperitoneal
Laparoendoscopic single-site surgery (LESS)
Robotic-assisted
Natural orifice transluminal endoscopic surgery (NOTES)

end-organ damage and cardiovascular disease are contraindications to kidney donation.[24,27]

Living donor nephrectomy is a low-risk procedure with perioperative mortality consistently reported at below 0.03%.[8,29,30] In a recent systematic review of 32 038 minimally invasive living donor nephrectomies, the overall intraoperative complication rate was 2.3% (mainly bleeding), postoperative complication rate 7.3% (mainly infective) and conversion rate 1.1%.[30] Although the long-term survival of kidney donors is equivalent to that of age- and comorbidity-matched controls,[8,31] there are emerging concerns regarding the long-term risk of ESRD post-donation. Previous studies demonstrated a lower incidence of ESRD in kidney donors compared with the general unscreened population.[31,32] However, two recent studies comparing kidney donors with healthy matched controls (who would have been considered fit enough for kidney donation) suggest up to an 11-fold increased risk of ESRD for kidney donors.[10,11] This risk is estimated to be higher for black than white donors.[10] Despite these results, the absolute incidence of ESRD amongst kidney donors remains low (<1%).[10,11]

Living liver donation

Living liver donation involves a partial hepatectomy in which a liver lobe or segment is resected. The optimal size of the graft is the smallest possible liver resection to minimise operative risk and ensure an adequate remnant liver volume for the donor, balanced with a graft volume that is sufficient to meet the metabolic demands of the recipient. A graft to body weight ratio of <0.8% increases the risk of small-for-size syndrome, which is associated with high recipient morbidity and mortality.[33-35] In adult-to-child transplantation, a left lateral segment graft (segments II and III) is most often used. In adult-to-adult transplantation, the full left lobe (segments II, III and IV) may be used, but more commonly the larger volume of a right lobe graft (segments V, VI, VII and VIII) is required. The higher operative risks of donor right hepatectomy must be considered. CT and magnetic resonance imaging (MRI) with intravascular contrast are necessary for volumetric analysis, determination of vascular and biliary anatomy and assessment for hepatic steatosis of the donor liver. It is generally accepted that the donor remnant liver volume should be at minimum 30%.[14,36-38] Most liver regeneration occurs rapidly within the first week after resection or transplantation.[39] Within 3 months, the donor liver remnant regenerates to around 80% of original liver volume, while the recipient graft reaches 93% of standard liver volume.[40] Donor hepatic steatosis increases both donor and recipient risk. Although no clear cut-off is defined, usually >30% steatosis precludes donation.[12]

There is insufficient evidence to define an upper age limit for living liver donation, but the increased risk of perioperative complications with older age must be given careful consideration, in conjunction with other risk factors. Obesity increases the risk of surgical complications and is associated with a higher frequency of hepatic steatosis, therefore a BMI >35 kg/m^2 is usually considered a contraindication to donation.[12]

Current data suggest the risk of donor mortality to be 0.2%.[9,41] The overall complication rate is reported to be between 16.1% and 39%, with the most common complications being biliary complications (e.g. leaks, strictures), infections (e.g. wound, urinary, lung) and incisional hernias.[9,41-43] Complications are more common and more serious in right than left lobe donors.[44,45] However, most donors return to normal activity within 3–6 months.[9]

In paediatric liver transplantation, there is evidence that living donor transplantation results in better survival compared with deceased donor transplantation.[46-48] In adult liver transplantation, living donor transplantation is associated with a higher rate of recipient complications, but no significant difference in mortality compared with deceased donor transplantation.[49] However, significant survival benefit has been demonstrated for patients who undergo living donor liver transplantation compared with remaining on the waiting list for deceased donor liver transplantation.[50,51]

Deceased organ donation

Deceased organ donation may occur after brain death (DBD) or after circulatory death (DCD). World-wide, the majority of organs transplanted from deceased donors are recovered from DBD donors. Deceased organ donation rates are influenced by many factors, including cultural, economic, legal and healthcare factors.[1] However, it is increasingly recognised that specialist and trained staff play an important role in deceased organ donation.[52] In the UK, when a Specialist Nurse in Organ Donation (SNOD) is involved in approaching families about donation, the consent rate is significantly higher than when a SNOD is not involved (70% vs 30%).[53] Similar findings have been shown in the United States and in Spain.[52,54-56]

Donor identification and referral

The identification and referral of potential deceased organ donors is a crucial step in the deceased donation process, and should be seen as a routine part of end-of-life care. All clinicians have a responsibility to recognise if a patient under their care becomes a potential organ donor, and to initiate discussions with specialist staff (i.e. SNOD) as early as possible. The General Medical Council (GMC) has published guidance for the responsibilities of doctors with respect to end-of-life care and organ donation (Box 10.3).[57]

Clinical triggers can aid the identification of potential organ donors. In the UK, National Institute for Health and Care Excellence (NICE) guidelines[58] recommend referral to the SNOD if either of the following criteria are met:

1. A patient with catastrophic brain injury **with**
   - the absence of one or more cranial nerve reflexes **and**
   - a Glasgow Coma Scale (GCS) score of 4 or less that is not explained by sedation.
2. A patient with a life-threatening or life-limiting condition **where**
   - a decision has been made to withdraw life-sustaining treatment **and**
   - this is expected to result in circulatory death.

Donation after brain death

Donation after brain death requires determination of death by neurological criteria. The concept of brain death was first proposed by Harvard Medical School in 1967.[59] Advances in intensive care techniques meant that comatose patients could be maintained on mechanical ventilation, despite loss of brainstem function and therefore loss of the capacity for spontaneous respiration and consciousness. Therefore, it was proposed that such cases of irreversible coma due to permanent damage to the brain could be defined as death.[59] Subsequently, the concept of brain death was gradually accepted elsewhere. In the UK,

a statement by the Conference of Medical Royal Colleges and their Faculties in 1979 concluded for the first time that brain death equated to the death of the whole person.[60,61] Current criteria for the diagnosis of brainstem death in the UK are shown in Table 10.4.[62] Brainstem death testing must be carried out by two doctors (at least one should be a consultant) who have been registered for more than 5 years and are competent in the procedure. Neither doctor should be a member of the transplant team. Testing should

Table 10.4 • Criteria for diagnosis of brainstem death in the UK

Preconditions

Patient is deeply comatose, unresponsive and apnoeic with his/her lungs being artificially ventilated
Patient's condition is due to irreversible brain damage of known aetiology

Exclusions

There should be no evidence that this state is due to:
   Depressant drugs
   Neuromuscular blocking drugs
   Hypothermia*
   Circulatory, metabolic or endocrine disturbance

Clinical examination

Absence of brainstem reflexes:
   Pupils are fixed and do not respond to sharp changes in the intensity of incident light
   No corneal reflex
   No oculo-vestibular reflex[†]
   No motor responses within the cranial nerve distribution by adequate stimulation of any somatic area
   No cough reflex response to bronchial stimulation by a suction catheter placed down the trachea to the carina
   No gag reflex to stimulation of the posterior pharynx with a spatula
   Apnoea despite an induced moderate hypercarbia and mild acidaemia[‡]

*Core temperature should be >34°C at the time of testing.
[†]Caloric test: no eye movements are seen during or following the slow injection of at least 50 mL of ice-cold water over 1 minute into each external auditory meatus in turn. Clear access to the tympanic membrane must be established by direct inspection and the head should be at 30° to the horizontal plane, unless this positioning is contraindicated by the presence of an unstable spinal injury.
[‡]The apnoea test should be the last brainstem reflex to be tested and should not be performed if any of the preceding tests confirm the presence of brainstem reflexes. A controlled rise in arterial $PaCO_2$ (>6.0 KPa or >6.5 KPa in the context of chronic CO_2 retention or intravenous bicarbonate) with corresponding acidaemia (pH <7.40) should be induced whilst maintaining a normal PaO_2 and blood pressure. The patient should be disconnected from the ventilator for 5 minutes to confirm no spontaneous respiratory response. A further confirmatory arterial blood gas sample should be obtained to ensure that the $PaCO_2$ has increased from the starting level by more than 0.5 KPa.
Source: Academy of Medical Royal Colleges. A code of practice for the diagnosis and confirmation of death. 2008. http://aomrc.org.uk/wp-content/uploads/2016/04/Code_Practice_Confirmation_Diagnosis_Death_1008-4.pdf. Reproduced with permission.

be undertaken by the doctors together and on two occasions. The diagnosis of brainstem death can generally be confirmed by clinical criteria alone, but on rare occasions where there is uncertainty over the completion or interpretation of clinical examination (e.g. extensive eye injuries, high cervical cord injury etc.) then ancillary tests may be required (e.g. cerebral angiography, electroencephalogram [EEG], evoked potentials etc.). There are considerable international differences in the definition of brain death. For instance, in the US, irreversible loss of all brain function (including the brainstem) must be confirmed, while in the UK confirmation of irreversible cessation of brainstem function is adequate (based upon the fact that the capacity for consciousness and cardiorespiratory function reside in the brainstem). There is also wide variation in the diagnostic criteria for brain death, including whether apnoea testing is required and the way in which it is conducted, the number and seniority of clinicians required for brain death testing and whether ancillary tests are mandatory.[63,64] Furthermore, in some countries brain death is not legally or culturally accepted as the death of an individual under any circumstances.

Brainstem death may be caused by intracranial or extracranial pathology. The most commonly reported causes include traumatic brain injury, intracerebral haemorrhage and subarachnoid haemorrhage.[65] Brainstem death triggers complex physiological changes that jeopardise organ function and ultimately lead to cardiac arrest. Effective management of DBD donors involves active care from the time of brainstem death to the point of organ retrieval in order to prevent organ damage, and is an essential part of the donation process that can substantially increase the number of transplantable organs.[66]

Around the time of brainstem death there is a rise in intracranial pressure, which limits cerebral perfusion and oxygen delivery. Cushing's reflex describes the compensatory hypertension that ensues as an attempt to restore cerebral perfusion, which stimulates arterial baroreceptors and causes reflex bradycardia. Subsequently there is a period of intense sympathetic activity (the catecholamine storm), followed by reduced vasomotor tone, hypotension, impaired cardiac output and a systemic inflammatory response.[67] Loss of central regulation results in haemodynamic instability, hypothermia and diabetes insipidus. Without adequate therapy, rapid deterioration and cardiac arrest follow. Optimal donor management is aimed at detecting and correcting the cardiovascular, respiratory and metabolic derangement of brainstem death. Therapy should be based on specific targets for physiological parameters (Box 10.4), and typically involves vasoconstriction, conservative fluid management, lung protective ventilation and the administration of hormonal therapy including methylprednisolone, vasopressin, thyroid hormones and insulin.[68]

Box 10.4 • Physiological targets in the management of brainstem death donors

- $Pao_2 \geq 10.0\,kPa$ ($Fio_2 < 0.4$ as able)
- $Paco_2$ 5–6.5 kPa (or higher as long as pH >7.25)
- MAP 60–80 mmHg
- CVP 4–10 mmHg (secondary goal)
- Cardiac index >2.1 L/min/m^2
- $Scvo_2 > 60\,\%$
- SVRI (secondary goal) 1800–2400 dyn*s/cm^5/m^2
- Temperature 36–37.5°C
- Blood glucose 4.0–10.0 mmol/L
- Urine output 0.5–2.0 mL/kg/h

Source: NHS Blood and Transplant. UK National Organ Donation Commitee. DBD donor optimisation extended care bundle. 2012. http://www.odt.nhs.uk/deceased-donation/best-practice-guidance/donor-optimisation/

Donation after circulatory death

In donation after circulatory death (DCD), donation occurs after the irreversible cessation of cardiorespiratory function. The clinical scenario in which cardiorespiratory arrest occurs can be classified into four different categories known as the Maastricht Classification, which were first described in 1995[69] and subsequently updated in 2013[70] (Table 10.5). These categories can be described as either 'controlled' or 'uncontrolled', referring to whether cardiac arrest was planned and expected or sudden and unexpected, respectively. In most countries, the majority of DCD donations are 'controlled' Maastricht category III. This is usually in the context of a critically ill patient with catastrophic brain injury who does not fulfil the criteria for brainstem death, but where life-sustaining cardiorespiratory support is no longer considered to be in the patient's best interests, and is withdrawn under controlled circumstances. 'Uncontrolled' donation is the predominant type of DCD donation in a few countries (e.g. Spain, France).[71] This occurs after unexpected cardiac arrest, when resuscitative measures fail to restore circulation.

After confirmation of circulatory death there is a mandatory 'no touch' observation period before DCD organ retrieval can commence. In most countries (including the UK) this period is 5 minutes, but it varies from 2 minutes in the US to 20 minutes in Italy.[70]

Despite a substantial increase in DCD donation over the past decade, its practice is not universally accepted. In some countries such as the UK and the Netherlands, DCD donation now accounts for around 50% of all deceased donors. However, in most countries DCD donation remains uncommon,[72] and in several countries is prohibited by the law (e.g. Germany, Greece, Finland).[73] A major concern over the use of DCD organs is the exposure to longer periods of warm ischaemia, leading to potentially inferior graft outcomes. Warm ischaemia

Table 10.5 • Modified Maastricht classification of donation after circulatory death

Type	Category	Circumstances	Scenario
Uncontrolled	I	Found dead Ia. Out of hospital Ib. In hospital	Sudden unexpected cardiac arrest, with no attempt at resuscitation by a medical team
Uncontrolled	II	Witnessed cardiac arrest IIa. Out of hospital IIb. In hospital	Sudden unexpected cardiac arrest, with unsuccessful attempt at resuscitation by a medical team
Controlled	III	Withdrawal of life-sustaining therapy	Planned expected cardiac arrest, following the withdrawal of life-sustaining therapy
Uncontrolled or Controlled	IV	Cardiac arrest while brain dead	Sudden unexpected or planned expected cardiac arrest after brain death diagnosis, but before organ recovery

Reproduced from Thuong M, Ruiz A, Evrard P, et al. New classification of donation after circulatory death donors definitions and terminology. Transpl Int 2016;29(7):749-59 with permission from John Wiley & Sons, Inc.

is a particular concern because at normothermic temperatures metabolic processes continue, thus ischaemic damage occurs more rapidly than under hypothermic conditions when metabolism is slowed. Despite its importance for graft outcomes, there is no consensus over the definition of warm ischaemic time in DCD donation. While the endpoint is defined as the start of cold perfusion, the start point has been variably defined as the beginning of treatment withdrawal, the beginning of circulatory arrest or the time of asystole. Increasingly it is recognised that periods of cardiovascular instability and organ hypoperfusion during treatment withdrawal should be considered as a functional warm ischaemic time. In the UK, this is defined as the time between a sustained (at least 2 minutes) fall of systolic blood pressure below 50 mmHg and the onset of cold perfusion.[74] Guidelines for maximum functional warm ischaemia times for specific organs are shown in Table 10.6.[75] Although it is recognised that the time during which donor oxygen saturation is low

Table 10.6 • Recommended maximum functional warm ischaemia times for donation after circulatory death

Organ	Stand-down time from the onset of functional warm ischaemia
Liver	30 minutes
Pancreas	30 minutes
Lungs	60 minutes
Kidney	120 minutes*

*Can be extended by a further 120 minutes in selected donors.
Source: The Intensive Care Society and the British Transplantation Society. Donation after Circulatory Death. Report of a Consensus Meeting. 2010. https://nhsbtdbe.blob.core.windows.net/umbraco-assets-corp/1360/donation-after-circulatory-death-dcd_consensus_2010.pdf.

(e.g. <70%) could be taken into account when assessing the suitability of donor organs, currently there is insufficient evidence to include it as a criterion for discarding organs.

A recent UK study of deceased donor kidney transplantation found that despite an increased risk of delayed graft function in DCD grafts, there was no difference in the long-term outcomes of DCD and DBD grafts in first-time kidney transplant recipients.[76] Similarly, outcomes of DCD and DBD lung transplantation are comparable.[77] In contrast, the liver and pancreas appear to be more susceptible to warm ischaemia. DCD pancreas transplantation is associated with a significantly higher risk of graft thrombosis,[78] and DCD liver grafts have inferior survival and higher rates of ischaemic biliary complications compared with DBD grafts.[79,80]

There is growing interest in the use of machine perfusion techniques (hypothermic or normothermic) to minimise the consequences of ischaemia. These technologies can be applied to the donor organ in situ, or ex situ during organ transport or preimplantation in the transplant centre. Normothermic regional perfusion (NRP) is a recent advance that is being investigated in DCD donation.[81] It involves perfusing the abdominal organs in situ with oxygenated blood at normal body temperature using a modified extracorporeal membrane oxygenator (ECMO) circuit. Initial results are promising[82] and evidence from further studies is awaited. Ex situ normothermic perfusion and preservation is also being explored for liver and kidney transplantation with encouraging early results.[83,84] These techniques allow for a more objective assessment of organ viability and enable 'resuscitation' of organs prior to transplantation.[85–87] Cold ex situ machine perfusion is increasingly used in kidneys as an alternative to cold static storage during transport. There is evidence that cold machine perfusion may reduce the overall risk of delayed graft function in kidney transplantation but results from randomised controlled trials are conflicting.[88–91]

Contraindications to deceased donation

Absolute contraindications to deceased organ donation are shown in Table 10.7. Any disease with the potential to be transmitted from donor to recipient and which could result in morbidity or mortality despite appropriate treatment (e.g. cancer, significant infections) requires careful risk assessment. It is the responsibility of the recipient transplant team to consider all relevant donor and recipient factors when deciding whether to accept an organ. Organs from all donors will carry some degree of risk, which must be balanced against the benefits of transplantation and the risks of awaiting a further offer of a donor organ.

Table 10.7 • Contraindications to deceased organ donation (UK guidelines)

General contraindications

Age $\geq$85 years
Primary intracerebral lymphoma
All secondary intracerebral tumours
Any active cancer with evidence of spread outside affected organ within 3 years of donation*
Melanoma (except completely excised stage 1 cancers)
Active (not in remission) haematological malignancy (myeloma, lymphoma, leukaemia)
Definite, probable or possible case of human transmissible spongiform encephalopathy, including CJD and variant CJD, individuals whose blood relatives have had familial CJD, other neurodegenerative diseases associated with infectious agents
Tuberculosis: active and untreated
West Nile virus infection
HIV disease (but not HIV infection[†])
A history of infection with Ebola virus

Liver specific contraindications

Acute hepatitis of viral, drug or other known aetiology
Serum AST or ALT >10000 IU/L (if of liver origin)
Cirrhosis
Portal vein thrombosis
Metabolic diseases that would be of harm to the recipient and not treatable (such as haemophilia A and B, inborn errors of metabolism such as oxaluria, tyrosinaemia)

Kidney specific contraindications

Chronic kidney disease (CKD stage 3B or worse, eGFR < 45)
Long-term dialysis (that is, not relating to acute illness)
Renal malignancy: Prior kidney tumours of low grade and previously excised would not necessarily exclude donation
Previous kidney transplant (>6 months previously)

Pancreas specific contraindications

Insulin-dependent diabetes (excluding ICU-associated insulin requirement)
Non-insulin-dependent diabetes (type 2)
Any history of pancreatic malignancy
Donor BMI >40 kg/m^2
Donors <15 kg (except where there is a small paediatric IFALD patient who requires donation of a pancreas with other abdominal organs)
DBD donors $\geq$66 years
DCD donors aged $\geq$56 years

CJD, Creutzfeldt–Jakob disease; HIV, human immunodeficiency virus; AST, aspartate transaminase; ALT, alanine transaminase; CKD, chronic kidney disease; eGFR, estimated glomerular filtration rate; ICU, intensive care unit; BMI, body mass index; IFALD, intestinal failure-associated liver disease; DBD, donor after brain death; DCD, donor after circulatory death.

*Active means not in remission; spread outside affected organ includes spread to lymph nodes. Localised prostate, thyroid, in situ cervical cancer and non-melanotic skin cancers are acceptable as possible organ donors.

[†]HIV infection means people who have infection with HIV but none of the associated complications. Organs from donors with HIV are highly likely to transmit the infection to the recipient and so are used only for those recipients who are already carriers of the virus. Such recipients must be informed and consented about the risks of possible super-infection and transmission of other infective agents that may be present in HIV-infected patients and whose effects may be exacerbated by immunosuppression.

Source: NHS Blood and Transplant. Policy POL188/5.2. Clinical contraindications to approaching families for possible organ donation. 2015. http://odt.nhs.uk/pdf/contraindications_to_organ_donation.pdf.

General surgery in the transplant patient

The management of transplant recipients requiring elective or emergency general surgery is complex and raises several key issues. Firstly, transplant recipients may have risk factors relating to their primary disease which need to be taken into account when estimating perioperative risk, e.g. renal transplant recipients have a three- to fivefold increased risk of premature cardiovascular disease compared with the general population.[92] Secondly, all transplant recipients require life-long immunosuppression, which impacts on both the presentation and management of general surgical conditions. Thirdly, the transplanted organ must be given due consideration in the planning of any general surgical procedure, as it may present technical issues and is at risk of functional injury in the perioperative period. A multidisciplinary approach is essential and the transplant team should be consulted as early as possible. This is even more relevant in hospitals with no on-site transplant team. The principles of perioperative management of transplant recipients are shown in Box 10.5.

Immunosuppression

Following a transplant, the most widely used immunosuppressive regimen is triple therapy with:

1. a calcineurin inhibitor (e.g. tacrolimus or ciclosporin);
2. an antiproliferative agent (e.g. azathioprine or mycophenolate mofetil);
3. a corticosteroid (e.g. prednisolone).

Other options include polyclonal antibodies (e.g. antithymocyte immunoglobulin – ATG) and monoclonal antibodies (e.g. interleukin-2 T-cell receptor antibody – basiliximab) for induction and mammalian target of rapamycin (mTOR) inhibitors (e.g. sirolimus or everolimus) for maintenance therapy.[93] Given the different immunosuppression options it is important that the general surgical team is aware of the temporal relationship between presentation and transplant, current patient medication and the correct dosages. These drugs have significant side-effects (Table 10.8) which may be responsible for surgical presentations (e.g. pancreatitis, peptic ulcer disease), increased perioperative risk (e.g. hypertension, diabetes) or complicated post-surgical recovery (e.g. impaired wound healing, pancytopenia, increased infection risk). Immunosuppression must be continued throughout the perioperative period. The calcineurin inhibitors tacrolimus and ciclosporin must be kept within their narrow therapeutic range and thus require regular monitoring. Calcineurin inhibitors, corticosteroids and mTOR inhibitors are metabolised through the cytochrome P450 pathway and therefore special attention should be given to any drugs that interfere with this pathway and could lead to either toxic or inadequate levels of immunosuppression (e.g. anticonvulsants, antimicrobials, calcium channel blockers etc.).[94] Corticosteroids diminish the stress response and may mask the clinical signs of peritonitis, thus a high

Box 10.5 • Principles of perioperative management of transplant recipients

- Careful assessment of perioperative risk
- Consider impact of immunosuppression on presentation and management
- Close monitoring of graft function throughout the perioperative period
- Avoidance of haemodynamic instability to maintain adequate perfusion to the graft
- Antibiotic prophylaxis required due to higher infection risk
- Anaesthetic drugs, analgesia and antibiotic choices and doses should be guided by graft function and potential interactions with immunosuppressive medication
- Gentle handling of tissues is particularly important due to the effects of immunosuppression on tissue integrity

Table 10.8 • Common immunosuppressive drugs used in transplant recipients and their main side-effects

Immunosuppressive drug	Side-effects
Tacrolimus	Nephrotoxicity
	Diabetes
	Hypertension
	Neurotoxicity
Ciclosporin	Nephrotoxicity
	Hypertension
	Gingival hypertrophy
	Hirsutism
Azathioprine	Pancytopenia
	Pancreatitis
Mycophenolate mofetil	Pancytopenia
	Diarrhoea
Prednisolone	Diabetes
	Pancreatitis
	Peptic ulcer disease
	Impaired wound healing
Sirolimus/everolimus	Hypertension
	Pancytopenia
	Impaired wound healing
	Hypertriglyceridaemia

index of suspicion is required in the assessment of transplant recipients with abdominal pain. It is also necessary to assess whether supplemental corticosteroids are needed during the perioperative period in cases of adrenal insufficiency. The combination of steroids with sirolimus or everolimus is associated with a higher risk of impaired wound healing,[95,96] which may also have implications for intestinal anastomoses.[97] Therefore the transplant team should be involved in assessing whether changes to the immunosuppressive regimen are indicated. Due to the increased risk of infective complications, all immunosuppressed patients should be given routine antibiotic prophylaxis for surgical procedures. Antibiotic dosages and selection should be guided by graft function and potential interactions with immunosuppressive medication (e.g. avoidance of cytochrome P450 antagonists such as clarithromycin). It is important to bear in mind that immunosuppression increases the risk of malignancy,[98] which could be the reason for presenting symptoms in transplant recipients.

Specific general surgical problems

Peptic ulceration

Peptic ulcer disease is common among transplant recipients. Immunosuppressive medication (in particular mycophenolate mofetil and corticosteroids)[99–101] increases the risk of peptic ulceration and predisposes to ulcerogenic infections such as *Helicobacter pylori*, *Candida* and *Cytomegalovirus* (CMV).[102] Since the introduction of H_2-blockers and proton pump inhibitors, morbidity from peptic ulceration after transplantation has significantly decreased.[103,104] However, a high index of suspicion remains essential, as the signs and symptoms of peptic ulceration may be diminished or absent in the immunosuppressed patient. In one study 61% patients with endoscopically proven ulcers were asymptomatic.[105] For this reason, a low threshold for investigation and treatment is indicated. Furthermore, the use of non-steroidal anti-inflammatory drugs (NSAIDs) should be avoided in transplant recipients due to the additional risk of peptic ulceration. It should be noted that immunosuppressed transplant recipients with *H. pylori* infection are also at increased risk of gastric mucosa-associated lymphoid tissue (MALT) lymphomas.[106,107]

Colonic perforation

Colonic perforations are the most frequent cause of gastrointestinal perforation in transplant recipients, and are associated with a severe clinical course and high mortality rate.[108–110] Diverticulitis is the commonest cause, but other causes include CMV colitis and malignancy.[102,111] Signs and symptoms may be atypical and not reflective of the severity of disease, leading to delay in diagnosis and treatment. Patients undergoing renal transplantation for polycystic kidney disease appear to be at higher risk of colonic perforation secondary to diverticulitis, though the mechanism for this is not known.[108,112,113] A systematic review of diverticulitis in immunocompromised patients reported an overall mortality rate of 23% for acute surgical management versus 56% for conservative treatment.[109] In this high-risk population, surgery should be considered early, along with antibiotics and involvement of the transplant team to consider a reduction in immunosuppression.

Cholelithiasis

The incidence of cholelithiasis is reported to be higher in transplant recipients compared with the general population.[114–118] The pathogenesis is not well understood, but thought to be related to the association of calcineurin inhibitors with cholestasis.[119,120] The management of gallstone disease in transplant recipients is controversial. Recommendations range from pre-transplantation screening of all patients with prophylactic cholecystectomy for asymptomatic gallstones (either pre- or post-transplantation), to expectant management with cholecystectomy only for symptomatic gallstones. The prophylactic approach has been prompted by reports of a high rate of progression to symptoms and complications, with the likelihood of requiring emergency cholecystectomy approximately 26% post-transplantation.[121] Moreover, the risk of mortality for emergency post-transplantation cholecystectomy is concerning, reported at 37% for cardiac transplant recipients and 5.6% for kidney or pancreas recipients.[122] A decision model analysis found that the preferred strategy for asymptomatic cholelithiasis in cardiac transplant recipients was prophylactic post-transplantation cholecystectomy before the development of symptoms (mortality risk 0.5%), while for kidney or pancreas transplant recipients, expectant management was favoured (mortality risk 0.2%).[121] Of note, these issues do not apply to liver transplant recipients as the gallbladder is routinely removed during transplantation.

Appendicitis

While appendicitis is one of the most common surgical emergencies in the general population, the reported incidence amongst transplant recipients is low (<0.5%).[123,124] Most patients present with abdominal pain, nausea and vomiting but not necessarily leukocytosis.[123,125] Clinical diagnosis may be particularly problematic in kidney transplant recipients, due to the potential for medial displacement of the appendix by the right lower quadrant position of the kidney graft, or misdiagnosis as graft-related complications such as rejection, infection or thrombosis.[126] Early surgery is advocated due to the high perforation and complication rate.[124]

🌐 Full references available at **http://expertconsult. inkling.com**

Key references

6. World Health Organisation Guiding Principles on Human Cell, Tissue and Organ Transplantation. 2010. PMID: 21235034.
   The World Health Organisation Guiding Principles provide a global ethical framework for the procurement and transplantation of human cells, tissues and organs. Most recently updated in 2010 in line with the changing challenges in transplantation, they have greatly influenced professional codes, practices and legislation around the world.

7. Steering Committee of the Istanbul Summit. Organ trafficking and transplant tourism and commercialism: the Declaration of Istanbul. Lancet 2008;372(9632):5–6. PMID: 18603141.
   The Declaration of Istanbul was the result of an international summit and presents clear definitions for organ trafficking, transplant commercialism and transplant tourism, as well as recommendations for fostering safe, ethical and accountable practices in transplantation.

8. Segev DL, Muzaale AD, Caffo BS, et al. Perioperative mortality and long-term survival following live kidney donation. JAMA 2010;303(10):959–66. PMID: 20215610.
   This US case-control study of 80 347 live kidney donors found that long-term risk of death was no higher for kidney donors than for age- and comorbidity-matched controls (n = 9364) from the NHANES III survey. Overall 90-day surgical mortality was 3.1 per 10 000 donors, but was higher in male, black and hypertensive donors.

9. Middleton PF, Duffield M, Lynch SV, et al. Living donor liver transplantation. Adult donor outcomes: a systematic review. Liver Transpl 2006;12(1):24–30. PMID: 16498709.
   This systematic review of living liver donor outcomes (214 studies) found overall donor mortality to be 0.2%

(13/6000 procedures, 117 studies), with mortality for right lobe donors (0.23–0.5%) higher than for left lobe donors (0.05–0.21%). The rate of donor morbidity was 16.1% (131 studies); most commonly biliary leaks and strictures (6.2%, 97 studies) and infections such as wound infections, urinary tract infections and pneumonia (5.8%, 50 studies). Median hospital stay was 9 days (58 studies) with return to normal activities within 3–6 months (18 studies.

10. Muzaale AD, Massie AB, Wang MC, et al. Risk of end-stage renal disease following live kidney donation. JAMA 2014;311(6):579–86. PMID: 24519297.
    This observational study from the US reported an 8-fold increased risk of end-stage renal disease in living kidney donors (n=96217) with a median follow up of 7.6 years, compared with matched healthy controls from the NHANES III study (n=9364) with a median follow up of 15.0 years.

11. Mjoen G, Hallan S, Hartmann A, et al. Long-term risks for kidney donors. Kidney Int 2014; 86(1):162–7. PMID: 24284516.
    This observational study in Norway reported an 11-fold increased risk of end-stage renal disease in living kidney donors (n = 1901) with a median follow up of 15.1 years, compared with healthy controls (n = 32621) with a median follow up of 24.9 years.

20. Terasaki PI, Cecka JM, Gjertson DW, et al. High survival rates of kidney transplants from spousal and living unrelated donors. N Engl J Med 1995; 333(6):333–6. PMID: 7609748.
    This landmark study demonstrated that despite a higher degree of HLA mismatching, the graft survival of living unrelated donor kidneys was superior to that of deceased donor kidneys.

33. Kiuchi T, Kasahara M, Uryuhara K, et al. Impact of graft size mismatching on graft prognosis in liver transplantation from living donors. Transplantation 1999;67(2):321–7. PMID: 10075602.
    Early animal studies and clinical reports of rapid hepatic regeneration of small-for-size liver grafts led to an increase in their use. This observational study demonstrated that small-for-size grafts (with a graft to recipient body weight ratio <1.0%) were associated

with insufficient metabolic and synthetic capacity and lower graft survival.

62. Academy of Medical Royal Colleges. A code of practice for the diagnosis and confirmation of death. 2008. http://aomrc.org.uk/wp-content/uploads/2016/04/Code_Practice_Confirmation_Diagnosis_Death_1008-4.pdf.

The UK code of practice for the diagnosis of death provides clear criteria for confirming brainstem death and circulatory death.

70. Thuong M, Ruiz A, Evrard P, et al. New classification of donation after circulatory death donors definitions and terminology. Transpl Int 2016;29(7): 749–59. PMID: 26991858.

The Maastricht classification is the universally accepted method for describing the four categories of donors after circulatory death.

76. Summers DM, Johnson RJ, Allen J, et al. Analysis of factors that affect outcome after transplantation of kidneys donated after cardiac death in the UK: a cohort study. Lancet 2010;376(9749):1303–11. PMID: 20727576.

This UK cohort study of 9134 kidney transplants found no difference in 5-year graft survival of kidneys from DCD versus DBD donors in first-time recipients.

95. Dean PG, Lund WJ, Larson TS, et al. Wound-healing complications after kidney transplantation: a prospective, randomized comparison of sirolimus and tacrolimus. Transplantation 2004;77(10):1555–61. PMID: 15239621.

This randomised trial found a higher incidence of wound-healing complications in sirolimus-based versus tacrolimus-based immunosuppressive regimens.

111. de'Angelis N, Esposito F, Memeo R, et al. Emergency abdominal surgery after solid organ transplantation: a systematic review. World J Emerg Surg 2016;11(1):43. PMID: 27582783.

This systematic review (39 studies, 71671 patients) found that the most common indications for emergency abdominal surgery after transplantation were gallbladder diseases (80.3%), gastrointestinal perforations (9.2%) and complicated diverticulitis (6.2%) with mortality rates of 3.4%, 17.5% and 13.6%, respectively.

11

Early assessment of the acute abdomen

Hugh M. Paterson

The acute abdomen can be defined as 'abdominal pain of non-traumatic origin with a maximum duration of 5 days'.[1] The list of potential causes is long and contains conditions ranging from the entirely benign, requiring no particular management other than reassurance, to the rapidly fatal where swift diagnosis and appropriate surgical treatment is life-saving. Abdominal symptoms may be manifested by conditions that are entirely extra-abdominal, and intra-abdominal conditions may present with extra-abdominal symptoms. Thus there are many pitfalls for the unwary, and many abdominal surgeons will readily attest that the emergency 'take' is the most challenging part of their activities. The majority of this chapter is written with current United Kingdom (UK) practice in mind, though the conclusions should be applicable to most developed countries.

Acute abdominal pain (for the purposes of this chapter the terms 'acute abdominal pain' and 'acute abdomen' are used interchangeably) remains a common cause for seeking medical attention. Between 5% and 10% of all United States emergency department (ED) consultations are for abdominal pain.[2] In the UK, there has been a substantial increase in emergency surgical admissions to hospitals in the last 15 years, reflecting the increase in all emergency admissions to secondary care.[3] The acute abdomen has long been the bread-and-butter of the general surgeon, with clinical experience in surgical decision-making honed in an era without recourse to extensive diagnostic investigations. However, much has changed in the last 15 years, and some of the old tenets have been modified. Although there has been no major change to the incidence of the common conditions (with the exception of a reduction in prevalence of peptic ulcer disease[4]), new challenges have arisen. As the population becomes more elderly, so frailty and multi-morbidity complicate surgical assessment and treatment. In many developed countries the hospital environment continues to evolve due to centralisation of services, reduced hospital inpatient capacity and limited resources; in the UK, substantial changes to primary care out-of-hours assessment have been associated with an increased workload for secondary care; and with the development of subspecialist training, surgeons themselves no longer have the breadth of surgical experience that characterised the previous generation.

Conditions associated with abdominal pain

The list of potential causes of the acute abdomen is extensive. An exhaustive account is not the purpose of this chapter, and readers will find the latest guidance on diagnosis and management of common conditions elsewhere in this book or within the Companion to Specialist Surgical Practice series. It is now more than 25 years since Irvin published an audit of diagnoses in 1190 patients presenting with acute abdominal pain to a UK general surgery department.[5] At that time, the most common diagnosis (over a third of the cohort) was non-specific abdominal pain (NSAP), twice as frequent as the next most common condition (acute appendicitis, 17%). NSAP is the most common diagnosis in numerous studies of acute abdominal pain from the developed world, varying from 20% to 60% of the cohort.[6–8]

NSAP may be defined as 'pain for which no immediate cause can be found following examination and baseline investigations and specifically does not require surgical intervention'. A variety of causes have been proposed (Box 11.1). Previously it was a source of anxiety to clinicians

Box 11.1 • Causes of non-specific abdominal pain[9]

Viral infections
Bacterial gastroenteritis
Worm infestation
Irritable bowel syndrome
Gynaecological conditions
Psychosomatic pain
Coeliac disease[10]
Abdominal wall pain[11]
* Peripheral nerve injuries
* Hernias
* Myofascial pain syndromes
* Rib tip syndrome
* Nerve root pain

Table 11.1 • Final diagnoses in 1021 patients with acute abdominal pain

Final diagnoses in 1021 patients	No(%)
Urgent	
Acute appendicitis	284 (28)
Acute diverticulitis	118 (12)
Bowel obstruction	68(7)
Acute cholecystitis	52(5)
Acute pancreatitis	28(3)
Gynaecological diseases	27(3)
Urological diseases	22(2)
Abscess	14(1)
Perforated viscus	13(1)
Bowel ischaemia	12(1)
Pneumonia	11(1)
Retroperitoneal or abdominal wall bleeding	9(1)
Acute peritonitis	3 (0.3)
Total urgent diagnoses	661 (65)
Non-urgent	
Non-specific abdominal pain	183 (18)
Gastrointestinal diseases	56 (5)
Hepatic, pancreatic and biliary diseases	43(4)
Inflammatory bowel disease	30(3)
Urological diseases	20(2)
Gynaecological diseases	9(1)
Malignancy	5 (0.5)
Hemia	2 (0.2)
Other	12(1)
Total non-urgent diagnoses	360 (35)

Reproduced from Lameris W, van Randen A, van Es HW, et al. Imaging strategies for detection of urgent conditions in patients with acute abdominal pain: diagnostic accuracy study. BMJ 2009;338: b2431. With permission from BMJ Publishing Group Ltd.

that a diagnosis of NSAP might mask an altogether more serious undiagnosed pathology. However, data from children with abdominal pain suggest NSAP is a safe diagnosis: a large retrospective study of >3000 admissions with NSAP in children over 20 years found a 'missed' appendicitis rate of only 0.2%.[12] A record linkage study of a cohort of >250 000 children with NSAP 1999–2011 from English national data found that only 5.8% were subsequently hospitalised for bowel disorders, the most likely conditions being appendicitis, inflammatory bowel disease (IBD) and irritable bowel syndrome (IBS).[13] In adults, the huge increase in use of diagnostic imaging in the past 10–20 years (see below) suggests that NSAP is likely to be much more secure than when de Dombal observed that 10% of patients over 50 years of age labelled as NSAP presented subsequently with an intra-abdominal malignancy (most commonly colorectal cancer).[14] Long-term follow-up of a group of adults diagnosed in 1985–6 with NSAP found a higher incidence of chronic pain and gastrointestinal disease than controls; they also demonstrated greater all-cause mortality.[15]

Table 11.1 shows the range and frequency of diagnoses from a 2009 multicentre study comparing diagnostic imaging strategies in a cohort of 1021 adult patients presenting with acute abdominal pain to emergency departments in the Netherlands. Compared to Irvin's 1989 audit the frequency of individual diagnoses has remained broadly similar over time. However, it is notable that the frequency of NSAP was substantially less in the Dutch study and no doubt reflects the more advanced imaging strategies employed.

A small number of medical conditions can present as acute abdominal pain, and, although uncommon, are mentioned here for the benefit of surgeons in training. Inferior myocardial infarction, lower lobar pneumonia and some metabolic disorders can all be excluded by examination and/or basic investigations (ECG, chest radiograph and serum glucose); failure to recognise them before embarking on exploratory surgery is associated with significantly increased morbidity and mortality.

Initial assessment: history, examination and simple tests

A careful medical history and clinical examination remains the keystone of initial assessment and should lead to formulation of a differential diagnosis from the conditions listed in Table 11.1. Age is an important determinant of likely diagnoses; the differential of, for example, right iliac fossa pain in teenagers is quite different in octogenarians. However, as previous generations of general surgeons knew well, in managing the acute abdomen there is an important distinction between assessing *urgency* and making an accurate *diagnosis*.

Although some conditions are recognised reliably at initial clinical assessment (particularly acute diverticulitis,[16] and small-bowel obstruction[17]), in general the accuracy of clinical diagnosis in the acute abdomen is only moderate. The Acute Abdominal Pain Study Group found that diagnostic accuracy was less than 50%, and qualified surgeons were no better than surgical trainees with substantial inter-observer variation, particularly in eliciting physical signs. Distinguishing urgent from non-urgent conditions was more reliable.[18] As with other aspects of clinical examination, there is good evidence that inter-observer agreement for eliciting signs in the acute abdomen is at best only moderate.[19,20] Nevertheless, a careful history is key to the subsequent direction of investigations: in a review of abdominal pain assessment errors in the ED, failure of history-taking was deemed one of the biggest contributors.[21]

In the previous era, the main decision for the general surgeon was when to operate immediately, when to observe and when not to operate at all. A precise diagnosis was less of a priority, partly because the diagnostic armamentarium was limited. Consequently, the prevailing negative laparotomy rate at the time was considerable ('better to look and see than wait and see'). In the patient with peritonitis and septic shock, it may still be argued that a precise diagnosis is less important than rapid intervention to resuscitate and achieve source control by laparotomy. However, for patients in whom the need for operation is less obvious, in modern practice a precise diagnosis has important implications:

- Subspecialisation in general surgery is now the norm in many countries, hence diagnosis is important for onward referral to the appropriate subspeciality (which may be in a different hospital). The emergence of the emergency general surgeon in UK practice has embedded this process in many hospitals.[22]
- Unnecessary admission to hospital needs to be avoided in an increasingly resource-limited service. Although time is a key determinant in the evaluation of the acute abdomen, and active observation is a well-established and safe practice, hospital bed occupancy is costly.
- Precise diagnosis allows selection of the appropriate treatment option depending on severity (operative vs non-operative; laparoscopic vs open surgery).

Prior to the current era of easy access to sophisticated diagnostic investigation, a variety of methods were described to improve the accuracy

of clinical diagnosis. Computer-aided diagnosis improved diagnostic accuracy from 45% to 65% in an oft-cited UK study, but the relevance to modern practice of these data acquired during an era with a negative laparotomy rate of up to 20% is questionable.[23] The main benefit of these types of studies was probably that the structured data collection ensured a comprehensive assessment of the patient by junior staff.[24] Systematic documentation of clinical variables has also been used to develop scoring systems, applied most frequently to acute appendicitis (e.g. Alvarado score,[25] Appendicitis Inflammatory Response score[26]). In current practice they probably have greatest application in allowing less experienced or non-surgical clinicians to triage patients that may safely be discharged and/or to select patients with unclear presentation for diagnostic imaging.[27–29]

The author remembers as a medical student in the previous century being told unequivocally that early administration of opiate analgesia did not mask abdominal signs in assessing the acute abdomen. It is therefore surprising that quite a number of clinical trials to re-answer this question seem to have been deemed necessary in the interim. It can be reiterated here that analgesia for patients suffering one of the most agonising events of their lives does not detrimentally affect surgical assessment or decision-making in the acute abdomen.[30–32]

✔✔ Analgesia does not mask clinical signs in assessment of the acute abdomen and should not be withheld.[30–32]

Initial investigations

Blood tests

'Routine' blood tests are useful for assessing the severity of illness in the acute abdomen (indeed the physiology component of the P-POSSUM risk stratification score relies heavily on these) but have a limited role as diagnostic tools. Serum amylase and/or lipase assays are requested routinely in assessment of abdominal pain in many centres. These tests are relatively cheap, but the yield is low. Serum lipase is the superior test, with a sensitivity and specificity of around 64% and 97%, respectively, compared to 50% and 99% for serum amylase.[33,34] It is important to note that both enzymes may be significantly elevated in non-pancreatic aetiologies of the acute abdomen, and a normal value does not always exclude acute pancreatitis.[35]

Serum glucose measurement is a cheap and reliable way of excluding serious diabetic complications such as diabetic ketoacidosis (DKA) or hyperosmolar hyperglycaemic state (HHS). DKA can mimic the acute abdomen; bear in mind, though, that occasionally DKA is associated with a primary abdominal pathology such as acute pancreatitis,[36] while HHS may be provoked by intra-abdominal sepsis.[37]

Although requested routinely, white cell count (WCC) and C-reactive protein (CRP) have almost no discriminatory value in assessment of acute abdominal pain, although trends over time may be of value in assessing response to treatment in some cases. Gans et al. summarised three large prospective studies examining the utility of WCC and CRP in acute abdominal pain: even at thresholds of $WCC > 15 \times 10/L$ and CRP >50 mg/L, over 80% of urgent diagnoses were missed.[38]

Some novel biomarkers have been evaluated in assessment of the acute abdomen. Plasma procalcitonin cannot yet be regarded as having other than experimental interest.[39] Biomarker panels may be of value in discriminating low-risk patients in some healthcare settings, particularly where over-reliance on radiological imaging is prevalent.[40,41] Perhaps surprisingly, given the prognostic value of elevated serum lactate in the assessment of sepsis, there are relatively few data examining its use as a triage test in the acute abdomen.[42] It has very limited discriminatory power in the diagnosis of acute mesenteric ischaemia.[43]

Diagnostic imaging

Contemporary surgical practice in the developed world is aided considerably by availability of sophisticated radiological investigations that would have been the envy of our predecessors. The use of plain and contrast radiology is diminishing as computed tomography (CT) becomes the dominant investigation of choice, but remains relevant to practice in developing countries and will be discussed here.

Plain radiography

Plain radiographs of the erect chest and supine abdomen have been embedded in assessment of the acute abdomen in the UK for decades. They are viewed as cheap and easy to obtain, but in fact consume time and resource, result in unnecessary radiation exposure and can be uncomfortable for patients. Their role in contemporary developed-world practice is almost redundant. The erect chest X-ray has very low yield and limited ability to identify a perforated intra-abdominal viscus by demonstrating free intraperitoneal air (**Fig. 11.1**).[44–46] It is useful if lower lobar pneumonia is being considered within the differential diagnosis (**Fig. 11.2**). Abdominal radiographs have very low yield if requested as part of the routine assessment of acute abdominal pain, although by most radiological guidelines this is inappropriate anyway. Its main indication is in the diagnosis of bowel obstruction (see **Fig. 11.3**).[47,48] Since bowel obstruction can be readily identified from the clinical assessment,[49] its primary function is to distinguish small- from large-bowel obstruction to guide early management, but even here CT is markedly superior.[50]

Contrast radiography

Only water-soluble contrast is discussed, as barium-based studies are relatively contraindicated in the emergency setting due to the presence or high possibility of developing intestinal perforation. The main indications are in the management of adhesive small-bowel obstruction, and in demonstrating the presence (or absence) of ongoing leakage from intestinal perforation. Use of water-soluble contrast enema in the diagnosis of colonic obstruction has now been superseded by CT in most institutions.

There is strong evidence from meta-analysis of a number of studies that water-soluble contrast reliably predicts the need for surgery in adhesive small-bowel obstruction. If contrast reaches the colon within 24 hours, obstruction will resolve in 99% of patients, significantly reducing hospital stay compared to conventional 'drip and suck'

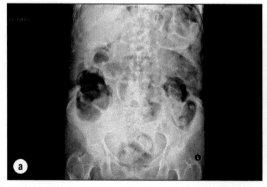
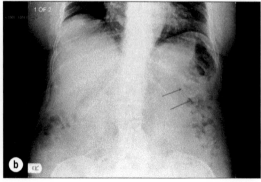

Figure 11.1 • Plain supine abdominal radiographs demonstrating free intraperitoneal air **(a)** in a patient with a perforated duodenal ulcer and retroperitoneal air **(b)** in a patient with perforated diverticular disease.

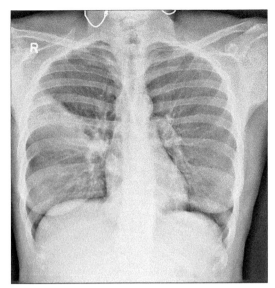

Figure 11.2 • Erect chest radiograph in a patient with acute right-sided pneumonia.

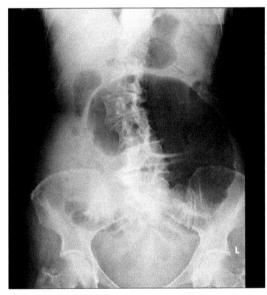

Figure 11.3 • Plain abdominal radiograph in a patient presenting with acute vomiting 1 week after closure of a defunctioning ileostomy. This is the characteristic appearance of caecal volvulus.
With thanks to Dr Tom Blankenstein, Specialty Trainee in Radiology, Western General Hospital, Edinburgh.

management (**Fig. 11.4**). Since the original Cochrane analysis, the addition of three further randomised trials has shown that this practice actually reduces the need for surgery (OR 0·62; $P = 0·007$).[51,][52] These studies form the basis for the Bologna guidelines for diagnosis and management of adhesive small bowel obstruction.[53]

The role of contrast radiography in suspected gastroduodenal perforation has largely been replaced in modern practice by oral contrast-enhanced CT. However, in resource-limited settings, patients diagnosed by erect chest X-ray to have a perforation may be selected for non-operative management by using a contrast study to demonstrate whether the leak has sealed or there is ongoing leakage.[54] This topic is discussed in further detail in Chapter 12.

✓✓ Early use of water-soluble contrast in adhesive small-bowel obstruction reduces the need for surgery, accurately selects patients for operative/non-operative management and reduces length of stay.[51,52]

Ultrasonography

Ultrasound is cost-effective, harmless, readily available and in experienced hands has high diagnostic accuracy in a variety of acute abdominal conditions. Its disadvantage is that accuracy is user-dependent and images lack the spatial resolution useful to surgical planning afforded by CT. In direct comparison with CT, ultrasound was less sensitive in diagnosis of appendicitis and diverticulitis (76% vs 94% and 61% vs 81%, respectively), though positive predictive values were similar.[55] Nowadays it is less frequently used as an unguided first-line investigation of the acute abdomen and is best targeted to confirm or refute specific diagnoses.

Ultrasound is the first-line investigation for acute biliary disease, with sensitivity of 90–95% in detecting gallbladder inflammation, gallstones and biliary dilatation, and is recommended as the first-line investigation in the Tokyo acute cholecystitis guidelines.[56,57] CT may be required in equivocal cases (see **Fig. 11.5**).[58,59]

In the assessment of right iliac fossa/lower abdominal pain, ultrasound is effective in evaluating the pelvic organs in women to triage acute ovarian/pelvic organ pathology requiring direct referral to gynaecology. The data available for its use in the diagnosis of appendicitis are more variable, reflecting user-dependency and limitations of patient habitus. The presence of specific diagnostic features (non-compressible appendix >7 mm, periappendiceal inflammation or abscess; see **Fig. 11.6**) is associated with high sensitivity (74%) and specificity (97%), but both a normal or perforated appendix can be difficult to visualise.[60] A multicentre observational trial in 870 patients concluded that there was no clinical benefit of ultrasound of the appendix in routine clinical diagnosis.[61]

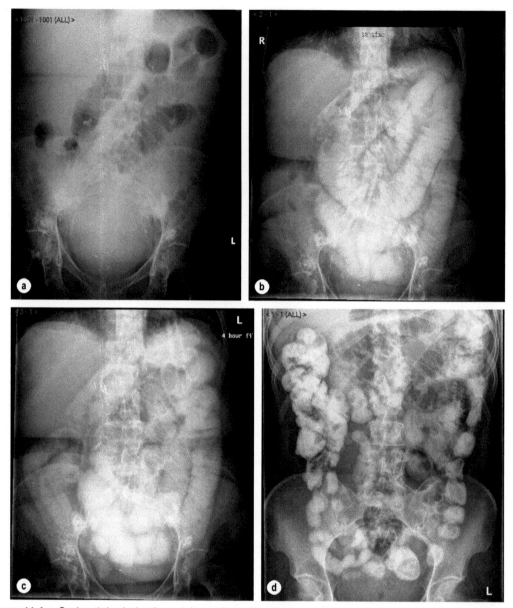

Figure 11.4 • Supine abdominal radiograph in a patient with adhesive small-bowel obstruction **(a)**, 90 minutes **(b)** and 4 hours **(c)** after oral administration of 50 mL of water-soluble contrast material. Note failure of contrast to reach the caecum and the obvious small-bowel obstruction. Laparotomy confirmed small-bowel obstruction due to adhesions. **(d)** A post-contrast 4-hour film in a patient with suspected small-bowel obstruction from the plain abdominal radiograph but on this occasion contrast has reached the colon by 4 hours and no surgery was required.

Ultrasound can also be useful in detecting abdominal wall problems such as hernias and rectus sheath haematoma (see **Fig. 11.7**). It may have a role in some settings for assessing the aorta and renal tract, but increasingly CT is the investigation of choice in these areas. Nevertheless, ultrasound can be an invaluable diagnostic aid in resource-poor healthcare and may be used by surgeons themselves with satisfactory results.[62,63]

Computed tomography

In the last 10–15 years, CT has become the diagnostic investigation of choice in the acute abdomen.[64] In some healthcare settings, notably the United States (USA), its use has become ubiquitous in assessing the acute abdomen in patients of all ages. In the UK, use of CT has increased as the test has become more readily available, but there has always been reluctance to subject younger patients,

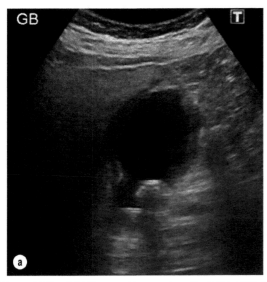

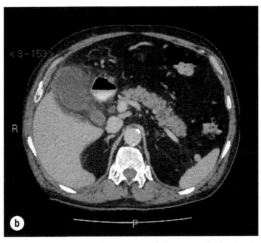

Figure 11.5 • (a) Ultrasound image of acute cholecystitis due to gallstones. Note the characteristic acoustic shadowing from the impacted gallstone, with associated features of gallbladder distension and wall thickening. There may also be evidence of pericholecystic fluid. **(b)** CT scan of patient with acute cholecystitis following equivocal ultrasound scan. This image demonstrates gallbladder distension, wall thickening and pericholecystic oedema.
With thanks to Dr Domenyk Brown, Consultant Radiologist, Western General Hospital, Edinburgh.

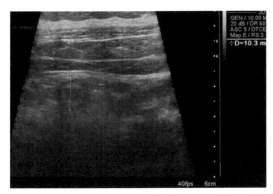

Figure 11.6 • Ultrasound examination on a patient with acute appendicitis. Note the non-compressible thick-walled hollow organ (appendix) beneath the probe.

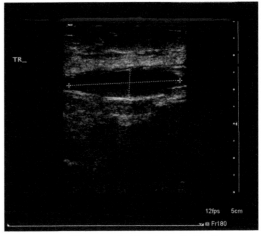

Figure 11.7 • Ultrasound of the abdominal wall demonstrating a rectus sheath haematoma.

particularly children, to the ionising radiation (IR) exposure of CT. In the USA, IR exposure concerns are less apparent, probably reflecting the high risk of litigation associated with misdiagnosis.[65] However, awareness of the risks associated with radiation exposure is growing. It has been estimated that a 10-mSV CT in a 25-year-old patient is associated with a risk of induced cancer of 1 in 900 individuals and a risk of fatal cancer in 1 in 1800 individuals.[66]

There is good evidence that CT is accurate across a range of diagnoses. It is sufficiently reliable to allow appropriate triage of acute abdomen patients in the ED (particularly by non-surgeons),[7] improves the accuracy of clinical diagnosis[67,68] and has been shown to have a demonstrable impact on patient management plans in a substantial proportion of cases, both by avoiding admission but also by prompting immediate surgery in equivocal cases (**Figs 11.8–11.10**).[69,70]

CT is highly accurate in diagnosing acute appendicitis. In one randomised trial, mandatory CT was associated with a negative appendicectomy rate of 3%, compared to 14% where CT was used selectively.[71] A recent meta-analysis comprising 26 cohort studies and 2 randomised trials concluded that CT was associated with a reduced negative appendicectomy rate compared to clinical assessment

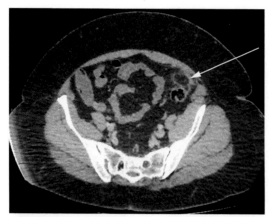

Figure 11.8 • This patient presented with left iliac fossa pain and localised tenderness to palpation suggestive of acute sigmoid diverticulitis. CT shows epiploic appendagitis (note the colon immediately below the arrowed area of inflammation is normal), which does not require hospital admission and is treated with simple analgesia.
With thanks to Dr Tom Blankenstein, Specialty Trainee in Radiology, Western General Hospital, Edinburgh.

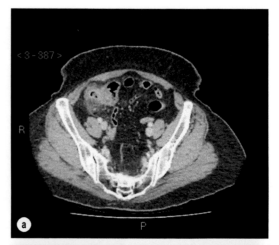

a

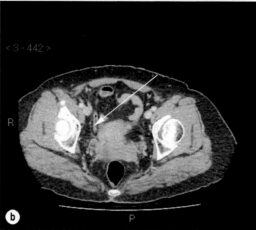

b

Figure 11.10 • CT images of caecal acute diverticulitis in a 56-year-old woman presenting with right iliac fossa pain; note clear views of the normal appendix (*arrowed*).

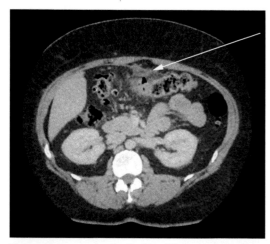

Figure 11.9 • Acute diverticulitis of the transverse colon. With thanks to Dr Tom Blankenstein, Specialty Trainee in Radiology, Western General Hospital, Edinburgh.

alone (8.7% vs 16.7%); this benefit was particularly apparent in women.[72] A USA single institution review over 10 years found that increased use of CT from 18% (1998) to 93% (2007) of cases was associated with reduced negative appendicectomy rate only in women under 45 years of age.[73] Although CT is accurate in acute appendicitis, in view of the concerns regarding radiation in a predominantly young patient group, selective use in cases where the clinical picture is unclear is a sensible policy. Despite increased imaging availability, the rate of negative appendicectomy does not seem to have altered

appreciably from the pre-CT era in which active observation with repeated clinical examination was the main diagnostic tool.[74]

The impact of widespread use of CT on some other clinical outcomes is less clear. In a comparison of CT diagnosis before and after emergency laparotomy in 361 adult patients, the CT report was judged inaccurate in 43 (12%) cases, which included five negative laparotomies.[75] Thus although CT is not infallible, the contemporary negative laparotomy rate is 10-fold lower than in series from 30 years ago.[5,76] This observation seems to be supported by other studies, in which much of the benefit of CT was to reduce the number of patients deemed to require urgent surgery compared to clinical assessment alone.[70]

However, diagnostic accuracy does not necessarily improve all aspects of patient management. A randomised trial of routine CT versus standard clinical assessment in 205 patients with acute abdominal pain found that although the diagnostic accuracy was higher in the CT group, there was no difference in length of hospital stay or mortality.[8] Other randomised studies of routine CT in abdominal pain have similarly failed to show any significant difference in length of stay; furthermore, treatment costs were significantly higher in the CT group.[77,78] The high diagnostic accuracy of routine CT may increase the confidence to treat operatively compared to selective imaging.[79]

As technological innovation continues, both IR dose and time delays in obtaining urgent CT are being reduced. Low-dose CT can give comparable results to standard CT protocols,[80,81] while some of the CT-associated delay can be reduced by avoiding administration of oral contrast; recent data suggest omitting oral contrast does not reduce diagnostic power in acute abdomen assessment[82,83]

Magnetic resonance imaging

Magnetic resonance imaging (MRI) is emerging as a highly sensitive and specific examination in acute abdominal pain. It avoids IR, but is more expensive and less readily available than CT in most settings. Patients with claustrophobia struggle to tolerate the examination and it is contraindicated in patients with implanted metal/devices. Most experience has been obtained in children and younger adults, including pregnancy, where it is effective in diagnosis of a range of conditions.[84,85]

In a UK series of 468 patients under 60 years of age with acute abdominal pain selected for further imaging after surgical review, overall diagnostic accuracy of MRI was 99%.[86] Early reports suggest it is highly accurate (sensitivity and specificity >95%) in the diagnosis of appendicitis in children.[87,88] As yet there are no randomised data on its use or cost-effectiveness in assessment of the acute abdomen.

Magnetic resonance cholangiopancreatography (MRCP) has a key role in evaluating the biliary tree in patients presenting with symptomatic gallstones who have abnormal liver function tests, being effective in demonstrating common bile duct stones with a sensitivity of >90%. It has the obvious advantage over endoscopic retrograde cholangiopancreatography (ERCP) of being non-invasive. MRCP is discussed in more detail in Chapter 14.

Diagnostic laparoscopy

Although diagnostic laparoscopy has been a useful tool in the past 15–20 years, its place has become less clear as accurate diagnostic imaging becomes more widely available[1] and laparoscopic techniques replace open surgery for appendicectomy. It has been used most frequently in the management of

women of child-bearing age presenting with lower abdominal or right lower quadrant pain, where NSAP and acute gynaecological conditions considerably lengthen the differential diagnosis compared to males of equivalent age. A Cochrane meta-analysis of four randomised trials (811 patients) comparing laparoscopy with active observation found that laparoscopy was associated with a reduced number of patients leaving hospital without a diagnosis but did not affect complications, readmission rates or length of stay.[89] Its role depends on availability of imaging locally, but in general it should be used only where imaging is inconclusive and high suspicion of an urgent cause remains (see **Figs 11.11** and **11.12**). This young and frequent patient group remains a challenge for the emergency general surgeon: routine CT scan would be very costly, is less accurate in diagnosing pelvic organ pathology and radiation dose remains a concern; diagnostic laparoscopy is invasive, costly and carries a (albeit low) risk of operative complications; active observation is time-consuming for the clinician and resource-heavy. An interesting observation comes from national data

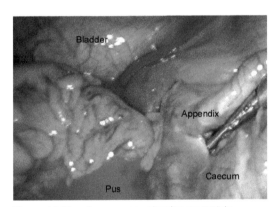

Figure 11.11 • Laparoscopy showing an acutely inflamed appendix with pelvic peritonitis.

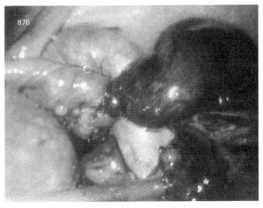

Figure 11.12 • Laparoscopic view of a torsion of the right fallopian tube with ischaemia of the distal tube and ovary.

from England comparing readmission rates after diagnostic laparoscopy alone versus laparoscopic normal appendicectomy: readmission within 1 year occurred in 33% of the whole cohort (19 000 patients), but laparoscopic normal appendicectomy reduced odds of readmission by 44%.[90]

Special populations

Two groups are worth highlighting for consideration: the pregnant patient and the elderly.

The acute abdomen in pregnancy is a relatively common presentation. Delay in diagnosis and treatment can have poor outcomes for mother and fetus. Assessment is complicated by the physiological and anatomical changes of pregnancy: uterine enlargement displaces other organs and may alter clinical signs; the abdominal wall is lax; pregnancy often induces a mild physiological leucocytosis; the patient herself and other clinicians may exhibit unwillingness to use radiological investigation due to concern about the fetal impact of ionising radiation. Ultrasound is the imaging modality of choice, but has limitations as noted above. MRI avoids IR and appears to be very accurate; its limitation is availability.[91,92] CT should be avoided if possible but if there is sufficient clinical concern, particularly given the factors above prejudicing clinical assessment, diagnostic imaging should not be withheld. The American College of Obstetricians and Gynecologists' Committee on Obstetric Practice has issued summary recommendations for diagnostic imaging procedures during pregnancy and lactation.[93]

Elderly patients may also be difficult to assess.[94] They may exhibit atypical presentations due to impaired ability to mount normal physiological responses such as tachycardia or abdominal guarding as a consequence of physical limitations, underlying comorbidity or the treatment thereof (e.g. beta-adrenoceptor antagonists, corticosteroids). Acute surgical illness may exacerbate pre-existing cognitive impairment or induce acute delirium. Because of the limitations of clinical assessment in these patients the clinician should have a low threshold for diagnostic imaging, particularly as the range of potential diagnoses in this age group is wide. CT scan is usually the investigation of choice in the elderly patient with acute abdominal pain. In patients with severe renal impairment, non-contrast CT should be considered.[95]

Pathways/guidelines for assessment

An institutional review of ED management of the acute abdomen from the USA over 35 years concluded that while diagnostic imaging had increased sixfold between 1993 and 2007 (increasing ED delays and patient charges), there had been no change in rates of hospital admission or missed surgical illness.[96] Routine CT does not appear to reduce length of stay.[8,77] Imaging costs continue to rise. Concerns about the risk of CT-associated IR have been noted above. Therefore, there is a need to optimise imaging strategies in patients with acute abdominal pain in order to achieve timely identification of urgent conditions, without using imaging unnecessarily.

An important recent prospective multicentre study examined a range of imaging strategies in acute abdominal pain in 1101 adults. Sensitivity and specificity for detecting urgent conditions were recorded for 11 diagnostic strategies, comprising single test strategies (e.g. CT alone), conditional strategies (e.g. CT if ultrasound inconclusive), strategies defined by patient characteristics (age, BMI) and strategies driven by location of pain. CT detected more urgent diagnoses than ultrasound (sensitivity 89% versus 70%, respectively). The highest sensitivity was obtained by a conditional strategy of CT after negative or inconclusive ultrasonography, missing only 6% of urgent cases. Alternative strategies guided by body mass index, age, or location of pain resulted in a loss of sensitivity.[97]

In the UK, emergency general surgery has become a topic of hot interest, with recognition that there is considerable variation in outcomes between centres in emergency laparotomy.[98] This was strikingly emphasised by a recent UK snapshot audit showing wide variation in management of acute appendicitis, in which the normal appendicectomy rate ranged from 3% to 36%.[99] Early assessment by experienced clinicians is seen as key to improving the results of emergency laparotomy, and that process begins with decision-making and rationalising use of investigations in the acute abdomen.[22,100] Reducing variation is also aided by following guidelines for effective practice: the Royal College of Surgeons of England and the Association of Surgeons of the Netherlands have developed guidelines for management of acute abdominal pain.[1,101] The American College of Radiologists publishes regularly updated guidance developed by consensus methodology on imaging strategies in a variety of clinical presentations.[102,103] In 2010 a national guideline for management of acute appendicitis was introduced in the Netherlands, mandating preoperative imaging in all suspected cases. A snapshot audit of national practice in 2015 found that over 99% of cases underwent preoperative diagnostic imaging, with a negative appendicectomy rate of only 2.2%.[104] When compared to the UK audit noted above, in which preoperative imaging took place in only one-third of patients, it is difficult to avoid the conclusion that the combination of practice guidelines based on confirmatory imaging has had a markedly beneficial effect in this condition. Future research will help to inform effective and appropriate imaging strategies, evaluating criteria based on patient subgroups, anatomical pain location, clinical scoring systems, or routine use.

✓✓ Clinicians are more accurate at distinguishing urgent versus non-urgent conditions than making an accurate diagnosis, and therefore imaging is an essential part of the diagnostic pathway.[97]

Key points

- The foundations for good management of the acute abdomen are accurate history and careful examination allied to an appreciation of the wide range of surgical and non-surgical conditions that may present with abdominal pain.
- Analgesia does not mask clinical signs in assessment of the acute abdomen and should not be withheld.
- Early use of water-soluble contrast in adhesive small-bowel obstruction reduces the need for surgery, accurately selects patients for operative/non-operative management and reduces length of stay.
- Although clinicians are able to distinguish urgent from non-urgent conditions on clinical grounds alone, they are less good at making an accurate diagnosis.
- Modern radiological imaging is highly accurate in identifying the correct diagnosis and informing choice of management by the clinician. The challenge in the acute setting is to use the available modalities effectively. Future research will seek to refine imaging strategies according to clinical presentation.

🌐 Full references available at **http://expertconsult. inkling.com**

Key references

8. Sala E, Watson CJ, Beadsmoore C, et al. A randomized, controlled trial of routine early abdominal computed tomography in patients presenting with non-specific acute abdominal pain. Clin Radiol 2007;62(10):961–9. PMID: 17765461.

   Early abdominal CT in patients with acute abdominal pain improved diagnostic certainty, but did not reduce length of hospital stay or 6-month mortality.

18. Acute Abdominal Pain Study group. Diagnostic accuracy of surgeons and trainees in assessment of patients with acute abdominal pain. Br J Surg 2016; 103(10):1343–9. PMID: 27465409.

    Diagnostic accuracy by senior clinicians was no better than by trainees and was less than 50% overall, illustrating the challenge of making a clinical diagnosis. Both groups were better at distinguishing urgent from non-urgent conditions.

30. Ranji SR, Goldman LE, Simel DL, et al. Do opiates affect the clinical evaluation of patients with acute abdominal pain? JAMA 2006;296(14):1764–74. PMID: 17032990.

31. Gallagher EJ, Esses D, Lee C, et al. Randomized clinical trial of morphine in acute abdominal pain.

    Ann Emerg Med 2006;48(2):150–60 160 e151–154. PMID: 16953529.

32. Manterola C, Vial M, Moraga J, et al. Analgesia in patients with acute abdominal pain. Cochrane Database Syst Rev 2011(1):CD005660. PMID: 21249672.

    Convincing individual studies and a meta-analysis confirming that early use of opioid analgesia does not adversely effect patient evaluation or management decisions in acute abdominal pain.

51. Branco BC, Barmparas G, Schnuriger B, et al. Systematic review and meta-analysis of the diagnostic and therapeutic role of water-soluble contrast agent in adhesive small bowel obstruction. Br J Surg 2010;97(4):470–8. PMID: 20205228.

52. Abbas S, Bissett IP, Parry BR. Oral water soluble contrast for the management of adhesive small bowel obstruction. Cochrane Database Syst Rev 2007;3. PMID: 17636770.

    Early use of water-soluble contrast in adhesive small-bowel obstruction reduces the need for surgery, accurately selects patients for operative/non-operative management and reduces length of stay.

97. Lameris W, van Randen A, van Es HW, et al. Imaging strategies for detection of urgent conditions in patients with acute abdominal pain: diagnostic accuracy study. BMJ 2009;338:b2431. PMID: 19561056.

    Carefully designed study seeking to evaluate a variety of imaging strategies in acute abdominal pain.

12

Perforations of the upper gastrointestinal tract

Ian Bailey

Introduction

The surgeon managing an acute illness due to foregut perforation will need to be prepared to manage a wide range of pathologies and utilise a number of therapeutic techniques and options. When making therapeutic decisions, the exact pathology may not be known, despite advanced imaging techniques. The patients are often old or comorbid and treatment might be palliative, non-operative, minimally invasive or maximally invasive. Evidence to support one treatment or another is often old and of questionable value. Much was generated before our understanding of the role of *Helicobacter pylori* in peptic ulcer disease and the availability of potent pharmacological acid suppression. Because of the diverse nature of these patients treatment is often based on 'first principles' and guided by case series and linked meta-analysis supported by a few, often small, randomised controlled trials.

Perforations may be due to benign or malignant disease in addition to iatrogenic causes which include both diagnostic and therapeutic endoscopy as well as the placement of both endoscopic and radiological feeding tubes. The acute surgeon must also be familiar with the complications related to bariatric, antireflux and hiatus hernia surgery.

Key principles of treatment

Anatomical consideration

The foregut includes oesophagus, stomach and duodenum. Perforation may therefore present with signs and symptoms in the neck, chest or abdomen. Some parts of the foregut pass through or are adjacent to large cavities (pleura, peritoneum) and others are anatomically confined by adjacent structures (neck, mediastinum and retroperitoneum). Perforations may therefore be:

(a) Contained with only localised contamination.
(b) Disseminated with widespread contamination into the peritoneum or pleura.
(c) Cross important anatomical junctions at the root of the neck or hiatus.

The oesophagus is a generally inaccessible organ with poor healing qualities. The stomach is an easily accessible organ with substantial muscular layers and an excellent blood supply. Its large lumen and structure makes surgical repair relatively simple. The duodenum is a surgically difficult organ. Its retroperitoneal structure, narrow lumen and intimate relationship to pancreas, bile duct, portal vessels and inferior vena cava make surgical repair challenging for all but small anterior perforations. Fortunately, the majority of peptic ulcer perforations are small and anterior!

Pathological considerations

How a perforation has been created is important in planning how to manage the patient. Perforations may be spontaneous or caused by trauma. They may be through normal tissue or diseased tissue. Normal tissue and benign ulcerated tissue should heal. Perforations through tumours are less likely to heal and hence more radical intervention is likely to be required to resolve the problem. Understanding these factors will help the surgeon plan appropriate treatment, which will include non-operative and/or palliative measures in some circumstances.

The illness caused by a perforation is dependent on the site of perforation, the level of contamination, the time between perforation and diagnosis, the patient's comorbidities and genetic factors that determine the response to an inflammatory insult. Therefore, in planning and delivering treatment, these factors will all need to be considered during the diagnostics phase of treatment planning. The surgeon will need to consider a range of treatment options:

1. Should the patient be simply palliated?
2. What are the risks of using non-operative techniques to manage the inflammatory and infected consequences of a perforation which is likely to seal or has sealed spontaneously?
3. Are there any endoscopic techniques that should be considered to achieve closure of the perforation (e.g. stents, clips and endo-sutures)?
4. Are there any radiological techniques that might help manage local contamination after a perforation to supplement antimicrobial chemotherapy and avoid more invasive surgery?
5. If surgical intervention is planned, can it be delivered effectively laparoscopically or thoracoscopically?
6. How and by whom should more complex surgical intervention be delivered when managing surgically difficult problems or perforated tumours?
7. After initial intervention to control the perforation and initiate decontamination, what is required to ensure rapid recovery and avoid re-perforation:
   i. How will healing be encouraged by acid suppression, pancreatic suppression and gut rest?
   ii. What is optimal antimicrobial therapy considering antibacterial and antifungal therapies?
   iii. How will nutritional support be established?

Diagnosis

Perforations may be large or small, resulting in variable levels of contamination. Perforations into the retroperitoneum or mediastinum may be locally contained and present with a more gradual development of symptoms. The classical story of sudden severe generalised abdominal pain with signs of generalised peritonitis ('board-like rigidity'), will alert the surgeon towards acute gastrointestinal perforation as a possible cause.

However, history and examination are frequently less clear. Foregut perforation should be considered in all patients presenting with acute chest, abdominal or thoracolumbar back pain and signs of sepsis. In addition, pain after foregut endoscopic or radiological interventions must be presumed secondary to perforation until proven otherwise.

Blood tests may show evidence of a systemic inflammatory response. This takes time to develop and may be absent or reduced in the elderly or immunosuppressed. Raised serum amylase may suggest a diagnosis of acute pancreatitis but does not exclude perforation and the surgeon needs to consider carefully the safety of a diagnosis of acute pancreatitis. Pneumoperitoneum is reported in 70% of patients with a perforated peptic ulcer.[1] Radiological signs other than subdiaphragmatic gas should be looked for on erect chest and abdominal films (**Fig. 12.1**) as well as ultrasound (US) and computed tomography (CT).[2]

Advanced imaging

CT is the investigation of choice in patients with a suspected foregut perforation and is highly sensitive for small volumes of free (extraluminal) gas. In addition, the exact site of perforation may be revealed and some staging information will help plan treatment in those with a tumour-associated

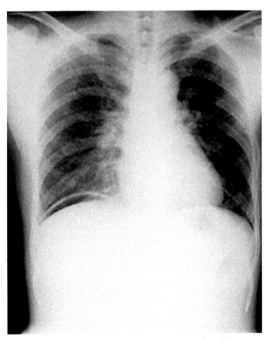

Figure 12.1 • Erect chest radiograph showing right subphrenic free gas shadow associated with a perforated peptic ulcer.

perforation. CT can, however, be falsely reassuring, particularly if performed early (within 6 hours) of the onset of the symptoms.[2] In critically ill patients with systemic sepsis and/or organ failure who have free peritoneal gas and/or who clearly require laparotomy or laparoscopy, requesting a CT must not cause an excessive delay in surgery. In such patients, evidence probably suggests rapid 'source control' of the sepsis improves prognosis, with mortality rates increasing with each hour of delay.[3]

Detailing CT protocols is beyond the scope of this chapter, but the surgeon should be aware that non-contrast CT is an effective technique to identify small volumes of extraluminal gas and may be useful in patients with contraindications to intravenous contrast (allergy and acute renal failure). Scans with intravenous contrast will give much better anatomical detail and will provide important staging information in patients with possible perforated tumours. Adding oral contrast may help localise the perforation and indicate if there is a continued leak from the intestinal lumen. While a positive scan is helpful and a negative scan may direct the surgeon to adopting a non-operative treatment plan, false negative scans are still seen in patients with an upper gastrointestinal perforations if a water soluble contrast is used.

Perforated peptic ulceration

Cause

This is the commonest type of foregut perforation with an estimated lifetime risk of perforation in peptic ulcer patients of 2–10%.[4] *Helicobacter pylori* and non-steroidal anti-inflammatory drugs are most frequently linked to this disease. A number of other risk factors are reported (Box 12.1).

Box 12.1 • Risk factors increasing the risk of peptic ulcer disease

- Non-steroidal anti-inflammatory drugs
- Smoking
- *Helicobacter pylori*
- Marginal ulcer after bariatric surgery
- Fasting
- Crack cocaine, cocaine and metamphetamines
- Gastrinoma
- Critical illness
- Steroids
- High salt diets
- Alcohol
- Chemotherapy with bevacizumab

Adapted from Soreide et al. Perforated peptic ulcer. Lancet 2015;386:1288–98. Soreide K, Thorsen K, Harrison E, et al. Perforated peptic ulcer. Lancet 2015;386:1288–98.

In addition, there is a clear correlation between socioeconomic deprivation and peptic ulcer disease.[5]

H. pylori

The link between *H. pylori* and peptic ulcer disease is well established.[6] Our understanding of this organism and how it causes disease continues to develop and is regularly reviewed.[7] The link between *H. pylori* and perforation is less clear although there are suggestions that strain virulence might be a factor,[8] and its prevalence varies in different populations. In a group of 73 patients with peptic ulcer perforation treated surgically, antral biopsy and testing confirmed *H. pylori* infection in 70% of patients.[9] Patients with ulcer perforation and confirmed *H. pylori* infection treated randomly with *H. pylori* eradication or no eradication had persistent or recurrent duodenal ulceration rates of 4.8% if eradicated and 38% if not eradicated.[10] Pooled data from three randomised studies showed 5.2% ulcer recurrence at 1 year in eradicated patients and 35.2% in non-eradicated patients.[11]

✓✓ All patients with a perforated peptic ulcer should receive eradication of *H. pylori*.[10,11]

Non-steroidal anti-inflammatory drugs (NSAIDs)

The association between NSAIDs and peptic ulcer disease has been known for many years.[12] Selective COX-2 inhibitors were developed to try to reduce the gastrointestinal side-effects of NSAID use and were shown to reduce annual risk from (1.27% to 0.44%).[13] Population-based studies reported in 2008[14] showed a significant increase in NSAID prescribing (44%) as COX-2 inhibitors became available, with a reduction in ulcer perforations from 17/100 000 per year to 12/100 000. Perforations in patients on NSAID medications are associated with a higher 30-day mortality than those not on NSAID medications,[15] probably reflecting an older and more comorbid population. However, increased evidence of a link between NSAIDs and cardiovascular-related death may be a factor.[16]

Systematic literature review and cost–benefit analysis suggest that patients with a condition such as osteoarthritis on long-term selective or non-selective NSAIDs should also take a proton pump inhibitor (PPI).[17,18]

Indications for surgery

Patients with perforated peptic ulceration represent a diverse group who present in a widely variable manner from the moribund to the remarkably well. Various groups have tried to develop reproducible risk predictor tools for these patients to assist clinical decision-making and outcome evaluation. Unfortunately none of these scoring systems appears to be an ideal risk prediction tool.[5]

- Preoperative factors that increase the risk of mortality after operation for perforated peptic ulcer are shown in Box 12.2.[5,19]
- Traditional surgical teaching has been that visceral perforation requires operative intervention for closure. However, clinical observation that some patients are remarkably well with little evidence of peritonitis on presentation and case series reports that in up to 50% of patients the ulcer has spontaneously sealed at the time of operation support non-operative treatment in some patients.[20]
- As long ago as 1946[21] a series of patients with perforated peptic ulcers treated non-operatively was reported and subsequent series[20,22] have demonstrated good outcomes in selected patients. A randomised study[23] suggested some caution with this approach, although the study was small and did not benefit from preoperative CT. Eleven patients (28%) in the observation group were converted to surgical intervention because of deterioration or failure to improve. In three of these patients the diagnosis was incorrect (two perforated gastric tumours and one perforated sigmoid colon). The outcomes in the two groups (early surgery or initial observation and delayed surgery if failing to progress) were similar. The authors suggested non-operative management was appropriate but raised concerns that it might disadvantage

Box 12.2 • Risk factors for mortality in perforated peptic ulcer

Acute kidney injury	2.4 (1.2–4.9)
ASA score 3–5	3.3 (2.0–5.3)
Comorbidity (undefined)	5.1 (3.5–7.4)
Diabetes	1.8 (1.2–2.8)
Low albumin	1.7 (1.2–3.5)
Malignancy	1.8 (1.4–2.4)
NSAID	1.7 (1.1–2.8)
Old age	3.2 (1.4–7.5)
Shock	4.9 (2.1–11.3)
Steroids	1.5 (1.2–2.0)
Surgical delay	3.6 (1.9–7.0)

Adapted from Soreide et al. Perforated peptic ulcer. Lancet 2015;386:1288–98. Soreide K, Thorsen K, Harrison E, et al. Perforated peptic ulcer. Lancet 2015;386:1288–98.

the over 70 age group due to their reduced ability to respond to sepsis. This study was under-powered to make this conclusion. A more pragmatic view would be that the study demonstrated that non-operative management is possible in selected patients. The main problem is making sure appropriate selection occurs.

- This view is endorsed by another study[24] which observed 82 consecutive patients without immediate surgery, where 54% improved and the group's overall mortality was only 1%, suggesting that good outcomes can be achieved with a period of observation, even if surgery is subsequently required.
- The difficulty with this strategy is that it conflicts with guidance from the Surviving Sepsis Campaign, with international guidelines advocating aggressive fluid resuscitation, early use of broad-spectrum antibiotics and early source control.[25] This would suggest that delaying surgery should be counter-productive and not in the patients' best interests. Data from large Danish and American population studies[26,27] showed progressive increases in postoperative mortality as the time to surgery increases, suggesting that 'every hour counts'. However, recently presented data from the UK National Emergency Laparotomy Audit (NELA) of over 2000 operations for perforated peptic ulcers showed no link between 30-day mortality and time to surgery (unpublished communication).
- This leaves the surgeon in a dilemma, particularly when dealing with sick, comorbid and elderly patients. This group are likely to struggle significantly after major surgery, have a high morbidity and mortality and use considerable resources. They are, however, likely to be the group who are most at risk if rapid source control is not established. Surgeons should be reassured that there is no 'right answer'. They need to rapidly and carefully assess each patient and demonstrate logical thought processes. Delaying surgery in all but the extremely unwell can be considered safe but requires regular review and active intervention if the patient is not recovering. A recent position statement from the World Society of Emergency Surgery[28] suggests that efforts should be made to show no continued contrast leak before adopting a non-operative approach. While

there is no strong evidence to support such a statement, it is recognised that lack of contrast extravasation may be falsely reassuring. It is not unreasonable in patients without generalised, or even local peritonitis, for a trial of non-operative treatment if an oral contrast CT does not confirm an ongoing leak.

✅ In a well patient with a suspected peptic ulcer perforation, a period of non-operative treatment is reasonable if there is no evidence of an ongoing leak and an absence of peritonitis. Failure to improve is an indication for surgery.

Open or laparoscopic surgery?

Surgical treatment of choice for a perforated peptic ulcer is now clearly established as omental patch repair to close the ulcer and peritoneal wash-out (**Fig. 12.2**). As our understanding of the pathogenesis of peptic ulceration has developed the emergency surgeon no longer needs to be concerned with considering a surgical intervention to reduce ulcer recurrence risks[29,30] (see also Chapter 13). Such guidance should now be removed from all surgical textbooks. Literature from the definitive ulcer healing surgery era identified that resectional surgery for simple ulcer perforations, in the form of a distal gastric resection, was associated with a higher than expected mortality.[31] Nowadays gastric resection should be avoided at all costs unless it is clearly impossible to repair a giant perforation.[32]

As a result of the technical simplification of surgery for perforated peptic ulcer, the laparoscopic approach has been widely reported. The utilisation of the laparoscopic repair, however, varies between health systems and within health systems, with some reporting up to 45% utilisation.[33] In the UK the rate is around 12% and reported as only 3% in a recent series from North America.[34] Studies comparing the laparoscopic and open approach are difficult to analyse due to the wide risk profile reported in patients with perforated ulcers. Randomised studies have been reported from Hong Kong[35,36] and systematic reviews in 2005, 2010 and 2013[37–39] all confirmed that there is little benefit in terms of mortality, morbidity or hospital stay. There is strong evidence that the laparoscopic approach takes longer and may actually be associated with more morbidity in patients with severe peritonitis.[40]

The surgeon managing a patient with a presumed perforated peptic ulcer should therefore not be concerned that performing an open operation will necessarily disadvantage the patient. If the surgeon has suitable skills a laparoscopic approach is probably as effective and, long term, has the benefits associated with avoiding a major abdominal incision.

- Laparoscopy may also be useful in managing a patient who might be managed more conservatively by confirming a low level of soiling and a sealed ulcer when there is doubt.
- Laparoscopic sutureless repair of an ulcer[41] using clips and/or glue is described and has been shown to be effective and more easily delivered by a less experienced laparoscopic surgeon. However, as there appears to be relatively little benefit to laparoscopic sutured repair over open sutured repair this seems to be of little direct clinical relevance. If the surgeon has approached the patient laparoscopically and a large

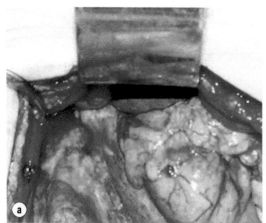 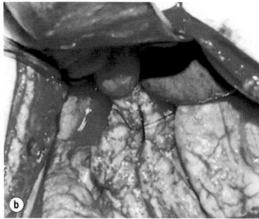

Figure 12.2 • (a) A small perforation at the juxtapyloric area. **(b)** Pedicle omental patch repair on the perforation site secured with absorbable sutures.

perforation found with significant peritoneal contamination or potential tumours seen, the operation should be converted to an open one.

> ✅ Laparoscopy and laparoscopic repair of small perforated duodenal ulcers in experienced hands is an acceptable treatment option. For larger perforations and significant peritoneal contamination the open approach is better.

New options

Technological developments in endoscopic surgical techniques have created new options to consider in sealing foregut perforations. These are likely to be of greater relevance in managing iatrogenic endoscopic perforations created during endoscopic therapy rather than in managing a pathological perforation with peritonitis. Stents,[42] endoscopic clips and suturing[43,44] and transluminal replication of omental patching[45,46] are all described. Unfortunately these only deliver 'source control' and do not allow peritoneal lavage. They may therefore apply mostly to the cohort of patients who could be managed non-operatively.

Giant duodenal ulcer

Most ulcers are small and relatively easily managed by closure with an omental patch. Duodenal ulcers >2 cm in diameter, however, present a more significant challenge. Simple closure has a higher failure rate and traditionally distal gastrectomy was advised for such.[47,48] However, in an era where gastric resection for ulcer disease is now rare, this is often an unfamiliar operation for the emergency surgeon particularly as the duodenal resection line will often present a significant challenge for closure. Surgeons should therefore be familiar with various techniques for managing a difficult duodenal stump closure.[49–51] Attempt at closing the duodenal stump should be made in all cases with a large tube drain (or two) left to control a leak if it occurs. An alternative technique used by some surgeons is to create a controlled duodenal fistula using a Foley catheter or T-tube duodenostomy (**Fig. 12.3**).

In many patients, however, there is reasonable evidence to support treating such large ulcers by closure as a Finney pyloroplasty or simply using an omental plug.[52] If the primary surgeon feels that a gastric resection may be, or may become, necessary 'damage control' surgery with a tube duodenostomy to provide source control is an acceptable treatment. This will allow stabilisation and urgent referral to an appropriate specialist surgeon if required.

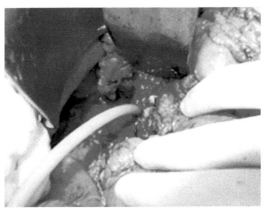

Figure 12.3 • A catheter duodenostomy for managing a difficult duodenal stump.

Pancreatic suppression with an octreotide infusion should be considered in patients with a high risk of a duodenal leak or an established fistula. There is evidence that this reduces fistula output making fluid and wound management easier but no strong evidence that it speeds up healing of an enterocutaneous fistula.[53]

Perforated gastric ulcers

This disease falls into two categories:

1. **Small classical peptic ulcers.** Gastric ulcers that perforate are usually small, prepyloric and associated with *H. pylori* and NSAID use. They are becoming more common[54–56] as a proportion of perforated ulcers, particularly in the elderly. A small proportion will be through a tumour and it is recommended that biopsies are taken from the ulcer edge in all gastric ulcer perforations. These ulcers can be managed in the same way as perforated duodenal ulcers by closure and omental patch repair.

2. **Perforated gastric tumours or large ulcers.** These present a surgical challenge and it is often difficult to decide if the patient has a giant benign ulcer or a neoplasm. It is easy to be negative about the longer-term outcome in such patients. The surgeon should remember that these tumours may be carcinomas, lymphomas or neuroendocrine tumours and therefore cure may be achieved despite the tumour perforation.

✅ Perforated gastric ulcers should be managed where possible with biopsy and omental patch repair. The only indication for resection is failure to close with patch repair.

For perforated gastric carcinomas evidence from nine observational studies gathered into a series of 127 patients[57] can help to create a surgical strategy:

1. It appears to be acceptable to simply close and cover the perforation with omentum having obtained a biopsy of the ulcer edge. In a specialist centre primary resection might be considered but as the diagnosis is often unclear this is rarely advisable.
2. Resecting the ulcer as a wedge gastrectomy is an ideal biopsy if it is relatively small and this is easily achieved.
3. Rapid postoperative staging studies and histological assessment will then allow clarity of diagnosis and disease stage.

Lymphoma and gastrointestinal stromal tumours (GISTs) or neuroendocrine tumours can also perforate either spontaneously or during chemotherapy.[58–60] The primary management of gastric lymphoma is dependent on the tumour type and stage and is now almost entirely non-surgical, with decisions regarding treatment best taken with multidisciplinary team input. Spontaneous perforations will present as above and should be biopsied and an omental patch repair carried out. Perforations that may occur during chemotherapy are very uncommon compared to lymphoma of the small bowel, which has a much higher rate of perforation during chemotherapy. However, as tumour necrosis is a major factor in lymphoma, perforation and healing of such a perforation if it occurs is unlikely, so resection will need to be considered in such instances.

Antimicrobial therapy

Patients with generalised peritonitis require urgent broad-spectrum antibacterial chemotherapy, ideally delivered at the time of clinical diagnosis. Blood cultures should be taken before the first dose but antibiotics should not be delayed until operation. The exact type and dosage of antibiotic will be determined by local guidelines, the patient's renal function and allergy profile. Positive fungal cultures from upper GI perforations are associated with a poorer prognosis.[61,62] Delayed diagnosis, perforations in patients on steroids and/or acid suppressive medication should be considered for antifungal therapy but there is no evidence to support its routine use.

Postoperative care

Critically ill patients or those identified at risk based on pre- and perioperative risk scoring (see also Chapters 4 and 5) should be managed in a critical care unit. Care bundles to ensure critical components of care are delivered improve results in patients with gastroduodenal perforations.[63] Nasogastric aspiration is commonplace until aspirates reduce and there is evidence of resolution of the peritonitis-induced ileus. This may take several days or longer and is usually the factor that slows discharge from hospital. Patients with minor peritoneal soiling and a laparoscopic surgical procedure studied in a randomised study in Turkey were safely managed along an 'enhanced recovery after surgery pathway' reducing length of stay from 4.8 to 1.5 days.[64]

There is no good evidence for intravenous proton pump therapy in this group of patients. Perioperative diagnosis of *H. pylori* is not easily achieved and as cohort studies show at least 70% of patients are *H. pylori*-positive, postoperative eradication therapy should be almost routine unless there is a clear contraindication.

Guidance from the UK National Institute for Health and Care Excellence (NICE)[65] recommends 6–8 weeks of PPI to ensure ulcer healing and continued PPI in higher-risk patients, eradication confirmed 6–8 weeks after therapy with a breath or faecal test. Patients with gastric ulceration should have healing confirmed by endoscopy as 13% of gastric ulcer perforations are malignant.[66] Patients with duodenal ulcers do not require follow-up endoscopy.

Oesophageal perforation

Oesophageal perforation should be regarded as a critical, life-threatening illness. Management advice is based on observational data and extrapolation from experience of managing surgical sepsis. As for other foregut perforations the surgeon will need to consider the specific problem, the patient, the site and type of perforation and surgical options that are available. Unfortunately diagnosis is often delayed, which affects both treatment and outcome.[67] The frequency of this problem is unclear, as in a whole population study perforation following endoscopy was reported to occur in 3.1/1 000 000/year;[68] however, it is likely that it is under-reported and as therapeutic endoscopy increases perforation as a complication will also increase, so overall rates of oesophageal perforation are probably higher than we realise.

Causes

Iatrogenic

The majority of oesophageal perforations are iatrogenic, most frequently occurring during therapeutic endoscopies, although perforation during diagnostic flexible endoscopy is reported in up to 2 or 3 per 10 000 procedures.[69,70] As therapeutic endoscopic procedures are increasing in frequency and complexity as instrumentation develops, more perforations will be seen. Perforation following stricture or achalasia dilatation is reported in 1–10% of patients.[71]

Endoscopic resection or ablation of Barrett's oesophagus or oesophageal tumours is increasingly frequent and associated with perforation in a small number of patients.[72]

If diagnosed at the time of endoscopy these perforations can often be managed with endoscopic closure,[73] simple gut rest and antibiotic therapy as there is little mediastinal or cervical soiling.

Late diagnosis or delayed perforation may require more active intervention. In addition, as endoscopic therapy of tumours or 'premalignant' conditions increases, oncological considerations may drive treatment. It appears that perforation during endoscopic resection of early oesophageal and gastric cancers does not adversely affect outcome by increasing the risk of disseminated malignancy.[74]

Peri- or postoperative oesophageal perforation is reported following neck and thoracic procedures. The author has treated patients with perforations following cervical spine surgery, parathyroid surgery, neck dissection, following endoscopic aortic valve replacement secondary to a transoesophageal echo probe injury and, most alarmingly, following descending aortic grafting, both open and radiological, with graft erosion into the oesophagus. Each of these cases will need to be managed with an individualised plan.

Spontaneous rupture (Boerhaave's syndrome)

The classical vomiting-induced condition of spontaneous oesophageal rupture accounts for about 15% of oesophageal ruptures. This condition is likely to produce substantial mediastinal and intra-pleural contamination and has a high mortality. Other situations with forceful oesophageal dilatation leading to perforation have been reported including labour, weight lifting, Heimlich manoeuvre, air blast injuries and blunt trauma.[75]

Caustic injury

This is either accidental or not. Oesophageal injury is rare with acidic substances, which usually cause injury to the oropharyngeal area and are less likely to penetrate the oesophagus. Alkali ingestion is more likely to penetrate to the oesophagus and causes a more extensive and deeper injury. Early endoscopic assessment and placement of a nasogastric tube secures the oesophageal lumen[76,77] and allows injury assessment.

Diagnosis of oesophageal perforation[78]

Early diagnosis is important as delayed diagnosis is associated with worse outcomes. Endoscopists should therefore investigate and manage possible iatrogenic perforations aggressively.

Mortality of oesophageal perforation reported in a review of 726 published patients was 18%.[79] This is likely to overestimate risk as minor endoscopic perforations are often excluded from case series and may actually go undetected in many patients. However, spontaneous rupture is a notoriously lethal condition. Delayed diagnosis and treatment significantly increases risk of mortality and morbidity and all clinicians need to consider the diagnosis in patients who present with acute chest pain, particularly if following vomiting and associated with surgical emphysema (Mackler's triad).[68,79,80]

Diagnosis only occurs at post mortem in 17% of patients,[68] but should be considered in all seriously unwell patients with sepsis, multi-organ failure and chest or upper abdominal symptoms.

Unexplained pain and/or sepsis after upper GI endoscopy should also lead to diagnostic tests to exclude perforation. Chest radiographs may reveal air in the mediastinum or neck (**Fig. 12.4**). Definitive diagnosis is usually based on imaging techniques to demonstrate the oesophageal perforation. Pneumomediastinum with or without a pleural effusion should raise concern (**Fig. 12.5**). If the patient is fit for a contrast swallow, water-soluble contrast studies will usually demonstrate the leak (**Fig. 12.6**). Often CT is performed, which adds additional information and diagnostic security (**Fig. 12.7**). Upper GI endoscopy as part of the investigation in a critically ill patient or in theatre during treatment is very useful and helps guide management (**Fig. 12.8**).

Treatment

As for infradiaphragmatic foregut perforations, treatment depends on the cause, site and condition

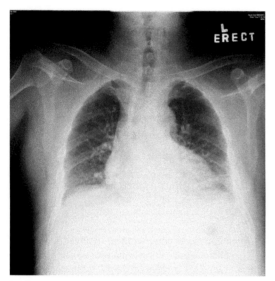

Figure 12.4 • Plain radiograph of a patient with surgical emphysema in the neck due to a mid-oesophageal perforation following endoscopic ultrasound examination and transmural biopsy.

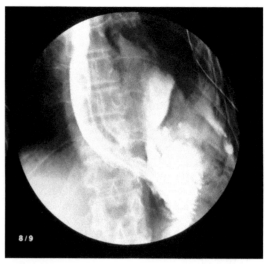

Figure 12.6 • A water-soluble contrast swallowing showing massive leak at the lower oesophagus in Boerhaave's syndrome.

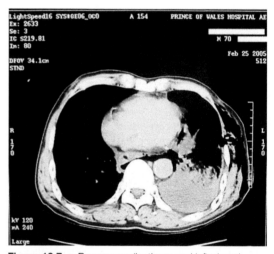

Figure 12.7 • Pneumomediastinum and left pleural effusion revealed by CT scan in a patient with lower oesophageal perforation.

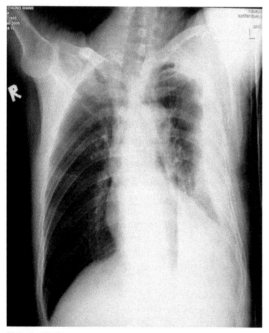

Figure 12.5 • Left hydropneumothorax revealed on decubitus chest radiograph in a patient with Boerhaave's syndrome.

of the patient. Evidence to specifically and accurately guide treatment is lacking and most is based on case series.

The principles driving therapies are those defined by the surviving sepsis guidelines[24] and by oncological considerations in the case of perforated tumours or premalignant conditions. The surgical dilemma is how aggressive and with what techniques should source control of the leak and associated septic focii be obtained.

Small contained perforations through healthy tissue, usually following endoscopy, often respond well to little more than antibiotics and gut rest. Nutrition is either provided via a parenteral route or an operatively placed jejunostomy tube.[81,82]

Observational data from Pittsburgh[83] utilised a severity scoring system based on old age, tachycardia, leukocytosis, pleural effusion, fever, non-contained leak, respiratory compromise, diagnostic delay, cancer and hypotension. Low-score patients treated

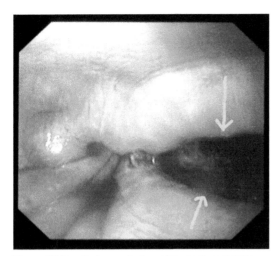

Figure 12.8 • Endoscopic view of lower oesophagus with perforation demonstrated with blue arrows on right side. The oesophageal lumen is central.

surgically appeared to do less well than those managed without surgery, suggesting that patients who are fit and 'less septic' should probably be treated without aggressive surgery.

The Newcastle group have published well-received clinical decision algorithms to support decision-making[84] which are described in Figs 12.9 and 12.10 (see also the Oesophagogastric Surgery volume in this Companion to Specialist Surgical Practice series).

Drainage

Mediastinal, pleural or cervical collections need to be aggressively and actively drained. The manner of this drainage will be determined by the situation and might be radiological or surgical. The surgical team must ensure that an adequate drain has been placed. Narrow bore radiological drains will often be inadequate and surgical lavage may be necessary

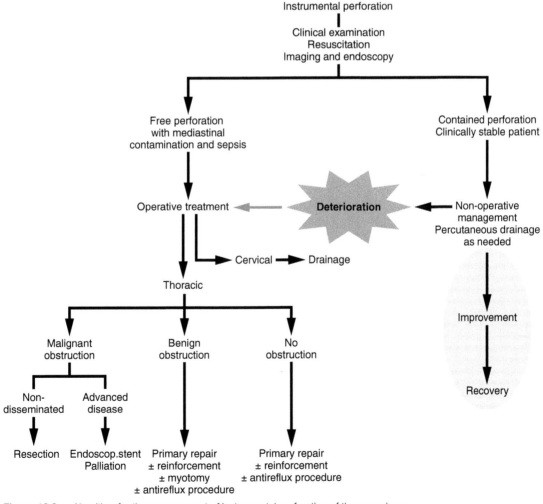

Figure 12.9 • Algorithm for the management of instrumental perforation of the oesophagus.

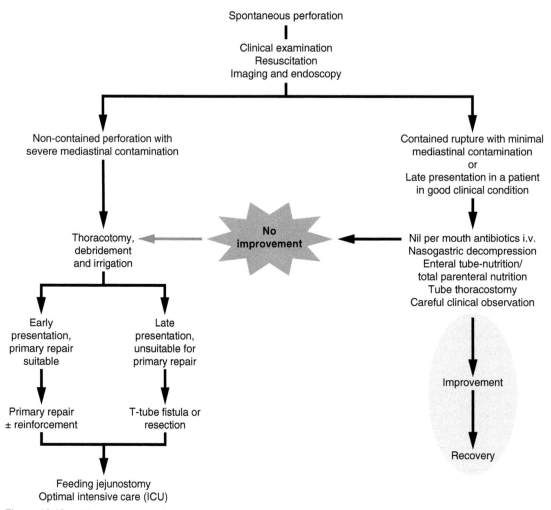

Spontaneous perforation

Clinical examination
Resuscitation
Imaging and endoscopy

Non-contained perforation with
severe mediastinal contamination

Contained rupture with minimal
mediastinal contamination
or
Late presentation in a patient
in good clinical condition

Thoracotomy,
debridement
and irrigation

No
improvement

Nil per mouth antibiotics i.v.
Nasogastric decompression
Enteral tube-nutrition/
total parenteral nutrition
Tube thoracostomy
Careful clinical observation

Early
presentation,
primary repair
suitable

Late
presentation,
unsuitable for
primary repair

Primary repair
± reinforcement

T-tube fistula or
resection

Improvement

Recovery

Feeding jejunostomy
Optimal intensive care (ICU)

Figure 12.10 • Management algorithm for spontaneous perforation of the oesophagus.

to achieve primary decontamination, particularly in patients with a vomiting-induced rupture.

Good drainage is an essential early element of managing serious perforations and can be achieved by all surgeons requiring no special skills even if pleural decontamination requires a simple thoracotomy. It should not be delayed.

Control of the perforation

Many perforations, particularly endoscopic perforations, will heal without any intervention other than treatment of sepsis, gut rest, drainage of collections and nutrition.

In patients with a significant leak, controlling this leak is likely to speed recovery and reduce morbidity and mortality. The surgical inaccessibiltiy of the oesophagus, however, creates a problem and extensive mediastinal dissection in a sick, septic patient is associated with high mortality and morbidity.

The surgeon has four options to control the oesophageal leak:

• endoscopic therapy;
• thoracotomy (or thoracoscopy) and direct repair;
• isolation of the oesophagus and diversion;
• oesophageal resection.

Endoscopic therapy

Permanent and removable stents that are self-expanding and covered now make coverage of a perforation a real option. A review of 276 patients from 25 case series with oesophageal perforations or anastomotic leaks, provides good evidence that this is often a successful technique for both controlling the leak and re-establishing early oral intake,[85] with patients often able to resume oral intake at 72 hours.[86] Stent deployment is successful in 99% of patients and achieves healing in 85% (**Fig. 12.11**).

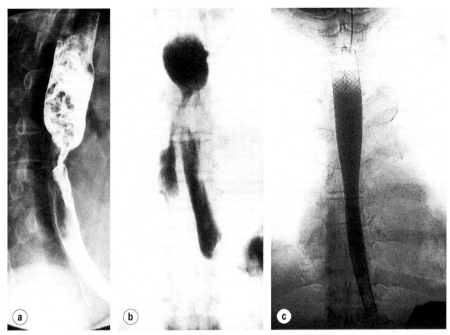

Figure 12.11 • Contrast radiography of the oesophagus. **(a)** Barium swallow demonstrating a tight malignant stricture. **(b)** Water-soluble contrast swallow after dilatation demonstrating a perforation. **(c)** Water-soluble contrast study in the same patient following insertion of an expandable metal stent, demonstrating no further leak.

Stent migration, however, remains the biggest problem reported and it is therefore essential that the stent is removed once healing has taken place, unless it has been inserted for a perforated tumour where subsequent management is palliative.

An alternative to stenting is endoscopic vacuum therapy. Increasing series are being reported with encouraging results. This requires multiple endoscopies with device changes every few days. In a series of 52 patients with mixed causes of upper gastrointestinal leaks (39 anastomotic defects, 9 iatrogenic injuries and 4 Boerhaave ruptures), 49 patients healed without further intervention. Two patients died of haemorrhage, possibly related to the vacuum device and patients required a mean of six sponge changes (1–25) and a mean duration of therapy of 22 days.[87]

Surgical repair

Direct repair of the oesophagus is achievable and encouraged if diagnosis is early (within 24 hours) although later repairs are still possible depending on the cause, site and state of the patient. Again, evidence to support this is largely anecdotal.[75] The surgeon should be aware that the perforation is often bigger than apparent from the adventitial side. Simple suture repair after excision of necrotic tissue is all that is required. Some advocate a pleural wrap to reinforce the repair in a similar manner to the use of a vascularised omental patch for gastroduodenal perforations.[88,89] However, care must be taken to avoid a circumferential wrap that is likely to increase the risk of stricture formation.

Primary repair even in favourable patients has a high failure rate and creation of a planned fistula over a T tube is common. It seems likely that as endoscopic technology progresses the majority of perforations will be controlled endoscopically in the future with the surgeon and interventional radiologists ensuring adequate drainage of the associated pleural contamination and collections. Surgical jejunostomy to establish enteral nutrition in patients who have a large leak or are requiring a surgical intervention should always be considered, as a long period of oesophageal rest may be necessary.

Resection and/or oesophageal exclusion

As for gastric perforation there are some circumstances when resection of the oesophagus might need to be considered. This will occasionally include patients with perforated tumours and those where the perforation is associated with a fistula to the airway or a mediastinal vessel.

Resection of the oesophagus with proximal exteriorisation as a cervical oesophagostomy and distal access with a surgical gastrostomy may be necessary in some circumstances. This is a challenging situation for patients and the clinical team but may be necessary to save a patient's life.

Intestinal continuity can then be re-established with a gastric tube or a colonic interposition graft, often placed in the retrosternal position, at a later date.

Perforation of an oesophageal tumour is a grave clinical situation and in the majority of patients indicates dissemination of tumour. While resection will not be curative in most patients it might be a reasonable option if localised, the patient's condition is favourable and the surgical team have the experience to perform the operation. As a result, the most common treatment in such instances is palliation with a stent.

Nutrition

Patients with an oesophageal perforation will often have a prolonged period of fasting to allow oesophageal healing. Early placement of an enteric feeding tube should be considered and may take the form of a feeding jejunostomy placed at the time of establishing drainage and source control.

Perforation after endoscopic retrograde cholangiopancreatography

Perforation occurs in 0.5–2% of patients during or immediately after endoscopic retrograde cholangiopancreatography (ERCP).[90,91] The risk is increased by sphincterotomy, in older patients and when the procedure takes a long time (presumably related to difficulty). Mortality can be as high as 15%.[92] Anatomical definition of the injury has been proposed[93] and allows the surgical team to plan the treatment strategy.

Intraperitoneal perforation

Duodenal wall injury

These injuries are classified as type 1. The lesion is likely to be intraperitoneal, is usually a traction-type injury and usually requires surgical repair. Repair of small tears is as for small perforations and larger tears may need more complex reconstruction. Duodenal mobilisation will be necessary for this type of injury to provide assessment and access to the whole duodenum.

Retroperitoneal perforations

These are classified as type 2 (sphincter of Oddi perforation), type 3 (bile duct perforation) and type 4 (retroperitoneal gas). These injuries should if possible be managed without surgery. The retroperitoneum will provide a natural sealing mechanism and the leak should heal provided that sepsis is controlled, there is no downstream obstruction and the perforation is not through a tumour. Operative repair is extremely difficult and the surgeon should be wary of duodenal mobilisation as this will convert a contained perforation into an uncontained perforation and often an enteric fistula, which can be very difficult to manage. Percutaneous drainage of collections, ideally through a retroperitoneal route, and gut rest are the mainstays of treatment. Severe injuries with big leaks and complex enterobiliary fistulas may require biliary diversion and duodenal exclusion.

Key points

- Early diagnosis and intervention of upper gastrointestinal perforations reduces morbidity and mortality.
- There are many conditions that cause foregut perforation but the principles of early treatment are remarkably standard.
- Treatment strategies range from non-operative to very major surgery.
- Treatment planning is greatly helped by easy and rapid access to CT with intravenous and oral contrast.
- Very major surgery is rarely required or indicated as a primary procedure.
- The key principles of treatment are those defined by the Surviving Sepsis campaign: aggressive fluid resuscitation, early broad-spectrum antibiotics and rapid source control.
- These key treatments can often be delivered with simple surgery, endoscopic therapy and/or interventional radiological placement of drains.
- Source control may not be necessary if a perforation has sealed spontaneously and there is little adjacent soiling.
- Evidence suggests that older, more frail patients may do better with earlier more rapid source control, though this may not need to involve surgery.
- Rapid source control is probably beneficial but evidence remains unclear.

- Patients with perforated tumours do not require immediate definitive surgical treatment. Damage control interventions allow patient stabilisation, diagnosis, staging and referral to a specialist unit if necessary.
- An increasing number of endoscopic therapies to control the perforations are coming into clinical practice and are likely to become increasingly used in these patients.
- In patients requiring abdominal surgical exploration there is little evidence that laparoscopic surgery has a major short-term benefit over open surgery.

🌐 Full references available at **http://expertconsult. inkling.com**

Key references

10. Ng EK, Lam YH, Sung JJ, et al. Eradication of Helicobacter pylori prevents recurrence of ulcer after simple closure of duodenal ulcer perforation: randomized controlled trial. Ann Surg 2000;231:153–8. PMID: 10674604.

This is the first randomised trial showing significant reduction in ulcer recurrence after eradication of H. pylori in patients undergoing simple omental repair of perforated duodenal ulcer.

11. Tomtitchong P, Siribumrungwong B, Vilaichone RK, et al. Systematic review and meta-analysis: Helicobacter pylori eradication therapy after simple closure of perforated duodenal ulcer. Helicobacter 2012;17(2):148–52. PMID: 22404446.

The pooled incidence of 1-year ulcer relapse from three prospective randomised trials was only 5.2% in patients treated with H. pylori eradication, which was significantly lower than that of the control group (35.2%).

13

Acute non-variceal upper gastrointestinal bleeding

Hon Chi Yip
James Lau

Introduction

A major audit of upper gastrointestinal (UGI) bleeding in the UK carried out over 20 years ago reported an incidence of 103 patients per 100 000 adults per year.[1] There is a twofold increase in the hospitalisation rate among those residents from the most deprived areas, according to a nationwide cohort study in the UK.[2] Overall mortality from an episode of UGI bleeding was 14% in the UK study[1] and a marked increase in mortality (33%) was observed if bleeding occurred following hospitalisation with another complaint. A more recent audit[3] covering patients admitted to UK hospitals during a 2-month period in 2007 demonstrated a marked reduction in the proportion of patients undergoing surgery, as well as an increase in the proportion of patients admitted with variceal bleeding. Overall crude mortality had fallen slightly at 10%, compared with 14% in the earlier UK audit, and the mortality of 26% for inpatients was also lower than in the previous study. However, mortality in patients admitted with peptic ulcer bleeding had fallen from 8.8% to 5.8% and the overall reduction in mortality from 14% to 10% occurred despite the increase in incidence of variceal bleeding. Mortality is now rare in the absence of comorbidity. The typical patient with severe peptic ulcer bleeding is now elderly, often with medical comorbidities and taking antiplatelet therapy and/ or on anticoagulants. Such patients are at greater risk of death despite skilled intervention and are less able to withstand surgery should this be necessary. Although the need for surgical intervention is now much reduced with the widespread availability of skilled endoscopic haemostasis, mortality following surgery remains high. As a result alternatives to surgical intervention are increasingly being employed and will be discussed in this chapter.

Aetiology

In the earlier study reported in 1995 by Rockhall,[1] only 4% of patients had UGI bleeding due to varices, with the majority (35%) being attributed to peptic ulcer disease. Of some concern was the 25% of patients in this study where no cause for bleeding was identified at all, particularly as this group had a mortality of 20%. Very similar figures were reported in the later study[3] where, in patients with a diagnosis made, approximately 25% were due to duodenal ulcer and 25% to peptic ulceration in the stomach, oesophagus or a combination of sites. The remainders were due to a number of other conditions, including oesophagitis, gastritis and duodenitis, with 10% of patients explained by malignancy or Mallory–Weiss syndrome (Table 13.1). In this later audit, the proportion of patients with variceal bleeding had increased to 11%, whereas the overall proportion with peptic ulcer remained unchanged.

Initial assessment and triage

Patients with acute UGI bleeding present with haematemesis, melaena or a combination of the two. Haematemesis is indicative of significant bleeding from a site proximal to the ligament of Treitz. Melaena usually indicates a bleeding site in the upper gastrointestinal tract, although bleeding from the small

Table 13.1 • Endoscopic diagnoses to patients who presented with acute upper gastrointestinal bleeding in the 2007 UK audit

Endoscopic diagnoses	Total number of patients (5004) % (n)
Peptic ulcer	36 (1826)
Varices	11 (544)
Malignancy	3.7 (187)
Oesophagitis	24 (1177)
Gastritis/erosions	22 (1091)
Erosive duodenitis	13 (640)
Mallory–Weiss tear	4.3 (213)
Others, including vascular ectasia	2.6 (133)
No abnormality seen	17 (865)

Modified from Hearnshaw SA, Logan RF, Lowe D, et al. Acute upper gastrointestinal bleeding in the UK: patient characteristics, diagnoses and outcomes in the 2007 UK audit. Gut 2011;60(10):1327–35.

bowel or even the right colon may present in a similar way, depending on speed of passage. Presentation with haematemesis is associated with an increased risk of mortality compared with melaena.[4] Coffee-ground vomiting is no longer considered a serious stigma of UGI bleeding. Patients with upper gastrointestinal blood loss may occasionally present with frank rectal bleeding (haematochezia), but this is indicative of major blood loss and, not surprisingly, is associated with an increased need for transfusion, surgery and mortality.[5] A good example of this would be a patient who has previously undergone aortic aneurysm surgery who subsequently develops an aortoduodenal fistula related to the aortic graft.

Scoring systems

Risk stratification in patients with UGI haemorrhage is important as it assists decision-making in the need for emergency intervention and feasibility of safe outpatient management. Published guidelines suggest routine use of validated stratification tools in these patients.[6,7] Multiple scoring tools have been previously reported, with the Rockall score and the Glasgow Blatchford Score (GBS) being most extensively validated. Using data from the first National UK Audit, Rockall and colleagues derived a scoring system based on five significant risk factors for mortality.[5] The Rockall system consists of an initial score from clinical parameters and a complete composite score after endoscopic assessment. Patients with an initial score of zero (i.e. age <60, no tachycardia, no hypotension and no comorbidity) had a very low mortality. The composite Rockall system, incorporating endoscopic information including

cause of bleeding and stigmata of haemorrhage, has been validated in prospective studies,[8-10] but is more accurate in predicting mortality than the risk of re-bleeding.[8,9]

The GBS, developed in the West of Scotland, aimed to allow early assessment of the need for intervention rather than risk of death (Table 13.2).[11] Based entirely on clinical risk markers before endoscopy, the GBS performed significantly better than the Rockall score at predicting the need for intervention and has now been validated in prospective studies from the UK[12] and Hong Kong.[11] In particular, the small proportion of patients with a GBS of 0 have minimal chance of requiring intervention as well as risk of re-bleeding and death, thus outpatient management of these patients is considered safe and cost-effective.[13] The proportion of patients who require endoscopic therapy increases with higher scores. There remains a small but significant proportion of patients with low to moderately high scores who require endoscopic therapy and it is difficult to define a cut-off score beyond which

Table 13.2 • Glasgow Blatchford score for predicting risk of re-bleeding or death in non-variceal UGI haemorrhage

Admission risk marker	Score component value
Blood urea (mmol/L)	
≥6.5 <8.0	2
≥8.0 <10.0	3
≥10.0 <25.0	4
≥25	6
Haemoglobin (g/L) for men	
≥120 <130	1
≥100 <120	3
<100	6
Haemoglobin (g/L) for women	
≥100 <120	1
<100	6
Systolic blood pressure (mmHg)	
100–109	1
90–99	2
<90	3
Other markers	
Pulse ≥100 (per min)	1
Presentation with melaena	1
Presentation with syncope	2
Hepatic disease	2
Cardiac failure	2

Modified from Blatchford O, Murray WR, Blatchford M. A risk score to predict need for treatment for upper-gastrointestinal haemorrhage. Lancet 2000;356(9238):1318–21.

urgent endoscopy becomes mandatory. Given the superiority of GBS in predicting the need for intervention over Rockall score, GBS is nowadays the preferred stratification system of choice in many centres.

Despite recommendations from guidelines, published nationwide registries consistently report a low adherence to the use of risk stratification tools in real-life practice. In the Canadian RUGBE study, only one of the 15 participating centres used the Rockall score to stratify patients with UGI bleeding, and not one was routinely using GBS.[14] In the 2007 UK audit, only 19% (1250/6750) of patients had either Rockall score or GBS recorded in the medical notes.[15] Risk stratification systems should be adopted into clinical management protocol for all patients presenting with UGI haemorrhage, as routine use of such a system would assist in detecting patients at high risk of re-bleeding or death, as well as increase cost-effectiveness by reducing unnecessary admission of low-risk patients. A GBS of 0 on presentation identifies a low-risk group of patients who may be safely discharged without the need for urgent UGI endoscopy.

✅ The most recently published comprehensive guidelines on the management of UGI bleeding based on studies published to date include data from published and new meta-analyses as well as expert opinion.[6,7]

Initial management

While it may be appropriate to consider discharge for young patients with no haemodynamic compromise and a GBS of zero, particularly where there has been no witnessed frank haematemesis, most patients with a history of UGI bleeding will be admitted for observation and endoscopy. This will entail insertion of a large-bore intravenous cannula, administration of pre-warmed fluid to expand the intravascular volume and immediate blood samples taken for crossmatch, biochemistry, full blood count, coagulation screen and arterial blood gases. There is also some evidence that admission to a dedicated UGI bleeding unit is associated with a reduction in mortality.[16] Such a unit requires a 24-hour on-call service for immediate endoscopy if required and early (within 24 hours) consultant-led endoscopy for all patients. Indications for urgent (out-of-hours) endoscopy vary, but the main factor determining the degree of urgency is the necessity for endostasis. Therefore patients with evidence of ongoing haemorrhage, declared either by fresh haematemesis or haemodynamic instability despite initial fluid resuscitation, require emergency endoscopy. Most stable patients will undergo UGI endoscopy within 24 hours (usually on the morning after admission). In such patients the purpose of endoscopy is twofold: firstly, patients with minor bleeds undergo full diagnostic assessment and if considered at low risk of re-bleeding can be discharged home; secondly, to identify the group of patients who have significant lesions and who require endoscopic therapy to reduce the risk of re-bleeding. This will be discussed in the next section.

Massive haemorrhage

In those patients who have evidence of haemodynamic compromise, initial resuscitation should follow the appropriate guidelines.[16] Early intensive haemodynamic resuscitation is recommended for such patients. In an observational study of patients suffering from UGI haemorrhage with haemodynamic instability, intensive haemodynamic resuscitation was associated with a lower risk of myocardial infarction and mortality than the control 'observation' group.[17] The type of intravenous fluid has always been a matter of dispute over the years. A Cochrane review of 55 trials found no evidence of any benefit of administering colloid rather than crystalloid solutions during resuscitation in critically ill patients.[18] As colloid solutions are more expensive, initial resuscitation with appropriate crystalloids is recommended.

Use of blood and blood products

Red cell replacement is likely to be required when 30% or more of the blood volume is lost. This can be difficult to assess, particularly in young patients, and clinical assessment of blood loss, coupled with the response to initial volume replacement, must guide the decision on the necessity of transfusion. While blood transfusion may achieve intravascular volume replenishment and enhance tissue oxygen delivery, a liberal transfusion strategy could be associated with worse clinical outcomes. In a recent randomised trial, 921 patients with acute UGI haemorrhage were randomised to restrictive transfusion strategy (target haemoglobin: 7–9 g/dL) and liberal transfusion strategy (target haemoglobin: 9–11 g/dL) groups.[19] The restrictive RBC transfusion group had a significantly improved 6-week survival (95% vs 91%; hazard ratio [HR] 0.55, 95% confidence interval [CI] 0.33–0.92) and reduced re-bleeding (10% vs 16%; HR 0.68, 95% CI 0.47–0.98). Of note, patients with massive exsanguinating haemorrhage as well as specific medical comorbidity were excluded from the trial. In patients with significant medical comorbidity, a higher target haemoglobin level should be considered in order to increase oxygen-carrying capacity. In patients with evidence of continuing haemorrhage, arrangements for emergency endoscopic intervention must be made in parallel with resuscitation.

Administration of platelets should aim to maintain a platelet count of more than 50×10^9/L, while coagulation factors are likely to be required when more than one blood volume has been lost. These are most commonly given in the form of fresh frozen plasma (FFP). The use of platelets, FFP and other agents, such as recombinant factor VIIa, should be guided by local protocols and early involvement of a haematologist.

Management of patients on antiplatelet agents and anticoagulants

Antiplatelet agents and anticoagulants are commonly used nowadays for different cardiovascular conditions and UGI haemorrhage is a serious complication for patients taking these drugs. Patients taking vitamin K antagonists (VKA) should be admitted with the drug withheld. In patients suffering from major bleeding with haemodynamic compromise, urgent reversal of VKA should be undertaken. This could be achieved by administration of prothrombin complex concentrates (PCC) or fresh frozen plasma (FFP). PCC contain clotting factors prepared from pooled and concentrated human plasma. The major advantages of PCC are faster onset of action and a smaller transfusion volume, thus a lower risk of fluid overload. PCC was associated with a quicker correction of International Normalised Ratio (INR) in a recent small-scale non-randomised study.[20]

In recent years, use of non-VKA oral anticoagulants (nOAC) is increasingly popular in patients with non-valvular atrial fibrillation and venous thromboembolism. The risk of UGI haemorrhage is at least similar to that of VKA. These agents have a short and predictable anticoagulation effect but rapid reversal in the setting of life-threatening haemorrhage is difficult. Vitamin K and FFP have not been found useful. The only reversal agent of dabigatran, idarucizumab, has been recently approved by the FDA. Administration of PCC or use of haemodialysis should be considered when urgent reversal of nOACs is necessary.

In patients with UGI haemorrhage who are taking antiplatelet agents, further management would depend on the severity of the bleeding, indication and the type of antiplatelet agents used. In general, patients on low dose aspirin for secondary cardiovascular prophylaxis should have the drug resumed as soon as satisfactory haemostasis is confirmed after endoscopy. In a randomised study, patients who received continuous aspirin had a significantly lower all-cause short-term mortality compared with placebo, with the difference being attributable to cardiovascular, cerebrovascular, or GI complications.[21] Patients who are taking dual antiplatelet agents should at least continue with low-dose aspirin to avoid cardiovascular events. Patients on other antiplatelet agents such as clopidogrel, prasugrel or ticagrelor should consider switching back to low-dose aspirin after an episode of clinically significant UGI haemorrhage.

Early pharmacological treatment

Upper gastrointestinal endoscopy is the mainstay of investigation and management of UGI bleeding, but there may also be a role for early treatment with acid suppression therapy. In vitro studies have shown that, at pH <6, platelet aggregation and plasma coagulation are markedly reduced,[22] a situation exacerbated by the presence of pepsin. It is therefore reasonable to expect acid suppression therapy to promote clot formation and stabilisation. Six randomised trials comparing pre-endoscopy proton pump inhibitor (PPI) therapy with histamine-2 receptor antagonist or placebo were analysed in a Cochrane review.[23] No significant impact of PPI therapy was demonstrated on mortality, surgery or re-bleeding rates. There was, however, a reduction in the proportion of patients with stigmata of recent haemorrhage at the time of endoscopy, and a reduction in the requirement for endoscopic therapy at the index endoscopy. A post-hoc cost-effective analysis was reported using data from a large randomised study in Asia.[24] The study concluded that the strategy of preemptive use of PPI infusion was cost-saving because of reduced endoscopic therapy and hospitalisation, offsetting the cost of PPI therapy.[25] It therefore seems reasonable to propose pre-endoscopic PPI therapy in patients admitted with UGI bleeding, but this should not delay or act as a substitute for early endoscopic intervention. There is no evidence to support the use of other agents such as somatostatin, octreotide or vasopressin in the pre-endoscopy setting, except where variceal bleeding is suspected.

✔✔ Pre-endoscopy treatment with PPIs is recommended as it reduces the number of actively bleeding ulcers and increases the number of clean-based ulcers seen at the time of endoscopy.[23]
Early use of PPI reduces the need for endoscopic intervention and hospitalisation.

The use of pre-endoscopy prokinetic agents has also been advocated to improve endoscopic visualisation by reducing blood clots within the gastrointestinal tract lumen. Earlier meta-analysis showed that prokinetic agents reduced the need for repeat endoscopy.[26] In another recent meta-analysis, pre-endoscopy erythromycin infusion significantly improved gastric mucosal visualisation, decreased the need for second-look endoscopy, red cell transfusion and duration of hospital stay.[27] Tranexamic acid, an antifibrinolytic agent, may also aid in haemorrhage control by reducing clot breakdown and its use in acute trauma has been proven in a recent large randomised study.[28] In a recently conducted Cochrane review, the use of tranexamic acid in UGI haemorrhage appeared to be associated with a reduction in overall mortality.[29] Unfortunately most of the included trials in the review were performed before the routine use of PPI and there was also a high dropout rate in some of the trials. A large multicentre randomised study of 8000 participants is currently under way and the results are eagerly awaited (NCT01658124).[30]

Endoscopy

Upper gastrointestinal endoscopy is required for any patient with significant UGI bleeding. Patients with haemodynamic instability or evidence of continuing haemorrhage require emergency endoscopy, whereas the majority of patients will undergo endoscopy within 24 hours of admission. A systematic review of the literature supports a policy of early endoscopy, as this allows the safe discharge of patients with low-risk haemorrhage and improves outcome for patients with high-risk lesions.[31]

✔✔ Early endoscopy is recommended for all patients with UGI haemorrhage.[31]

Endoscopic technique

Endoscopy for UGI bleeding requires the support of a dedicated endoscopic unit with trained nursing staff, availability of additional endoscopes and equipment, ready access to anaesthetic staff and operating theatre, and, increasingly, access to interventional radiology services. These procedures are not ideal for the unsupervised trainee and should be performed or supervised by experienced consultant staff.

For the majority of stable patients, procedures can be safely carried out using standard diagnostic endoscopes. In the unstable patient or where continuing haemorrhage is suspected, the twin-channel or large (3.7mm) single-channel endoscope is preferable and allows better aspiration of gastric contents as well as more flexibility with regard to the use of heater probes and other instruments. In unstable or obtunded patients, anaesthetic support is mandatory as an endotracheal tube should be passed before endoscopy to guard against aspiration. Reported studies on the use of pre-endoscopy gastric lavage were disappointing as it did not improve visualisation of the stomach at endoscopy or improve clinically relevant outcomes such as re-bleeding, need for second-look endoscopy or blood transfusion requirements.[32–34] The use of a tilting trolley allows repositioning of the patient, which can facilitate visualisation of the proximal stomach when obscured by blood and clot. Initially, placing the patient in a head-up position may suffice, and if necessary rolling the patient into a right lateral and head-up position may be needed for complete visualisation of the gastric fundus. In general, lavage is more successful in achieving visualisation than endoscopic aspiration, as endoscope working channels rapidly block with clot. Lavage can be achieved using repeated flushes of saline down the endoscope working channel or with the use of the powered endoscopic lavage catheters such as that provided with the heater probe. With experience, it should rarely be necessary to proceed to surgery or angiography because of inability to visualise the bleeding site due to blood and clot in the stomach or duodenum.

Bleeding gastric ulcers are most likely within the antrum or at the incisura (77%), or less commonly higher on the lesser curve (15%), with ulcers at other sites within the stomach being uncommon. Ulcers at the incisura and proximal lesser curvature can be readily overlooked unless the endoscope is retroflexed within the stomach. The most common site for a bleeding duodenal ulcer is the posterior wall, sometimes with involvement of the inferior and superior walls of the first part of the duodenum. Superficial anterior duodenal wall ulcers can ooze, but usually these ulcers perforate. Ulcers elsewhere in the duodenum are seen in less than 10% of patients.[35] The presence of active bleeding at the time of endoscopy and the size of the ulcer, rather than its anatomical site, are the main endoscopic determinants of the risk of therapeutic failure.

Management of bleeding due to causes other than peptic ulceration

Gastritis/duodenitis

Bleeding due to gastritis or duodenitis may be associated with non-steroidal anti-inflammatory drug (NSAID) therapy or ingestion of alcohol. It may also be due to *Helicobacter pylori* and can be severe enough to cause superficial erosions. Such bleeding, however, is almost always self-limiting in the absence of bleeding disorders and therapeutic intervention is not required at the time of endoscopy. Treatment with appropriate acid suppression therapy and early discharge is usually appropriate in the absence of other comorbid illness.

Mallory–Weiss syndrome

Mallory–Weiss syndrome was first described in 1929 and refers to haematemesis following repeated or violent vomiting or retching. It is caused by a linear tear of the mucosa close to the oesophagogastric junction. It accounts for approximately 5% of patients with UGI haemorrhage and most will settle without the need for therapeutic intervention. However, if bleeding is seen at the time of endoscopy, several approaches have been described. The simplest and most readily available technique is the injection of 1:10000 adrenaline, as for bleeding peptic ulcers, which is sufficient in the great majority of patients.[36] Mechanical methods of endostasis such as endoscopic band ligation or clip application have not been shown to be superior to adrenaline injection alone but are appropriate alternatives, particularly when major bleeding or shock has occurred or where adrenaline injection fails to achieve endostasis.[36,37]

Oesophagitis

Gastro-oesophageal reflux disease is responsible for approximately 10% of cases of UGI haemorrhage and is rarely severe. Following diagnosis treatment is with oral PPI therapy.

Neoplastic disease

Major bleeding is occasionally associated with oesophageal, gastric or duodenal tumours. Gastro-intestinal stromal tumours (GISTs) may present with bleeding, which can be severe in some patients. Malignancies of the UGI tract commonly cause occult, chronic bleeding but major bleeding can occur and may be difficult to control endoscopically. Management will be dependent on the specific circumstances and may include endoscopic techniques such as argon plasma coagulation, angiographic embolisation or, as a last resort, surgical resection. Where possible, however, if a malignancy is suspected, non-operative methods of achieving haemostasis should be employed, allowing full staging investigations to be organised to guide appropriate management. Some patients with ongoing but slow blood loss from non-curable gastric malignancy can be helped by a single treatment of radiotherapy.

Dieulafoy's lesion

This rare cause of UGI bleeding is due to spontaneous rupture of a submucosal artery, usually in the stomach and often within 6 cm of the cardia. The characteristic endoscopic appearance is of a protruding vessel with no evidence of surrounding ulceration. They are commonly missed due to their small size and relatively inaccessible position. Endoscopic clip application or band ligation offers durable and definitive treatment when the lesion is identified. In a small randomised trial,[38] haemoclip

application was associated with a lower rate of re-bleeding than adrenaline injection, although both achieved similar rates of initial haemostasis.

Endoscopic management of bleeding peptic ulcers

Endoscopy has a central role in the management of non-variceal UGI bleeding. It enables an early diagnosis and allows for risk stratification. Endoscopic signs or stigmata of bleeding are of prognostic value and, in patients with actively bleeding ulcers or stigmata associated with a high risk of recurrent bleeding, endoscopic therapy stops ongoing bleeding and reduces re-bleeding.[6] When compared to placebo in pooled analyses, endoscopic therapy has been shown not only to reduce recurrent bleeding, but also the need for surgery and mortality.[39,40]

Endoscopic stigmata of bleeding

Forrest et al.[41] categorised endoscopic findings of bleeding peptic ulcers into those with active bleeding, stigmata of bleeding and a clean base and a modified nomenclature has been in common use in the endoscopy literature since then. Laine and Peterson[42] summarised published endoscopic series of ulcer appearances in which endoscopic therapy was not used and provided crude figures for both the prevalence and rate of recurrent bleeding associated with these stigmata of bleeding. In ulcers that are actively bleeding (**Fig. 13.1**) or exhibit a non-bleeding visible vessel (NBVV; **Fig. 13.2**), endoscopic treatment should be offered. There has, however,

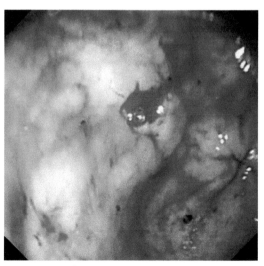

Figure 13.1 • Bleeding vessel in base of ulcer.

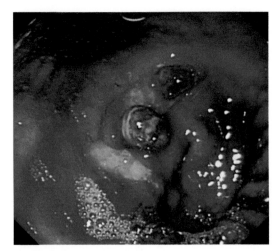

Figure 13.2 • Visible vessel.

been observer variation in the interpretation of endoscopic signs[43] and the National Institutes of Health Consensus Conference[44] defined an NBVV as 'protuberant discoloration' (**Fig. 13.2**). The endoscopist should search the ulcer base diligently in patients judged to have bled significantly or when there is circumstantial evidence of ongoing or recent bleeding, e.g. presence of fresh blood or altered blood or blood clot in the gastroduodenal tract. There has been until recently a controversy whether to wash away adherent clot overlying an ulcer (**Fig. 13.3**). Endoscopists vary in their vigour in clot irrigation before declaring a clot adherent. There have been several randomised studies and a pooled analysis has demonstrated that recurrent bleeding is reduced following clot elevation and treatment to the underlying vessel when compared to medical therapy alone.[45] Techniques for clot elevation include target irrigation using a heat probe and cheese-wiring using a snare with or without pre-injection with diluted adrenaline. One should, however, be cautious in elevation of clots overlying large deep bulbar and lesser curve ulcers as some of these may have eroded into large arteries. A recourse to angiographic embolisation without clot elevation and possible provocation of bleeding may be a better option in such patients. Ulcers with flat pigmentation and a clean base (**Fig. 13.4**) are associated with minimal risk of recurrent bleeding. Stable patients with such ulcers can be discharged home early on medical treatment (Table 13.3).

✓✓ Endoscopic therapy should be applied where there is active bleeding or a non-bleeding visible vessel in the ulcer base.[6] Adherent clot should be removed and endoscopic therapy applied to the underlying vessel.[45]

Endoscopic treatment

Modalities of endoscopic treatment can be broadly categorised into: injection, contact thermocoagulation, clipping and, recently, the use of topical haemostatic powder.

Injection

Injection therapy has been widely used because of its simplicity. Injection therapy works principally by volume tamponade. Aliquots (0.5–1 mL) are injected near the bleeding point at four quadrants using a 21- or 23-gauge injection needle. Adrenaline 1:10 000 has an added local vasoconstrictive effect. There is no role for the use of a sclerosant as there have been fatal case reports of gastric necrosis following its injection and the added injection of a sclerosant such

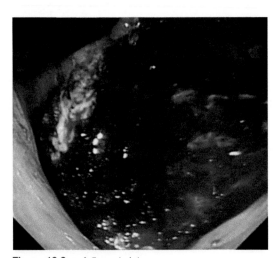

Figure 13.3 • Adherent clot.

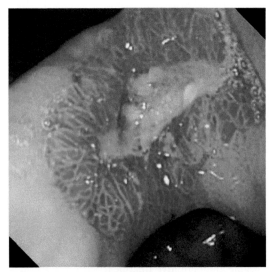

Figure 13.4 • Ulcer with clean base.

Table 13.3 • Prevalence and outcomes of ulcers based on endoscopic appearance

Endoscopic signs	Prevalence (%)	Further bleeding (%)	Surgery (%)	Death (%)
Clean base	42	5	0.5	2
Flat spot	20	10	6	3
Adherent clot	17	22	10	7
Non-bleeding visible vessel	17	43	34	11
Active bleeding	18	55	35	11

Data from Laine L, Peterson WL. Bleeding peptic ulcer. N Engl J Med 1994;331(11):717–27.

as polidocanol or sodium tetradecylsulphate after pre-injection of diluted adrenaline does not confer any advantage over injection of diluted adrenaline alone. Injection of fibrin or thrombin has been shown to be effective in some studies but repeated injections are required. These products are costly.[46,47]

Thermal methods

In a canine mesenteric artery model, contact thermocoagulation is superior to injection therapy and non-contact coagulation such as laser photo-coagulation in securing haemostasis. Contact thermocoagulation using a 3.2-mm probe consistently seals arteries up to 2mm in diameter in ex vivo models. Johnston and colleagues emphasised the need for firm mechanical tamponade before sealing of the artery with thermal energy, introducing the term 'coaptive thermocoagulation'. Mechanical compression alone stops bleeding, reduces heat-sink effect and dissipation of thermal energy. The footprint after treatment provides a clear endpoint to therapy. Non-contact thermocoagulation in the form of laser photocoagulation is no longer used as a laser unit is bulky and difficult to be transported. At least in animal experiments, non-contact coagulation in the form of laser photocoagulation is not as effective as contact thermocoagulation. There has also been interest in the use of argon plasma thermocoagulation, with a meta-analysis that summarised clinical trials comparing this to injection sclerotherapy or heat-probe treatment, respectively.[49] No significant difference in outcome was demonstrated.

Mechanical methods

Haemoclips are commonly used. Their application may be difficult in awkwardly placed ulcers such as those on the lesser curvature of the stomach and the posterior bulbar duodenum. In a meta-analysis of 15 studies with 390 patients[50] that compared haemoclipping versus injection and thermo-coagulation, successful application of haemoclips (81.5%) was superior to injection alone (75.4%) but comparable to thermocoagulation (81.2%) in producing definitive haemostasis. In this pooled analysis, haemoclipping also led to a reduced need for surgery when compared to injection alone.

Hemospray®

Recently the endoscopic use of a haemostatic nano-powder has been developed following its approval in the USA for external use in traumatic injuries. During endoscopy, the tip of a catheter is placed 1–2 cm from the ulcer. With the push of a button, the powder is then sprayed onto the bleeding ulcer using a canister pressurised with carbon dioxide. In a small series of 20 patients with actively bleeding peptic ulcers[51] it was successful in the control of bleeding in 19 of the 20 patients. In a European registry, 63 patients with non-variceal UGI haemorrhage received endoscopic haemostasis with Hemospray®.[52] Primary haemostasis was achieved in 85% but re-bleeding occurred in 15%. Comparative studies are required to determine the efficacy of this haemostatic powder, but the simplicity of its application certainly appeals to endoscopists.

'Over-the-scope clip (OTSC)'

The over-the-scope clip (OTSC) is a large-size clip that has the ability to grasp the full thickness of the wall of the gastrointestinal tract. It is attached to a cylindrical cap that can be mounted onto the tip of the endoscope. Before deployment of the OTSC, gentle suction is applied to allow approximation of the target lesion and the application cap. An additional anchoring device is also available for adequate tissue accumulation during clip application. Initial small case series using OTSC after failure of conventional endoscopic techniques showed a high rate of successful primary haemostasis (85.4–97%).[53,54] The exact role of OTSC in the management algorithm of UGI haemorrhage is yet to be defined.

Single versus combined methods

Soehendra introduced the concept of combination treatment that involved pre-injection with adrenaline allowing a clear view of the vessel, which then permitted targeted therapy using a second modality to induce thrombosis. In a meta-analysis of 16 studies and 1673 patients,[54] adding a second modality after adrenaline injection further reduces bleeding from 18.4% to 10.6% (odds ratio [OR] 0.53, 95% CI

0.4–0.69), emergency surgery from 11.3% to 7.6% (OR 0.64, 95% CI 0.46–0.90) and mortality from 5.1% to 2.6% (OR 0.51, 95% CI 0.31–0.84). In an independent meta-analysis of 22 studies (2472 patients),[56] dual therapy was shown to be superior to injection alone. However, treatment outcomes following combination treatments were not better than either mechanical or thermal therapy alone. Based on the above pooled analyses, adrenaline alone should no longer be considered an adequate treatment for bleeding peptic ulcers. The current evidence suggests that after initial adrenaline injection to stop bleeding, the vessel should either be clipped or thermocoagulated. In ulcers with a clear view to the vessel, direct clipping or thermocoagulation should yield similar results.

✓✓ Endoscopic therapy for bleeding peptic ulcers should use dual therapy or mechanical therapy rather than adrenaline injection alone in order to reduce the risk of re-bleeding.[55,56]

Limit of endoscopic therapy

As mentioned previously, the size of the bleeding artery is a critical determinant in the success of endoscopic treatment. In an ex vivo model, a vessel size of 2 mm could be consistently sealed by a 3.2-mm contact thermal device.[49] In clinical studies that examined factors that might predict failure of endoscopic treatment, ulcer size greater than 2 cm, ulcers on the lesser curvature of the stomach and ulcers on the superior or posterior wall of the bulbar duodenum were consistently identified as major risk factors for recurrent bleeding.[6] These ulcers erode into large artery complexes such as the left gastric and the gastroduodenal artery, which are usually sizeable. Consideration should therefore be given to prophylactic measures against recurrent bleeding in these ulcers judged endoscopically to be at significant risk of re-bleeding. This will be discussed later.

Second-look endoscopy

Many endoscopists re-scope their patients the next morning and re-treat ulcers that have remaining stigmata of bleeding. In a pooled analysis on the role of second-look endoscopy,[57] the authors found a modest 6.2% reduction in the absolute risk of re-bleeding (number needed to treat [NNT] to reduce one episode of recurrent bleeding). The NNT for reduction of re-bleeding and then surgery was 58 and 97, respectively. A subsequent meta-analysis and a third meta-analysis carried out for an international consensus conference confirmed that routine second-look endoscopy did reduce the incidence of re-bleeding, with the findings strongest in studies that included a high proportion of high-risk ulcers. However, in many of these trials, adrenaline injection alone was used and the role of second-look endoscopy following dual therapy or mechanical therapy remains unclear. In addition, adjuvant treatment with PPI therapy following endoscopic haemostasis can be expected to reduce the benefit of second-look endoscopy even further. With aggressive first endoscopic treatment, the risk of complications, especially perforation, with second treatment is substantial. There may, however, be a role for second-look endoscopy in selected high-risk patients, although this would require further studies and the most recent international consensus guidelines did not recommend this approach on the basis of the available evidence.[6,7]

✓✓ Second-look endoscopy is not indicated as a routine if primary optimum endoscopic haemostasis has been performed.[6,7]

Pharmacological management of bleeding peptic ulcers

Acid suppression

It has been shown in an in vitro study that platelet aggregation is dependent on plasma pH. It is thought that a pH of 6 is critical for clot stability and an intragastric pH above 4 inactivates stomach pepsin, preventing the digestion of clots.[22] To raise intragastric pH consistently above 6, a high-dose PPI given intravenously is required. The antisecretory effect of histamine receptor antagonists, due to tolerance, is less reliable than PPIs. In a study from the Hong Kong group,[58] a 3-day course of high-dose omeprazole infusion given after endoscopic therapy to bleeding ulcers reduced the rate of recurrent bleeding from 22.5% to 6.7% at day 30. The majority of recurrent bleeding occurred within the first 3 days of endoscopic treatment. This trial demonstrated the importance of early endoscopic triage, selecting only the high-risk ulcers for aggressive endoscopic treatment followed by profound acid suppression. In a Cochrane systematic review of 24 controlled trials and 4373 patients,[59] PPI treatment was shown to reduce re-bleeding (pooled rate of 10.6% vs 17.3%, OR 0.49, 95% CI 0.37–0.65) as well as surgery (pooled rate of 6.1% vs 9.3%, OR 0.61, 95% CI 0.48–0.78) when compared with placebo or histamine-2 receptor antagonist. There was no evidence of an effect on all-cause mortality, although when the analysis was confined to patients with high-risk stigmata (active bleeding or visible vessels) there was an associated reduction in mortality with PPI therapy. A multicentre study randomised study of 767 patients from 91 hospitals in 16 countries compared intravenous esomeprazole to placebo following successful endoscopic haemostasis.[60] Esomeprazole was associated with significant reductions in re-bleeding and endoscopic re-intervention rates and non-significant reductions in mortality and the need for surgery.

✓✓ High-dose intravenous PPI therapy (80 mg omeprazole followed by 8 mg/h for 72 hours) is recommended for patients with active bleeding or visible vessels at the time of endoscopy.[60]

Surgical management of bleeding peptic ulcers

The first UK audit revealed a mortality of 24% in those patients (251 of 2071, 12%) who required surgery for bleeding peptic ulcers.[1] However, in 78% of these patients, no previous attempt at endoscopic haemostasis had been made. In the most recent UK audit,[3] surgery was required in only 1.9% of patients but mortality remained high in this group (30%). The high mortality is probably related to a combination of an aged population with high incidence of comorbidity, as well as surgery being utilised as a salvage therapy after failed endoscopic haemostasis. Bleeding ulcers that fail endostasis are typically 'difficult' ulcers – larger chronic ulcers that erode into major arterial complexes. The decline in elective ulcer surgery also means the atrophy of surgical expertise in dealing with these ulcers. Ideally, a specialist team with an experienced upper gastrointestinal surgeon should be involved in managing these patients.

Although emergency ulcer surgery has diminished significantly, it has an important gatekeeping role in the management algorithm. The clear indication for surgery is loosely defined as 'failure of endoscopic treatment'. In a patient with massive bleeding that cannot be controlled by endoscopy, immediate surgery should obviously follow. However, the difficulty lies in deciding the exact role of surgery in ulcers judged to have a high risk of recurrent bleeding (e.g. >2 cm and at difficult locations), in which endoscopic haemostasis has been initially successful. Increasingly, angiographic embolisation is replacing emergency surgery in these circumstances.

Choice of surgical procedure for bleeding peptic ulcers

The choice of surgical procedure for bleeding peptic ulcers, when required, has not been adequately examined in the era following routine eradication of *Helicobacter pylori* and high-dose PPI therapy. Many surgeons maintain that under-running of ulcers alone combined with acid suppression using high-dose PPI therapy is safer than definitive surgery by either gastric resection or vagotomy. Two randomised studies looking at the different surgical procedures used to control bleeding peptic ulcers have been reported,[61,62] but both predate the PPI and routine *H. pylori* eradication era and therefore their results must now be considered totally unhelpful. However, it is of some interest to review the results as they do support the current 'minimalist' surgical approach. One of these studies was a multicentre one comparing minimal surgery (under-running the vessel or ulcer excision alone plus intravenous histamine receptor antagonist) versus definitive ulcer surgery (vagotomy and pyloroplasty or partial gastrectomy) in patients with gastric and duodenal ulcers.[61] The trial was terminated, however, because of the high rate of fatal re-bleeding in the minimal surgery group (6 of 62 vs 0 of 67, P = 0.02). The other trial was carried out by the French Association of Surgical Research and included only bleeding duodenal ulcers.[62] The patients in this trial were randomly assigned to either under-running plus vagotomy and drainage (58 patients) or partial gastrectomy (60 patients). Recurrent bleeding occurred in 10 of 58 patients (17%) after under-running and vagotomy. In the group assigned to partial gastrectomy, only two patients (3%) re-bled and both recovered without the need for further surgery. The rate of duodenal stump leak in the gastrectomy group was 8 in 60 (13%). When the results were analysed on an intention-to-treat basis, and those with duodenal leaks after re-operations for re-bleeding in the under-running and vagotomy group were included, duodenal leak rate was similar in both groups (7/58 vs 8/60). The mortality in both groups was similar (22% after vagotomy and 23% after gastrectomy). In the era of PPI therapy, the role of vagotomy has now completely disappeared. A proper ligation of the gastroduodenal artery complex including the right gastroepiploic and the transverse pancreatic branches is the key to avoid recurrent bleeding.

In a survey of UK surgeons reported in 2003, more than 80% of respondents rarely or never perform vagotomy for bleeding peptic ulcer.[63] Despite the absence of recent randomised evidence, surgeons have clearly adopted a more conservative approach based on the efficiency of PPI treatment and *H. pylori* eradication in the healing of peptic ulceration. With improvements in endoscopic therapy and the increasing age and comorbidity of patients, the risks of definitive ulcer surgery may outweigh any potential benefit from reduction in re-bleeding. For duodenal ulcer haemorrhage, longitudinal duodenotomy is carried out and control of bleeding achieved by digital pressure or by grasping the posterior duodenal wall in tissue forceps. If possible, preservation of the pylorus is preferred, but extension of the duodenotomy to include the pylorus may be required if access is difficult. Control of bleeding may be aided by mobilisation of the duodenum (Kocher's manoeuvre), allowing pressure to be applied posteriorly. In the majority of patients, simple under-running of the bleeding vessel can be achieved using 0 or 1/0 absorbable sutures above and below the bleeding point, ensuring deep enough tissue penetration to completely occlude the vessel. Due to the variation in anatomy of the gastroduodenal artery (**Fig. 13.5**), four or five sutures should be placed to ensure enduring haemostasis. The duodenotomy can then be closed longitudinally or converted into a formal pyloroplasty if the pylorus has been divided.

In cases of a massive duodenal ulcer, it may be necessary to exclude the ulcer, perform a distal gastrectomy and close the duodenum distal to the ulcer. This can be a challenging procedure in an elderly, unstable patient, particularly where duodenal thickening and scarring prevent safe stump closure. In this situation it is reasonable to attempt duodenal closure as best as possible, leaving large drains to the area, which will permit a leak to be managed non-operatively. Some surgeons advocate forming a controlled duodenal fistula by closing the duodenal stump around a Foley catheter or drain rather than attempting more complex closures. In either scenario, a Roux-en-Y partial gastrectomy is to be preferred to a Bilroth II reconstruction, as oral nutrition can then be maintained while still managing the duodenal stump leak.

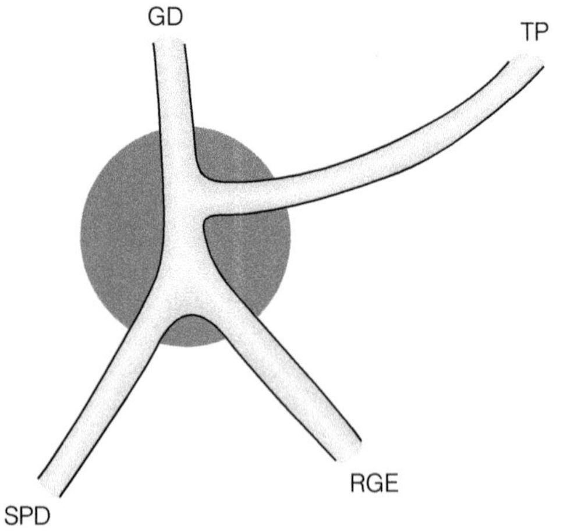

In the case of surgery for a bleeding gastric ulcer, the common scenario is for the ulcer to be located high on the lesser curve of stomach. Anterior gastrotomy, identification of the bleeding site and simple under-running of the ulcer (with biopsy of the ulcer edge) is the procedure of choice, and is also suitable for rare cases of Mallory–Weiss tear or a Dieulafoy lesion that does not respond to endoscopic management. In the rare case of a distal gastric ulcer that does not respond to endoscopic therapy, there may occasionally be a case for ulcer excision or even distal gastrectomy, but it is difficult to justify such a course of action in the hands of a non-specialist surgeon, and simple under-running should be the aim in the majority of patients.

✔ The choice of operation in patients with bleeding peptic ulcers who have failed endoscopic treatment should involve, where possible, simple under-running of the bleeding ulcer, without either vagotomy or gastric resection. Biopsies should be taken from the edge of a gastric ulcer.

Management of recurrent bleeding

The decision on management of patients who re-bleed after initial endoscopic control can be difficult. In a randomised study that compared endoscopic re-treatment to surgery in such patients,[64] endoscopic re-treatment secured bleeding again in 75% of patients. With intention-to-treat analysis, complications following endoscopic re-treatment were significantly less in patients when compared to those who received surgery. The gastrectomy rate in the surgery group was 50%. In a subgroup analysis, those re-bleeding with hypotensive shock from ulcers greater than 2 cm were less likely to respond to a repeat endoscopic treatment. It is therefore suggested that a selective approach can be used in re-bleeding patients. Patients with smaller ulcers and subtle signs of re-bleeding should undergo repeated endoscopic therapy, with surgery reserved for those who fail haemostasis. Patients with large chronic ulcers who are unstable should go straight to surgery without recourse to endoscopic re-treatment. Some of these patients identified at a 'high risk of re-bleeding' may, however, benefit from early 'elective/preemptive' surgery or (increasingly) angiographic embolisation.

Figure 13.5 • The anatomy of the gastroduodenal (GD) artery complex with confluence of several branches into the artery itself. RGE, right gastroepiploic; SPD, superior pancreatico-duodenal; TP, transverse pancreatic. Reproduced from Berne CJ, Rosoff L. Peptic ulcer perforation of the gastroduodenal artery complex: clinical features and operative control. Ann Surg 1969; 169: 141–4. With permission from Lippincott, Williams & Wilkins.

✅ Management of re-bleeding following successful endostasis will depend on the specific circumstances. Further endoscopic haemostasis may be appropriate for many patients,[64] but high-risk ulcers, particularly those where good endostasis was difficult to achieve at the first procedure, may be better considered for surgery or even transarterial angiographic embolisation.

The role of angiographic embolisation

Angiographic embolisation is an alternative rescue procedure for bleeding gastroduodenal ulcers and the technique has been in use for over two decades. In the 1980s there were reports of visceral infarcts[65,66] following angiographic embolisation, and its use was restricted to a small group of patients with refractory bleeding considered unfit for surgical intervention. With advances in embolisation techniques and specifically the use of coils and other agents (**Fig. 13.6**), the success rate in the control of bleeding has been reported to be between 64% and 91%, and mortality between 5% and 25%. A meta-analysis of these retrospective cohort studies, involving 423 patients of whom 182 had angiographic embolisation and 241 underwent surgery, demonstrated a significant failure rate with angiographic embolisation (relative risk of 1.82). However, no difference in mortality or need for re-intervention was found.[67] In one of the series from Hong Kong,[68] although overall mortality was similar, surgery was associated with a significantly higher complication rate. These findings suggest that angiographic embolisation may be at least as good an option as surgery in the management of refractory ulcer bleeding, especially in those patients at advanced age with high risk of surgical morbidities. The potential role of angiographic embolisation as a prophylactic measure following successful endostasis for patients considered at high risk of re-bleeding or death is also a subject worth investigating. Results of a randomised study

of 222 patients with high-risk peptic ulcers, of whom 109 were randomised to receive prophylactic angiographic embolisation were recently reported.[69] On per-protocol analysis, there was a trend of reduced re-bleeding after angiographic embolisation (4.4% vs 10.9%, $P = 0.08$). Subgroup analysis of those with ulcer size ≥ 1.5 cm demonstrated a significant risk reduction in re-bleeding after prophylactic angiographic embolisation (5.0% vs 23.2%, OR 0.173, 95% CI 0.036–0.850, $P = 0.027$). These large ulcers are likely to be associated with subserosal erosion to larger gastric supplying vessels, therefore embolisation of such feeding vessels would be particularly effective in securing adequate haemostasis.

✅ Angiographic embolisation should be considered in patients who re-bleed following surgery for bleeding peptic ulcers and as an alternative to surgery when endoscopic haemostasis has failed, provided appropriate facilities and expertise are available. This may be particularly useful in elderly patients with medical comorbidity. It should also be considered as a possible preemptive treatment option in high-risk surgical patients who are at high risk of re-bleeding after endostasis.

Helicobacter pylori eradication

A Cochrane review[70] concluded that *H. pylori* eradication was associated with a significant reduction in the risk of re-bleeding compared with no *H. pylori* eradication, from 20% to 2.9%. If antisecretory therapy was continued, the risk was 5.6%, still significantly higher than achieved with *H. pylori* eradication. The overall risk of re-bleeding following *H. pylori* eradication was less than 1% per year. While it was indeed a concern that in a UK review of consultant surgical behaviour reported in 2003, fewer than 60% routinely tested patients for *H. pylori* following treatment for complicated peptic ulcers,[63] the same is very unlikely to still be the case now.

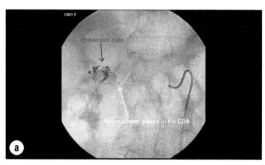
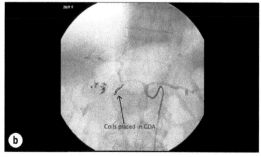

Figure 13.6 • **(a)** Active bleeding from the gastroduodenal artery complex during transfemoral angiography. **(b)** Coils were used to embolise the artery leading to cessation of bleeding.

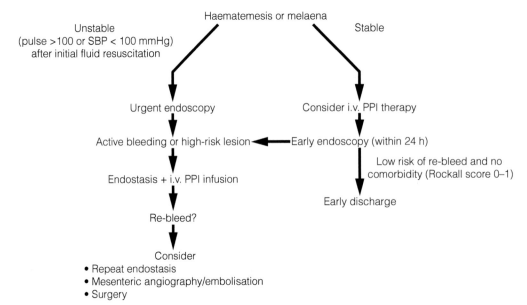

Figure 13.7 • Management algorithm. SBP, systolic blood pressure.

✅✅ Following treatment for bleeding duodenal ulcer, patients should be tested for *H. pylori* and receive eradication therapy where appropriate. Patients should have further testing to ensure successful eradication.[68]

Use of NSAIDs

In patients who continue to require NSAIDs, co-therapy with PPI reduces recurrence in peptic ulcers and bleeding. In these patients, *H. pylori* should first be tested and treated if confirmed. A randomised controlled trial compared the use of a traditional NSAID plus a PPI to COX-2 inhibitors and found that the rate of further ulcer complications is from 4-6% in 6 months.[71] A subsequent randomised trial combined the use of COX-2 inhibitor to PPI and compared them to the use of a COX-2 inhibitor alone.[72] At 1 year, the use of COX-2 inhibitor alone was associated

with a rate of 8.9% in recurrent bleeding. The risk of recurrent bleeding was completely abolished in those who received the combined treatment. COX-2 inhibitor plus PPI appears to offer the best protection to these high-risk patients.

Summary

The challenge posed by peptic ulcer bleeding has altered with the increasing age of the population at risk and the increasing availability of skilled therapeutic endoscopy. Failure of endoscopic haemostasis is increasingly uncommon but the surgical challenge presented by the elderly patient with refractory bleeding from a large ulcer is considerable. Successful management of UGI bleeding will involve the close cooperation of a multidisciplinary team, which will increasingly include interventional radiologists, aided by local protocols based on evidence-based best practice (**Fig. 13.7**).

Key points

- A risk stratification system should be utilised for all patients with UGI bleeding.
- Pre-endoscopy treatment with PPIs is recommended as it reduces the risk of active bleeding at the time of endoscopy and may reduce the need for endoscopic intervention.
- Early endoscopy should be performed on all patients with UGI bleeding/haemorrhage.
- Endoscopic therapy should be applied where there is active bleeding or a non-bleeding visible vessel in the ulcer base. Adherent clot should be removed and endoscopic therapy applied to the underlying vessel.

- Endoscopic therapy for bleeding peptic ulcers should involve use of dual therapy or mechanical therapy rather than adrenaline injection alone in order to reduce the risk of re-bleeding.
- High-dose intravenous PPI therapy (80 mg omeprazole followed by 8 mg/h for 72 h) is recommended for patients with active bleeding or visible vessels at the time of endoscopy.
- The choice of operation in patients with bleeding peptic ulcers who have failed endoscopic treatment should involve, where possible, simple under-running of the bleeding ulcer, without gastric resection unless it is not possible to close the duodenotomy. There is no longer any place for vagotomy.
- Management of re-bleeding following successful endoscopic haemostasis will depend on the specific circumstances. Further endoscopic haemostasis may be appropriate for many patients but those with high-risk ulcers, particularly where good endostasis was difficult to achieve at the first procedure, may be better considered for surgery or transarterial angiographic embolisation.
- Following treatment for bleeding duodenal ulcer, patients should be tested for *H. pylori* and receive eradication therapy where appropriate. Patients should have further testing to ensure successful eradication.

▶ Recommended videos:

- Hemoclip application for bleeding gastric ulcer – https://youtu.be/DwF_yyWWTvQ
- OTSC application for bleeding duodenal ulcer – https://youtu.be/VJTFxyFf654

🌐 Full references available at **http://expertconsult. inkling.com**

Key references

6. Barkun AN, Bardou M, Kuipers EJ, et al. International consensus recommendations on the management of patients with nonvariceal upper gastrointestinal bleeding. Ann Intern Med 2010;152(2):101–13. PMID: 20083829.

7. Gralnek IM, Dumonceau JM, Kuipers EJ, et al. Diagnosis and management of nonvariceal upper gastrointestinal hemorrhage: European Society of Gastrointestinal Endoscopy (ESGE) Guideline. Endoscopy 2015;47(10):a1–46. PMID: 26417980.
These are the most recently published comprehensive guidelines on the management of UGI bleeding based on studies published to date and include data from published and new meta-analyses as well as expert opinion.

23. Sreedharan A, Martin J, Leontiadis GI, et al. Proton pump inhibitor treatment initiated prior to endoscopic diagnosis in upper gastrointestinal bleeding. Cochrane Database Syst Rev 2010;(7). CD005415. PMID: 20614440.
This systematic review of randomised trials found no effect of pre-endoscopy PPI therapy on mortality but there was a significant reduction in active bleeding and the need for intervention at the time of endoscopy.

31. Spiegel BM, Vakil NB, Ofman JJ. Endoscopy for acute nonvariceal upper gastrointestinal tract hemorrhage: is sooner better? A systematic review. Arch Intern Med 2001;161(11):1393–404. PMID: 11386888.

This systematic review of 23 studies concluded that early endoscopy improved outcome in patients with UGI bleeding in all risk categories.

45. Kahi CJ, Jensen DM, Sung JJ, et al. Endoscopic therapy versus medical therapy for bleeding peptic ulcer with adherent clot: a meta-analysis. Gastroenterology 2005;129(3):855–62. PMID: 16143125.
A pooled analysis of several randomised studies demonstrated that recurrent bleeding is reduced following clot elevation and treatment to the underlying vessel when compared to medical therapy alone.

55. Calvet X, Vergara M, Brullet E, et al. Addition of a second endoscopic treatment following epinephrine injection improves outcome in high-risk bleeding ulcers. Gastroenterology 2004;126(2):441–50. PMID: 14762781.

56. Marmo R, Rotondano G, Piscopo R, et al. Dual therapy versus monotherapy in the endoscopic treatment of high-risk bleeding ulcers: a meta-analysis of controlled trials. Am J Gastroenterol 2007;102(2):279–89 quiz 469. PMID: 17311650.
These two meta-analyses provide compelling evidence that addition of a second endoscopic therapy is better than adrenaline alone.

59. Leontiadis GI, Sharma VK, Howden CW. Proton pump inhibitor treatment for acute peptic ulcer bleeding. Cochrane Database Syst Rev 2006;(1). CD002094. PMID: 16437441.
This Cochrane review of randomised trials found that high-dose PPI therapy reduced re-bleeding, surgery and mortality rates following endotherapy for high-risk ulcers.

70. Gisbert JP, Khorrami S, Carballo F, et al. Meta-analysis: Helicobacter pylori eradication therapy vs. antisecretory non-eradication therapy for the prevention of recurrent bleeding from peptic ulcer. Aliment Pharmacol Ther 2004;19(6):617–29. PMID: 15023164.
This Cochrane review included seven studies and a reduction in re-bleeding rates following *H. pylori* eradication compared with antisecretory therapy and no eradication.

14

Pancreatico-biliary emergencies

Saxon Connor

Introduction

Complications of gallstone disease are a major component of an acute general surgeon's workload and as a general surgeon it is important to be competent in the management of the common emergency presentations associated with calculous biliary disease. In addition, it is important to recognise the patients who will benefit from specialised hepatobiliary-pancreatic (HPB) surgical care and transferring them after appropriate initial management has been initiated. The aim of this chapter is to provide an evidence-based approach to the management of acute calculous biliary disease and acute pancreatitis (AP), appreciating that the management of severe or complicated acute and chronic pancreatitis, pancreatic tumours and pancreatico-biliary trauma are dealt with in the Hepatobiliary and Pancreatic Surgery volume of this Companion to Specialist Surgical Practice series (6th edition).

Gallstones

The cumulative incidence of gallstones in the Western world has been reported as 0.6% per year with an overall prevalence of 9% in females and 10% in males.[1,2] Risk factors identified include increasing age, female gender, obesity, elevated non-HDL cholesterol and gallbladder polyps.[1] Given the high prevalence within the population, complications of gallstone disease represent a significant workload for acute surgical services.[3] The underlying contributing aetiologies and risk factors are shown in **Fig. 14.1**. It is important to understand the differences in stone composition by geographical area or ethnicity. In parts of Asia

pigment stones predominate, while in Western countries mixed-type or cholesterol-based stones predominate. Although most gallstones remain asymptomatic, acute presentation can be divided into complications from local obstruction of the gallbladder due to cholecystolithiasis or migration of stones into the bile duct (choledocholithiasis) via the cystic duct. Occasionally, large stones can erode through the gallbladder into the duodenum through a cholecysto-duodenal fistula and present as gallstone ileus. This is discussed later here, and also in Chapter 15.

Cholecystolithiasis and associated complications

Clinical presentation and diagnosis

The underlying aetiology and pathogenesis of biliary colic and its sequelae are shown in **Figs 14.2** and **14.3**, respectively. The commonest presentation is right upper quadrant (RUQ) pain with nausea or vomiting.[4] Clinical examination reveals tenderness in the RUQ made worse by inspiration during palpation (Murphy's sign) and is associated with acute cholecystitis (AC).[3] Biliary colic usually has a short history without signs of clinical or biochemical inflammation. As the disease progresses RUQ peritoneal inflammation develops and systemic inflammation can be present either clinically or biochemically. Following development of a mucocele or empyema a RUQ mass may be palpable although this is uncommon.[4] The 2013 Tokyo Guidelines (TG-13) have defined a diagnosis of AC as requiring a combination of clinical and

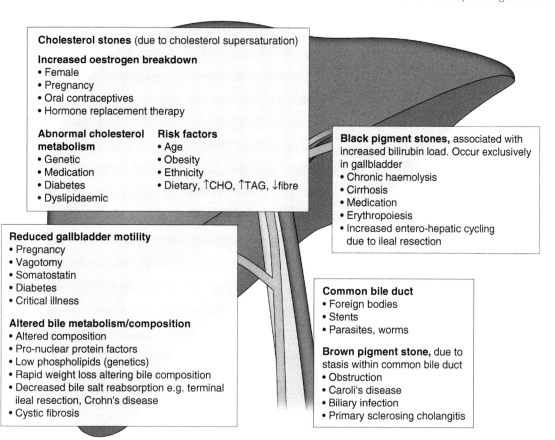

Cholesterol stones (due to cholesterol supersaturation)

Increased oestrogen breakdown
• Female
• Pregnancy
• Oral contraceptives
• Hormone replacement therapy

Abnormal cholesterol metabolism
• Genetic
• Medication
• Diabetes
• Dyslipidaemic

Risk factors
• Age
• Obesity
• Ethnicity
• Dietary, ↑CHO, ↑TAG, ↓fibre

Black pigment stones, associated with increased bilirubin load. Occur exclusively in gallbladder
• Chronic haemolysis
• Cirrhosis
• Medication
• Erythropoiesis
• Increased entero-hepatic cycling due to ileal resection

Reduced gallbladder motility
• Pregnancy
• Vagotomy
• Somatostatin
• Diabetes
• Critical illness

Altered bile metabolism/composition
• Altered composition
• Pro-nuclear protein factors
• Low phospholipids (genetics)
• Rapid weight loss altering bile composition
• Decreased bile salt reabsorption e.g. terminal ileal resection, Crohn's disease
• Cystic fibrosis

Common bile duct
• Foreign bodies
• Stents
• Parasites, worms

Brown pigment stone, due to stasis within common bile duct
• Obstruction
• Caroli's disease
• Biliary infection
• Primary sclerosing cholangitis

Figure 14.1 • Aetiology and risk factors for cholelithiasis and choledocholithiasis.

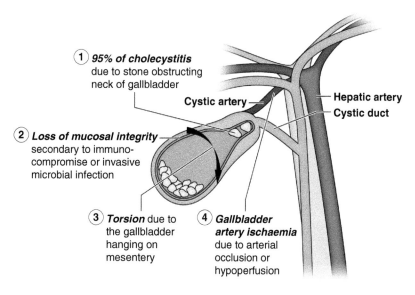

① *95% of cholecystitis* due to stone obstructing neck of gallbladder

Cystic artery —

— Hepatic artery
— Cystic duct

② *Loss of mucosal integrity* secondary to immuno-compromise or invasive microbial infection

③ *Torsion* due to the gallbladder hanging on mesentery

④ *Gallbladder artery ischaemia* due to arterial occlusion or hypoperfusion

Figure 14.2 • Aetiology of acute cholecystitis and its complications.

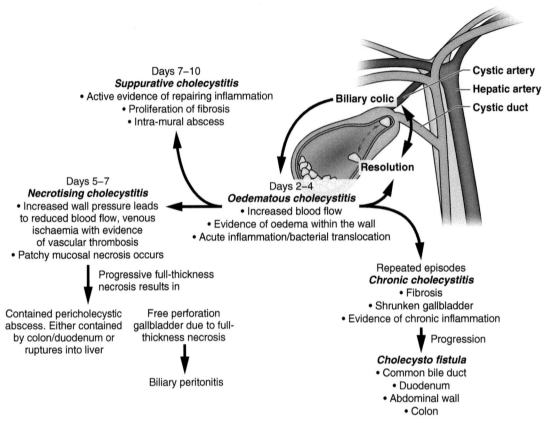

Figure 14.3 • Pathogenesis of acute cholecystitis and its complications.

imaging findings (Table 14.1).[4] The sensitivity and specificity of the TG-13 criteria for AC are 91% and 96%, respectively, although the World Society of Emergency Surgery (WSES) guidelines have questioned the generalisability of these figures given the limitations of the supporting study.[2,3] Ultrasound (US) is the investigation of choice given its availability, although the sensitivity and specificity in diagnosing AC are only moderate, with ranges reported between 50–88% and 80–88%, respectively.[4] In contrast, the sensitivity and specificity of US for detecting

cholecystolithiasis is 84% and 99%, respectively.[2] The key ultrasonographic findings of AC are a thickened gallbladder wall (>5 mm), pericholecystic fluid and tenderness on gallbladder compression (radiological Murphy's sign).[4] Ultrasonographic tenderness of the gallbladder has been shown to be highly specific (>90%) in confirming AC.[4] Although nuclear medicine imaging has been shown to have higher sensitivity and specificity than US it is not widely used given its limited availability and practicality.[2] More common alternative investigations include cross-sectional imaging such as computed tomography (CT) or magnetic resonance cholangio-pancreatography (MRCP). CT findings indicating AC include gallbladder distension, wall thickening, subserosal oedema, mucosal enhancement or pericholecystic fat stranding.[4] Other findings include transient focal enhancement of the liver adjacent to the gallbladder.[4] This is due to increased blood flow and subsequent venous drainage through the draining cholecystic veins.[4] Occasionally gas will be seen within the gallbladder or within a pericholecystic abscess in event of a contained perforation,[4] while loss of gallbladder wall enhancement suggests gangrenous cholecystitis.[5] However, CT definitions of definitive AC are scarce.[2] Similarly, magnetic resonance imaging

Table 14.1 • Tokyo Guidelines 2013 (TG-13) criteria for diagnosis of acute cholecystitis[4]

Local signs of inflammation	Murphy's sign, right upper quadrant tenderness, pain or mass
Systemic signs of inflammation	Fever, raised C-reactive protein or white blood count
Imaging findings	Characteristics of acute cholecystitis

Suspected diagnosis = one item each from local and systemic signs of inflammation.
Definitive diagnosis = one item from each category.

(MRI) is thought to be comparable with abdominal US in terms of accuracy but the data are based on only 59 patients and therefore the level of evidence is low.[2] The TG-13 guidelines classified the severity of AC into three grades in an aid to guide management.[4] Mild AC is defined as a healthy patient with no organ dysfunction or local complications. Moderate AC is defined as AC with local complications secondary to marked inflammation but without organ dysfunction. Local inflammatory complications include gangrenous or emphysematous cholecystitis, pericholecystic or hepatic abscess or biliary peritonitis. Markers of moderate AC include grossly elevated white count ($>18\,000/mm^3$), palpable mass or symptoms >72 hours. An elevated C-reactive protein (CRP) has also been associated with severe inflammation. In a large retrospective study ($n = 1843$) a CRP of $>67\,mg/L$ predicted moderate and severe histological changes of AC with a 96% sensitivity and 100% specificity with an AUC of 100%.[6] Severe AC is defined as AC with associated organ dysfunction.

Management of acute cholecystitis

The various choices of surgical management of AC have been proposed by the TG-13 severity classification.[7] In an evidence-based review of the literature, the authors of TG-13 recommend patients with mild AC undergo acute cholecystectomy.[7]

✓✓ Both TG-13 and WSES guidelines strongly recommend a laparoscopic approach for those with mild AC based on several randomised controlled trials (RCTs) and a meta-analysis showing better short-term outcomes with laparoscopic cholecystectomy (LC) as compared with open cholecystectomy.[2,7]

However, the authors of TG-13 acknowledge that a lot of these data were collated prior to enhanced recovery programmes and more recent data may suggest that the differences between the two techniques are less marked.[7] However, the point of surgical equipoise would appear to have passed and a laparoscopic approach is now widely regarded as the standard of care. The WSES guidelines[2] do, however, acknowledge the low level of evidence to support cholecystectomy *per se* as the standard of care and made the following statements with regard to other options in management of AC:

✓ • Antibiotics should be suggested as supportive care; they are effective in treating the first episode of AC but a high rate of relapse can be expected. Surgery is more effective than antibiotics alone in the treatment of AC.
• Surgery is superior to observation of AC in the clinical outcome and shows some cost-effectiveness

advantages due to the gallstone-related complications and to the high rate of readmission and surgery in the observation group.
• Since there are no reports on surgical gallstone removal (cholelithotomy) in the setting of AC, surgery in the form of cholecystectomy remains the main option.
• There is no role for gallstones dissolution, drugs or extracorporeal shock wave lithotripsy or a combination in the setting of AC.

✓ For patients with moderate AC and whose symptoms are of less than 72 hours duration, LC remains the treatment of choice in experienced centres.[7]

The authors of TG-13[7] rightly highlight some of the limitations of the data that were used to come to the above conclusion. Many of the trials had strict exclusion criteria based on patient comorbidity or complicated biliary disease and availability of surgeons skilled in laparoscopic cholecystectomy. Therefore when using this evidence to support such an approach it is important that these factors are considered. Surgeons should also be aware that although clinical and financial short-term outcomes are improved from an early approach to cholecystectomy, the trials and meta-analyses are underpowered to detect whether the incidence of bile duct injury (BDI) remains equivalent. A recently published population study from a region of Sweden showed that overall the risk of BDI doubled (OR [95%CI] 1.97 [1.05–3.72]) for those with AC.[8] However, when stratified by TG-13 severity there was no increase in BDI for those with mild AC (OR [95%CI] 0.96 [0.41–2.25]), twofold (OR [95%CI] 2.41 [1.21–4.80]) increase for moderate AC and an eightfold (OR [95%CI] 8.43 [0.97–72.9]) increase for those with severe AC.[8]

WSES guidelines also address the issue of timing and question the short cut-off period mentioned above. There is considerable heterogeneity with regard to definition of early versus late LC, especially with regard to duration of symptoms versus time from admission. The WSES guidelines[2] make the following statements:

• Early LC is preferable to delayed LC in patients with AC as long as it is completed within 10 days of onset of symptoms. Earlier surgery is associated with shorter hospital stay and fewer complications.
• LC should not be offered for patients beyond 10 days from the onset of symptoms unless symptoms suggestive of worsening peritonitis or sepsis warrant an emergency surgical intervention. In patients with more than 10 days of symptoms, delaying cholecystectomy for 45 days is better than immediate surgery.

For those with severe local inflammation or severe AC then urgent gallbladder drainage should be carried out.[7] In those with systemic organ dysfunction critical care will need to be provided. However, it is important to be aware that in the presence of bile peritonitis, gallbladder torsion, emphysematous, gangrenous or purulent cholecystitis, urgent surgery is required[7] (**Fig. 14.4**). The low threshold used to commence antibiotics within medical practice has come under sharp focus as the emergence of multidrug resistant organisms gathers pace. As part of TG-13 the need for antibiotics in treating AC was reviewed.[9] The authors acknowledge levels of evidence remain poor and the antibiotic of choice will be dependent on the local resistance patterns and severity of cholecystitis. Common organisms associated with biliary infections include *Escherichia coli*, *Klebsiella* spp., *Pseudomonas* spp., *Enteroccus* spp.[9] For mild AC, ampicillin with aminoglycoside-, cephalosporin-, carbapenem- or fluroquinolone-based therapies are all potential options.[9] Blood cultures are not required and antimicrobial therapy can be stopped once source control is achieved for mild AC.[2,9] For more severe infections bile and blood cultures are recommended.[9] Piperacillin may be used instead of ampicillin.[8] Duration should be extended for 4–7 days.[9] Of note, anti-anaerobic cover is only required if a biliary enteric anastomosis is present while vancomycin may need to be considered if concern over enterococci is suspected in those patients with severe infection or if hospital-acquired.[9] A recent systematic review of the true role of antibiotics in AC also failed to come to definitive conclusions given the low quality of evidence despite 12 randomised trials.[10]

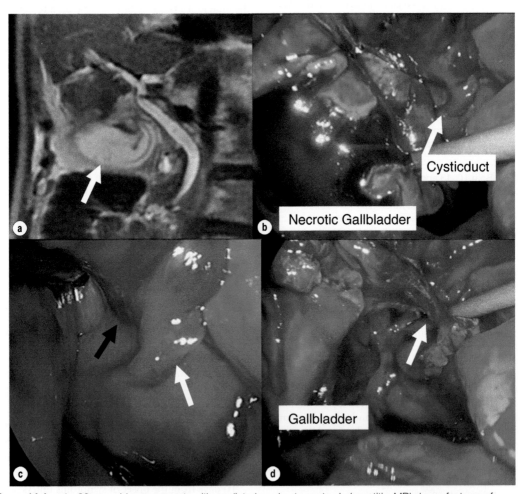

Figure 14.4 • An 86-year-old man presents with predicted moderate acute cholecystitis. MRI shows features of cholecystitis. Note transverse orientation of gallbladder on MRI (**a**, *white arrow*). At surgery a necrotic gallbladder secondary to acute torsion is observed (**b**). The cystic duct is twisted (**c**, *white arrow*) and a narrow mesentery can be seen (**c**, *black arrow*) and the gallbladder lies free of the hepatic surface. With the gallbladder detorted and small mesentery divided the gallbladder can be seen attached by cystic duct alone (**d**, *white arrow*). Caution is required given lack of classical landmarks to guide safe cholecystectomy.

In patients whose disease burden or comorbidity meets criteria for percutaneous drainage it is important to realise the importance of the effect of time to drainage on short- and long-term outcomes. Increasing time to drainage increases both inpatient and 30-day mortality,[11] while an increase in operative difficulty and conversion is seen in those patients in whom drainage is delayed >74 hours from onset of symptoms.[12]

✅ Early decision-making regarding surgery or percutaneous drainage is required for patients with AC.

TG-13 recommends percutaneous drainage for frail elderly patients or those who are critically ill, based on historical mortalities of 4% associated with acute cholecystectomy in these groups of patients.[13] However, the authors acknowledge that with modern perioperative care this could be challenged and a randomised trial is warranted.[13] Since publication of the TG-13 recommendations, Fuks et al.[5] retrospectively analysed 414 patients who had been enrolled in a non-related randomised trial and underwent laparoscopic cholecystectomy for mild or moderate AC of <5 days duration. Patients were divided by those greater than ($n=78$) or less than ($n=336$) 75 years of age. There was no difference in postoperative outcomes by age group, even in those greater than 85 years of age ($n=20$) or by performance status. There was only one death in the elderly group.

✅ Fuks et al. concluded that acute LC is safe in elderly patients with early mild or moderate AC.[5]

WSES guidelines simply acknowledge age >80 years as a risk factor for greater severity of disease, morbidity and mortality.[2]

✅ For those with severe AC, TG-13 recommends percutaneous transhepatic gallbladder drainage (PTGD) as the standard of care but acknowledges that both direct gallbladder puncture and endoscopic approaches have also been described.[13]

There is a lack of high-level evidence to strongly support one technique over another but one should be cognisant of the differing complication profiles. Direct gallbladder puncture is associated with an increased risk of dislodgement[11] and subsequent bile leak, while PTGD has an increased risk of hepatic haemorrhage. Endoscopic techniques remain the domain of highly specialised units and outcomes still need to be formally compared with PTGD.

Long-term management options of PTGD will depend on an individual's comorbidity. In those who return to good health, delayed cholecystectomy is the obvious solution. In a retrospective study of 46 patients in whom the indication appeared to be the severity of AC rather than patient comorbidity,

delaying elective surgery by >14 days resulted in a reduced incidence of severe adhesions (defined as the inability to establish the critical view of safety or remove gallbladder from liver bed) but did not alter operation time or rates of conversion. However, there was significant risk of type II error within this study.[12] In a study of 103 patients[11] with a median age of 80 years in whom PTGD was used, short- and long-term outcomes were described. The inpatient mortality was 13%, indicating the severity of disease and comorbidity in this group of patients. Eventually only 41% underwent cholecystectomy, with a 15% rate of conversion. One study describes 279 patients who presented with AC and underwent PTGD.[14] Of these patients, 3% died during initial illness and 31% underwent delayed cholecystectomy. Thus 184 (66%) patients were deemed symptom-free (drainage into cystic duct and no symptoms after clamping) at follow-up and underwent PTGD removal. At 1 year 60 (33%) patients had undergone LC and 5 (3%) patients had died and 17 (9%) patients developed recurrent AC. Factors associated with recurrent AC were complicated cholecystitis, antibiotic duration <10 days and percutaneous drainage >32 days.

Although specific complications, such as emphysematous cholecystitis, mucocele, empyema, pericholecystic abscesses and cholecysto-duodenal/colonic fistula can develop as sequelae of AC, acute LC remains the standard of care.[7] The exception is Mirizzi syndrome and gallstone ileus, both of which deserve further consideration as the management differs.

Mirizzi syndrome is due to a large gallstone compressing or eroding into the common bile duct (CBD). It usually presents with symptoms and biochemical signs of AC or cholangitis. If suspected on US (by the presence of intrahepatic duct dilatation with normal distal CBD and a large stone impacted in Hartmann's pouch) then further imaging in the form of MRCP and MRI liver should be considered. The MRI liver should be added as the differential will include gallbladder malignancy. Mirizzi syndrome has been classified into four types[15] based on absence (type 1) or presence of a fistula (types 2–4). Types 2–4 are split by degree of erosion of circumference of the bile duct: <1/3, <2/3 or complete destruction, respectively.[15] The key concept here is that there is a high probability that the hepatobiliary triangle has been obliterated due to fibrosis and so the surgeon must be aware that pursing the critical view of safety and complete cholecystectomy may be dangerous and lead to a BDI. The surgeon should consider a preoperative MRCP to provide a detailed preoperative road map of the biliary and vascular anatomy so that a planned approach to the hepatobiliary triangle can be formulated. In type 1 a subtotal cholecystectomy can be performed, while types 2–4 are likely to require a hepatico-jejunostomy. Thus referral to a hepatobiliary surgeon is recommended for the more advanced disease, especially if malignancy cannot be excluded. In a recent study by Kumar et al. of 169 patients with Mirizzi syndrome, the incidence was 2.1% of all cholecystectomies.[16] Median duration of symptoms was 8 months. Presentation by type 1–4 was 20%, 57%, 17%, 6%, respectively.[16] Of concern, only 32% of patients were diagnosed preoperatively. Important coexistent findings were 41% incidence of CBD stones, 14% incidence of coexisting fistula into adjacent hollow organs, 33% incidence of xanthalomatous cholecystitis and 5% incidence of gallbladder cancer.[16] Those patients with Mirizzi type 2–3 that were treated without hepatico-jejunostomy had higher rates of bile leak and a non-significant doubling of morbidity.[16]

✅ The study by Kumar et al. concluded in favour of hepatico-jejunostomy for type 2–3 Mirizzi's syndrome.[16]

Gallstone ileus occurs after formation of a cholecysto-duodenal fistula and migration of a large stone (>2 cm) into the small-bowel lumen.[17] The incidence is 0.3–0.5% of patients with cholelithiasis and is more common in female elderly patients.[17] Because the distal ileum is the narrowest part of the gastrointestinal tract, presentation is usually in the form of a small bowel obstruction although proximal obstruction at the duodenal bulb can occur (Bouveret syndrome). Radiological signs include pneumobilia and possibly a luminal calcified mass at the point of obstruction. Management of the bowel obstruction is not controversial, with enterotomy and stone extraction the standard approach. However, it is worth noting that if possible the stone should be milked proximally to perform an enterotomy as the obstruction point is likely to be oedematous and potentially partially ischaemic secondary to pressure from the offending stone. A thorough search for upstream stones should be conducted. In the acute setting nothing further requires to be done to the gallbladder or cholecysto-duodenal fistula. More recently a single definitive procedure has been advocated given high reported rates of recurrence and cholangitis.[17] However, most recommendations are based on small patient series.[17] In the frail, elderly or unstable patient at high risk of perioperative mortality a simple enterolithotomy should be performed. Definitive simultaneous or metachronous management of the gallbladder may be determined by symptoms and presence or absence of cholecystolithiasis or choledocholithiasis. In those with a clear CBD and empty gallbladder spontaneous closure of the fistula may occur. Endoscopic management of choledocholithiasis by stone extraction with or without temporary covered stenting of a patent cystic duct may be appropriate for those with choledocholithiasis only. In those patients with persistent cholecystolithiasis the gallbladder is likely to be shrunken and therefore formal dissection

of the hepatobiliary triangle may be hazardous. Simply opening the fundus, extracting the stones, performing a cholangiogram (to ensure a clear CBD), closing the cystic duct if patent from within and then closing the duodenal fistula either primarily or with an omental patch would be the standard of care. Failure to assess the common duct may result in cholangitis once the fistula is closed if distal CBD obstruction remains.

Patient-specific factors for consideration in acute cholecystitis

There is an increased incidence of gallstones in patients with cirrhosis and such patients are at risk of increased morbidity and mortality from liver failure in the postoperative period, which is proportional to the severity of the liver disease.[2] In addition, in patients with portal hypertension, cholecystectomy exposes the patient to significant risk of haemorrhage. Therefore consideration should be given to referring patients with cirrhosis and AC to HPB units familiar with the perioperative management of liver failure and techniques associated with minimising bleeding during cholecystectomy, including laparoscopic subtotal cholecystectomy.

During pregnancy up to 0.8% of patients will present with symptomatic gallstone disease.[18] Two recent systematic reviews and meta-analyses have reported no increased risk of preterm labour (3.8%) or fetal mortality (1.5%) associated with cholecystectomy and improved maternal and fetal outcomes with LC as compared to open cholecystectomy.[18,19] The data were unable to be analysed by presentation type, comorbidity or by gestational age.

✅ In a well patient with non-complex disease, LC in 1st and 2nd trimester would appear to be treatment of choice.[18,19]

Clearly, involvement and support of obstetric, neonatal teams and ensuring the patient is well-informed of the risks of all treatment options is a must.

Investigation for suspected choledocholithiasis in acute cholecystitis

Although the incidence of choledocholithiasis is lower in AC than other presentations of gallstone disease it still can be present in 5–15% of patients.[2] Normal liver function tests (LFTs) have been shown to have a very high negative predictive value (97%); however, an accurate positive biochemical predictor remains elusive.[2] The strongest preoperative predictor is evidence of CBD stones in AC by abdominal US.[2] The surgeon's individual opinion and preference with regard to intraoperative cholangiography (routine vs other) and managing CBD stones will determine the algorithm for subsequent investigation (see below).

Acalculous acute cholecystitis

This is defined as AC without the presence of gallstones and is said to contribute 14% of all patients presenting with AC.[20] The aetiology is not well understood but thought to be due to a combination of change in bile salt composition, loss of mucosal integrity and microcirculatory disturbances.[20] Patients tend to be older with associated complications of atherosclerosis.[19] Although traditionally associated with critically ill patients, up to 88% of patients will present from the community.[20] Importantly, there are higher rates of gangrenous cholecystitis (31%) as compared to gallstone-induced AC (6%).[21] For those who are fit enough for surgery LC is the treatment of choice, otherwise PGTD is recommended.[21]

> ✔ Importantly, the recurrence rates following conservative treatment are less than 2% so delayed cholecystectomy is not usually indicated once the acute episode has settled.[21]

Choledocholithiasis and associated complications

Gallstones can migrate into the bile duct via the cystic duct or form within the CBD primarily (primary duct stones). Primary duct stones may form in response to foreign bodies (including parasitic infection), stasis or abnormal bile metabolism. In Western populations part of the traditional definition for a primary duct stone was for the gallbladder to be absent for >2 years although this is not relevant when associated with foreign bodies or Asiatic cholangio-hepatitis. Complications of CBD stones usually result from biliary obstruction leading to acute bacterial cholangitis (ABC) or AP, which occasionally may coexist.

The incidence of CBD stones in the presence of cholelithiasis is between 5% and 20%.[2] Many are found incidentally while others cause transient obstruction resulting in disordered liver function or clinical jaundice. Although RUQ or back pain may be present it is not always a symptom.[22] The level of bilirubin may fluctuate as the obstruction can be transient and does not tend to be as high (<180 μmol/L) or as unrelenting as that seen with malignancy.[22] The alkaline phosphatase (ALP) and aspartate aminotransferase (AST) tend to rise proportionally (2× upper limit normal) with stone disease, while ALP is more markedly raised (4× upper limit of normal) in those with malignant obstruction.[22] The AST rise in stone disease is associated with biliary pain and can rise and fall very quickly at a rate much greater than seen with ALP.[22] Normal LFTs have a high negative predictive value (>95%) for CBD stones.[2,23] While elevated LFTs may increase the clinical suspicion of underlying choledocholithiasis, they lack clinically useful levels of sensitivity or specificity to proceed directly to therapeutic intervention (endoscopic retrograde cholangiopancreatography [ERCP] or surgery) without further diagnostic confirmation.

Abdominal US does not accurately assess for the presence or absence of CBD stones. At a median pre-test probability of 41% for a CBD stone the post-test probability (95% CI) associated with a positive US was 0.85 (0.75–0.91) and a negative US was 0.17 (0.08–33).[23] Appreciating how these figures will change with the pre-test probability based on a selected group of patients is an important consideration with regard to utility and cost-effectiveness of further investigations. Further radiological investigation of the CBD can be performed either metachronously or synchronously with regard to cholecystectomy depending on the clinical situation. In the metachronous scenario (pre- or post-cholecystectomy) MRCP or endoscopic ultrasound (EUS) have replaced ERCP as the investigation of choice given the risks associated with diagnostic ERCP.

> ✔✔ Both MRCP and EUS have been shown to be highly accurate in the assessment of the presence or absence of CBD stones. At a median pre-test probability of 41% the post-test probabilities associated with positive or negative results have been reported between 0.94–0.96 and 0.03–0.05, respectively.[24] Therefore either can be used depending on availability and individual patient preference or coexisting contraindications.

However, resource utilisation is often an important consideration for such specialist tests. Therefore in the precholecystectomy setting one has to consider whether a synchronous approach is actually as effective which has been a subject of much debate, especially when combined with the subsequent management of synchronous cholecysto- and choledocholithiasis. At a median pre-test probability of 35% for a CBD stone the post-test probability of a positive and negative intraoperative cholangiogram has been shown to be 0.98 and 0.01, respectively.[25] Therefore pre- and intraoperative investigations can be considered equivalent tests and their place in the management of patients with suspected CBD stones will be dependent on the planned management strategy (see below). Although laparoscopic ultrasonographic assessment of the CBD has long been available its use has generally been restricted to those surgeons with a strong HPB interest. However, with the increasing availability of the hardware this may change, particularly because a recent cost analysis supports laparoscopic US use over intraoperative cholangiography or expectant management in those with silent CBD stones and an underlying prevalence of CBD stones >3%.[26] Fluorescent intraoperative cholangiography has been described as a potential method of reducing bile duct injuries by demonstrating the anatomy in real time;

however, there are no data regarding its effectiveness in detecting CBD stones.

Management of choledocholithiasis

To optimise the management of any condition it is important to understand the natural history. For patients with 'silent' or incidental stones the seminal and definitive paper is by Collins et al.[26] A total of 962 patients with cholelithiasis and no current suspicion of CBD stone (defined as normal CBD on US, absence of jaundice) underwent LC and successful intraoperative cholangiogram. Acute patients and those with altered LFTs or a history of AP were included. At the completion of the cholangiogram the catheter was left in situ with no attempt to manage the CBD stones if detected. A follow-up cholangiogram at 48 hours and 6 weeks was performed. Of the 962 patients 46 (4.7%) were found to have filling defects. At 48 hours 12 patients had normal cholangiograms (these patients were interpreted as having false-positive intraoperative cholangiogram). At 6 weeks 12 of the 34 patients with an abnormal cholangiogram at 48 hours had a normal cholangiogram. None of these 12 patients had complications from passage of stones and only 2 described an episode of pain. Twenty of the remaining 22 patients underwent successful ERCP while 2 did not and neither developed any symptoms after 5 years of follow-up. This study highlighted several important points. Although increasing age and raised ALP predicted the presence of CBD stones, no factors (including bile duct size or number of stones) predicted those CBD stones that were more likely to pass spontaneously. The data also showed that in a group of patients without complications of CBD stones, the potential long-term morbidity is low and likely less than 2.5%, which was at least <50% of those diagnosed if systemically looked for. This needs to be considered against the morbidity of intervention either surgically or endoscopically. Expectant management has been recommended if the pre-test probability of a CBD stone is <3% or less than ideal intraoperative imaging can be performed.[27]

For those patients with CBD stones that warrant intervention then the options can be divided as surgical or endoscopic. Either procedures may be performed metachronously or synchronously with regard to cholecystectomy. There has been considerable literature dedicated to whether an endoscopic or laparoscopic approach is superior. A systematic review was published in 2013 examining all possible combinations (one-stage or two-stage, endoscopic or laparoscopic approaches and open surgery).[28] This review included 16 randomised controlled trials with a total of 1758 patients. The key findings were that laparoscopic and endoscopic options appeared equivalent in terms of short-term outcomes. Although the authors reported open CBD exploration having lower rates of retained stones than ERCP, these data

were gathered early in the endoscopic era. However, the authors noted there were significant systematic and random errors associated with the available data and therefore further trials were warranted with those factors controlled.

✅ At this point it would seem reasonable that the treatment option be tailored by the individual patient (duct size, stone size or position, difficulties of endoscopic or laparoscopic access, gallbladder in situ) and service (such as local skillset and availability of endoscopic or laparoscopic equipment) factors (**Fig. 14.5**).

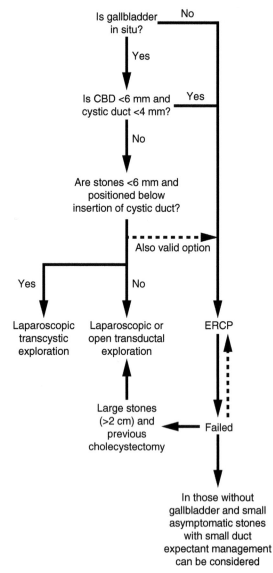

Figure 14.5 • Possible algorithm for management of common bile duct (CBD) stones.

Long-term outcomes after laparoscopic common bile duct exploration have shown recurrence rates to be low (2%) and importantly even in a series where a transverse choledochotomy and T tube were used routinely, no biliary strictures were reported (46 patients, median follow-up of 17 years).[29] Long-term outcomes following ERCP and sphincterotomy have raised the possibility of association with cholangiocarcinoma but the level of evidence is poor.[30] However, because of this potential association some authors have recommended caution in using this approach in very young patients.[30]

Acute bacterial cholangitis

Similarly to AC, the definition, investigation and management of acute bacterial cholangitis (ABC) has been subjected to expert systematic review.[9,31–34] It has been defined as acute inflammation and infection of the bile duct and requires a combination of biliary obstruction and the presence of bacteria. Therefore ABC as a presentation of malignancy is unusual in the absence of biliary tree instrumentation. The obstruction generates increased intraductal pressure allowing translocation of bacteria and toxins into the venous or lymphatic systems. The incidence of ABC in those with asymptomatic gallstones is 0.3–1.6% at 5–10 years.[31] The diagnosis of ABC has been refined (Table 14.2). In revising the diagnosis the authors acknowledged the high specificity associated with the traditional diagnosis of Charcot's triad but its low sensitivity prohibited it as a useful definition.[32] Validation studies have shown a 92% sensitivity and 78% specificity with the described diagnostic criteria.[32] The importance of the inflammatory component is that it is rarely seen in acute hepatitis but if there is concern virology and serology should be performed.[31] In terms of diagnostic imaging, although US is inaccurate in detecting the underlying aetiology, it will confirm biliary dilatation (or differential diagnoses such as hepatic abscess or AC), providing evidence to support the diagnosis and facilitating early intervention, particularly in those patients with moderate or severe ABC. Both MRI and CT will show evidence of periportal inflammation and altered perfusion within hepatic parenchyma due to reduced portal venous flow and increased hepatic arterial flow. MRI is more useful

for determining aetiology.[32] ABC can be graded into three grades of severity: severe (any associated organ dysfunction, including haematological (INR > 1.5, platelets < 100 000/mm³), moderate (any two of the following: white cell count <4 or >12×10³/mm³, temperature >39°C, age >74 years, bilirubin >85 μmol/L, albumin <0.7×lower limit of normal), and mild without any of the above.[32]

> ✔✔ The recommended treatment is antibiotics for all grades of severity with the addition of urgent biliary drainage in those classified with moderate or severe disease.[33]

Importantly, reassessment of severity should be performed regularly as patients can deteriorate rapidly. Subsequent to the publication of TG-13 guidelines, it has been shown that an elevated procalcitonin is highly accurate in predicting those with bacteraemia and therefore can identify those who would benefit from emergency biliary drainage.[35] If this can be confirmed in further studies it may simplify the grading and subsequent management of ABC. In those with severe disease the principles and interventions associated with managing severe sepsis should be included in the treatment algorithm.[33] Antibiotics of choice are similar to those discussed for management of AC (see preceding section) and are dependent on local patterns of resistance.[9] Once source control is achieved then a short course of 4–7 days is indicated. In those patients with bacteria associated with bacterial endocarditis, a 2-week course is recommended, but the level of evidence to support the practice of ongoing antibiotics after source control remains poor.[9]

> ✔ In terms of biliary drainage, endoscopic drainage has been recommended; however, in a proportion of patients percutaneous transhepatic biliary drainage (PTBD) will be required when drainage via the papilla cannot be obtained.[34] Surgical drainage has been associated with a higher mortality and should be reserved when all other options have been explored. In performing an endoscopic approach the overriding aim is to achieve drainage with the use of an endoscopic stent or nasobiliary drain.[34]

Table 14.2 • Tokyo Guidelines 2013 (TG-13) criteria for diagnosis of acute cholangitis[32]

Systemic signs of inflammation	T > 38°C and/or shaking/chills
	Abnormal white count (<4,or >10/mL) or raised C-reactive protein (>10 mg/L)
Biochemical evidence of cholestasis	Bilirubin >34 μmol/L or
	Raised (>1.5xupper limit normal) liver function tests
Imaging findings	Biliary dilatation or evidence of aetiology (e.g. stones, stricture, stent)

Suspected diagnosis = one item systemic signs of inflammation and one from either biochemistry or imaging.
Definitive diagnosis = one item from each category.

Whether the underlying aetiology is treated definitively will be dependent on the clinical stability of the patient and the skill of the endoscopist. Newer treatment options include the use of endoscopic ultrasound to access the biliary tree in event of failure to cannulate the papilla. Mortality associated with cholangitis has steadily decreased and is now <2% in most reported series.[32]

Acute pancreatitis

Acute pancreatitis (AP) is a common reason for patients to present to acute general surgical services, with an underlying incidence of 13–45/100 000 population.[36] It ranges from a mild self-limiting illness to a fulminant and rapidly fatal disease that affects all age groups. Its aetiology is multifactorial with alcohol (ETOH) and gallstones being the commonest causes, although hypertriglyceridaemia is now reported to account for 9% of AP.[37] The pathophysiology of AP is complex and there is a lack of a unifying theory, possibly due to the multifactorial aetiology.[38] Although a detailed description of the underlying pathophysiology for each aetiology is beyond the remit of this chapter, it is important for the clinician to have an understanding of the time-dependent changes that determine the severity of the disease. It is thought that the aetiological stimulus results in intracellular activation of pancreatic enzymes such as trypsin.[38] This then triggers a local inflammatory response resulting in release of both pro- and anti-inflammatory mediators and chemokines.[38] This results in microcirculatory disturbance including increased capillary permeability and microcirculatory intravascular coagulation and ischaemia.[39] If the inflammatory response is confined to a local response the outcome is mild pancreatitis and usually resolves within a week without systemic or local complications.[38] However, if a systemic inflammatory response (SIRS) is mounted then moderate or severe pancreatitis ensues. If sustained, multi-organ dysfunction will develop.[38] After a week to 10 days there is transition through to a compensatory response syndrome.[38] In this phase there is downregulation of the immune system thus explaining why pancreatic infection peaks in weeks 2–5 after onset.[38] Understanding this cascade of events is important so that early accurate recognition of stratification into those with mild and severe disease can occur. This serves to ensure timely and appropriate treatment for those patients with mild disease but also prompt consideration and recognition of the likely time-dependent complications in those patients with severe disease. This facilitates optimal and timely intervention which may include transfer to a specialised HPB unit for those patients with severe disease.

Although there is an extensive guideline-based literature, much is of variable quality. In 2013 the International Association of Pancreatology (IAP) and the American Pancreatic Association (APA) collaborated to produce a systematic and evidence-based guideline compiled by a group of international multidisciplinary experts.[36] This highly readable document provides the best available evidence-based summary of the literature and forms the basis for many of the recommendations in this section.

AP has been defined as requiring two of three of the following criteria: clinical (upper abdominal pain), biochemical (3× upper limit of normal lipase or amylase), imaging (ultrasound, CT, MRI).[36] It is important to note, however, that routine cross-sectional imaging is not usually required for the diagnosis particularly in those with mild disease. It should be used only in the initial phase if there is diagnostic uncertainty or there has been a prolonged period prior to presentation, in which case the enzyme rise may have passed.[36] Although other biochemical markers have been described, their use has been limited by availability.[38]

Initial assessment, investigations and management

Initial investigations are structured around predicting severity or identifying aetiologies or complications that require urgent intervention. In those with a SIRS response and obstructive LFTs with or without jaundice, or a dilated bile duct with evidence of gallstones on abdominal US, coexisting cholangitis (Table 14.2) can be diagnosed.

✅✅ For patients with suspected coexisting cholangitis, antibiotics should be commenced and urgent ERCP should be performed.[36]

✅✅ ERCP is not indicated for those patients with non-biliary pancreatitis or mild biliary pancreatitis without cholangitis.[36]

✅ In those with predicted severe biliary pancreatitis and cholestasis without cholangitis a prospective, multicentre study[40] has shown early ERCP (within 72 hours) to be associated with a reduction in the incidence of complications (54% vs 25%, $P = 0.020$) and patients with >30% necrosis (31% vs 8%, $P = 0.010$).

Serum triglycerides (TAG) should be measured, especially in those with lipaemic specimens. Although mildly elevated TAG are commonly associated with AP, grossly elevated levels (>1000 mg/dL) indicate hypertriglyceridaemia as an aetiology.[37] However, it should be acknowledged there is no uniformly accepted cut-off to act as a definition.[37] Early diagnosis of hypertriglyceride-induced pancreatitis is important as rapid reduction in serum TAG levels can be achieved with a combination of insulin infusion, anti-hyperlipidaemic medication, dietary manipulation and plasmapheresis.[37] Plasmapheresis has been shown to reduce abdominal pain and APACHE II scores but not morbidity or mortality, although the possibility of a type II error exists.[37] These patients are complex in terms of physiology, nutritional requirements and management and so a multidisciplinary approach with lipid and transfusion specialists, interventional radiologists and dietitians is required. Randomised data are, however, lacking about the true effect of any of these interventions.

Although abdominal US is the mainstay for the diagnosis of a biliary aetiology, an ALT >150 within 48 hours has been shown to have a positive predictive value of a biliary aetiology of >85%.[36]

Taking a history for ETOH intake, recent ERCP, trauma and family history of pancreatitis are also important but do not necessarily change immediate management other than management of ETOH withdrawal and vitamin supplementation.

There have been multiple proposed predictors of severity; however, the IAP/APA guidelines have taken a pragmatic approach in using SIRS criteria (Table 14.3) given its ease of use, early applicability and widespread uptake.[36]

It is important to emphasise that early cross-sectional imaging is not required in patients where the diagnosis of AP is confirmed. For those with predicted severe disease early CT does not alter management or improve prediction of outcome and may in fact be harmful due to contrast toxicity to both the pancreas and kidneys. Exceptions to this include those patients in whom bowel ischaemia or hollow viscera perforation is suspected. It has been estimated that it takes 72 hours for pancreatic necrosis to become radiologically evident, although in the future CT perfusion scans may allow earlier detection.

✅ Contrast-enhanced (arterial and portal venous phase) CT can be delayed at least for 96 hours after onset of symptoms of AP.[36]

Early management of severe disease

Fluid management

Appropriate resuscitation has come into focus in recent times as an increased understanding of the iatrogenic harm caused by over-resuscitation through the enhanced recovery literature. It is becoming clearer that there exists a 'Goldilocks zone' for resuscitation in AP. It is important to keep in mind the reason for fluid resuscitation in AP. The aim is restore and maintain the macrocirculation but also restore the microcirculation in terms of stabilising the capillary permeability, reducing the inflammatory reaction and sustaining the intestinal barrier function.[39] The purpose is to restore homeostasis with the hope of minimising the development of pancreatic necrosis. However, it should be realised that many of the microcirculatory changes are time-dependent and irreversible changes may have occurred by the time the patient presents.[39] The effect of time to presentation on the outcome of fluid resuscitation has not been well studied within the literature.

✅✅ Currently it is recommended that an isotonic semi-balanced crystalloid solution (Ringer's lactate or Hartmann's solutions) rather than normal saline or colloid be used for the initial resuscitation.[36]

This recommendation is based on evidence that balanced crystalloid solutions reduce the incidence of SIRS as compared to normal saline while colloid solutions have been associated with increased mortality in patients with severe sepsis.[36] Yet there may be some evidence that AP differs from sepsis and that colloids may help protect and stabilise the microcirculation by preventing inflammatory mediators reaching the acinus.[39] Some authors would suggest limited use of colloids to those patients with AP and low haematocrit (<25% or albumin <20g/L).[39] There is now also some evidence to support use of hypertonic saline.[39] Clearly this area is fraught with confounding factors and further evidence will be required.

✅✅ The infusion rate is important, with goal-directed therapy of 5–10 mL/kg/hr to be used until resuscitation goals are met. This has been shown to reduce incidence of SIRS, need for mechanical ventilation, sepsis and mortality as compared to higher (10–15 mL/kg/hr) rates of resuscitation.[36]

Table 14.3 • Definitions that predict severity in acute pancreatitis based on variables contributing to systemic inflammatory response syndrome[36]

Variable	Criteria
Temperature	<36°C or >38°C
Heart rate	>90/min
Respiratory rate	>20/min
White blood cell count	<4×10⁹/L or >12×10⁹/L or 10% bands

Terminology	Criteria	Outcome
SIRS	2 or more of above criteria	
Transient SIRS	SIRS <48 hours	25% mortality
Persistent SIRS	SIRS >48 hours	8% mortality

The evidence for the proposed resuscitation goals as the ideal physiological endpoints to resuscitation remains poor. It has been recommended that the non-invasive goals be defined as heart rate <120/min, mean arterial pressure 65–85 mmHg, urine output 0.5–1 mL/kg/hr and maintain haematocrit between 35% and 44%, while invasive measures include stroke volume variation.[36] This concept is not, however, easy to implement in the ward setting as traditional intravenous fluid prescribing is based on time not by response. Therefore new prescribing algorithms are required (Fig. 14.6).

Epidural analgesia may also have an important role to play in helping improve pancreatic perfusion but further trials are needed.[41]

Nutrition

The need for nutritional support is widely adopted as the standard of care for those with established severe acute pancreatitis and is covered in detail within the Hepatobiliary and Pancreatic Surgery volume of this series. However, the aim of this section is to discuss the role of early feeding in both mild and severe pancreatitis. Historically, non-randomised data had suggested that early (<48 hours from admission) nasoenteric feeding could reduce infectious complications and mortality.[42] This concept has now been tested in two randomised controlled trials.[42,43] The first study selected patients within 24 hours of

admission with APACHE II score ≥6 and AP. Patients were randomised to nil by mouth (NBM) or enteral nutrition (EN) with the primary endpoint being a reduction in incidence of persistent (>48 hours) SIRS. The trial was powered to detect a reduction in SIRS incidence of 60–40% and enrolled 214 patients. The incidence of persistent SIRS at 48 hours was 45% in the EN group versus 48% in the NBM group ($P=0.681$). None of the secondary outcome measures of severity of inflammation, local pancreatic specific complications, organ failure or mortality showed a reduction in the treatment arm, although the possibility of type II error existed. It is worth noting that prophylactic antibiotics were used in this trial and the patients in the NBM group received higher volumes of IV fluid resuscitation. No measure of time from onset of symptoms was provided. The low APACHE II score for admission into the trial may have diluted any potential difference for those with severe AP. However sub-group analysis did not alter the outcomes although it would seem that the trial may be underpowered in that regard. The second RCT by the Dutch pancreatitis study group enrolled 208 patients to either early nasoenteric feeding (within 24 hours of admission) versus NBM for 72 hours (unless patients requested food) and then oral diet with nasoenteric supplementation if required. The primary endpoint was a composite of major infection or death within 6 months. Inclusion

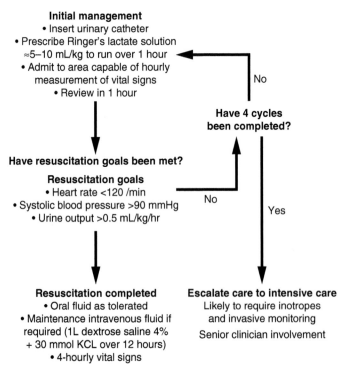

Initial management
- Insert urinary catheter
- Prescribe Ringer's lactate solution ≈5–10 mL/kg to run over 1 hour
- Admit to area capable of hourly measurement of vital signs
- Review in 1 hour

No

Have 4 cycles been completed?

Have resuscitation goals been met?

Resuscitation goals
- Heart rate <120 /min
- Systolic blood pressure >90 mmHg
- Urine output >0.5 mL/kg/hr

No

Yes

Resuscitation completed
- Oral fluid as tolerated
- Maintenance intravenous fluid if required (1L dextrose saline 4% + 30 mmol KCL over 12 hours)
- 4-hourly vital signs

Escalate care to intensive care
Likely to require inotropes and invasive monitoring
Senior clinician involvement

Figure 14.6 • Goal-directed resuscitation for patients with systemic inflammatory response syndrome (SIRS) and acute pancreatitis (predicted severe).

criteria were limited to those with APACHE II score >7 or CRP >150 mg/L. Patients were stratified by APACHE II score < or ≥13. There was no difference in the primary endpoint (30% in early enteral feeding vs 27% in oral diet group, $P = 0.76$) or secondary outcomes such as incidence necrosis or amelioration of the inflammatory response. No benefit was seen in the subgroup analysis based on the APACHE II score.

✓✓ There is no current evidence to support the statement that early EN will reduce SIRS or mortality in severe AP.[42,43]

Any future work in such patients will also need to address the issue of feed type as early use of polymeric formulas has been associated with chylous ascites.[44] Currently there is insufficient evidence to support a specific EN formulation including immunomodulatory agents or probiotics.[45]

✓✓ Probiotics have not been recommended outside trial conditions given the potential for increased harm.[45]

For those with mild disease the relevant clinical question relates to NBM versus allowing early institution of normal diet. There are three RCTs[46–48] that have tested clear liquid diets against solid diets, all showing reduced length of stay (2 days) in those who were allowed to eat normally. In addition a further RCT comparing early nasogastric feeding in those patients with mild to moderate AP showed reduced pain scores and need for opiates in those fed early.[49]

✓✓ There is strong evidence that allowing patients with mild or moderate acute pancreatitis to eat early and on demand is beneficial.[46–48]

Preventing secondary infectious complications

Prophylactic antibiotics have been extensively studied in a systematic review of 14 trials consisting of 841 patients.[50] There was no reduction in infectious complications, surgical intervention or mortality associated with prophylactic antibiotic use and so they cannot be recommended.[50] Continuous regional perfusion with protease inhibitors, antibiotics or microcirculatory promoters has been more popular in Japan than in Western countries. In a recent systematic review, six RCTs using variable treatment combinations were reviewed.[51] Only two trials reported infectious complications as an endpoint and the combination of continuous regional arterial infusion of a protease inhibitor and antibiotics did not reduce infectious rates compared to the control group.[51] However, in one RCT the mortality was reduced by the use of continuous regional arterial infusion of protease inhibitors and

antibiotics (2/39 vs 9/39; $P = 0.04$), therefore further trials are justified.[51]

Management of mild biliary pancreatitis

The recently published PONCHO trial[52] randomised 266 patients to same admission cholecystectomy or interval (25–30 days) cholecystectomy. Inclusion criteria were CRP <100 mg/L, pain free and eating and ASA <4 or if >75 years, ASA < 3. The composite primary endpoint was readmission for gallstone related complications or mortality within 6 months. The primary endpoint was reduced from 17% to 5%, $P = 0.002$. There was no difference in operative safety endpoints between the groups. In those patients who underwent interval cholecystectomy 51% reported gallstone pain during the interval that did not bring them to hospital. It is worth observing that 31% of patients underwent ERCP and sphincterotomy and intraoperative cholangiography was not routinely performed. The median time to randomisation was 5 days. Therefore it may be possible to improve on the time to randomisation if a more liberal approach to intraoperative cholangiography is taken.

✓✓ Patients with mild biliary pancreatitis should undergo laparoscopic cholecystectomy on the same admission.[52]

It clear that early LC is highly desirable for patient-centred care but it important to be aware of those patients who may harbour acute peripancreatic fluid collections or an acute necrotic collection. In patients who are systemically well with raised inflammatory markers or blood urea nitrogen >20 mg/dL or packed cell volume >44% cross-sectional imaging should be considered to identify those with acute fluid or necrotic collections.[53] Such patients should be excluded from early LC as this has been associated with increased infectious pancreatic complications and need for intervention.[54] The natural history of acute peripancreatic fluid collections is resolution while acute necrotic collections may become infected early (5/80), resolve (33/80) or develop walled-off necrosis (30/80) which may become infected (8/39), remain sterile (7/39) or resolve (23/39).[53]

✓ Patients with acute peripancreatic fluid collections should be left for 6–10 weeks prior to cholecystectomy.

✓ A small group of patients may not be fit enough for laparoscopic cholecystectomy in which case they should be considered for definitive endoscopic sphincterotomy as it results in significant reduction in risk of recurrent pancreatitis.[55]

When should a patient with severe acute pancreatitis be transferred?

This will be dependent on the local services (interventional and endoscopic) and the critical care and surgical skill sets at the local hospital. The IAP/APA guidelines have defined which patients should be admitted to an intensive care unit and what determines a tertiary centre for management of AP.[36]

> ✓ The authors of IAP/APA guidelines recommend patients with severe AP be managed in a specialist centre based on population data suggesting improved outcomes from high-volume centres.[36]

Many health systems face physical and resource constraints with regard to the ability to transfer all patients into regional intensive care units especially with the increasing centralisation of HPB cancer services. To get around this some services have developed the concept of a regional 'hub and spoke' model with remote advice and management given by the tertiary centres; however, no data exist on the outcomes of this approach as compared to early physical transfer. If such an approach is to be taken, close links between the referring and receiving centre will be required with ability for efficient and timely transfer as necessary.

Follow-up for non-biliary, non-ETOH-induced pancreatitis

Although a rare cause of AP, hypercalcaemia should be screened for as further attacks can be prevented by early diagnosis. Other aetiologies include medications that can be difficult to prove given the latency of exposure and presentation with AP. Sphincter of Oddi dysfunction should be considered in those with disordered LFTs. An interval MRI pancreas should be considered looking for structural abnormalities such as pancreatic divisum or neoplasms, including pancreatic intraductal papillary mucinous neoplasms (see Chapter 17 in the Hepatobiliary and Pancreatic Surgery volume in this series). Endoscopic ultrasound is also useful to detect occult gallstones or structural changes of chronic pancreatitis. In patients with family history or recurrent attacks at an early age genetic screening should be considered in conjunction with a genetic service.

Recent literature also raises an important issue with regard to long-term outcomes for all patients irrespective of severity of the AP. In a systematic review[55] of 24 prospective clinical studies involving 1102 patients who presented with their first attack of AP the prevalence of prediabetes, diabetes and treatment with insulin was 16%, 23%, 15%. By 5 years there was a 2.7-fold increase in the diagnosis of new onset diabetes.

> ✓ Patients and primary practitioners should be informed of this to ensure appropriate long-term follow-up and awareness of symptoms of diabetes.

Implementation and compliance with the evidence base

Although there are many published evidence-based guidelines for the management of acute pancreatitis there is considerable evidence that compliance is poor.[57,58] To achieve the optimal management and outcomes of patients with pancreatitis requires a multidisciplinary team following complicated decision-based algorithms. Therefore considerable thought needs to be given at a local level how to optimise the correct decision-making to ensure patients receive appropriate and timely treatment.[58]

> ✓ Availability of evidence, feedback to clinicians regarding appropriate metrics and, increasingly, use of technology and bundles of care or clinical pathways are all required to assist decision-making and optimise patient management.[58,59]

Technical considerations of cholecystectomy, laparoscopic bile duct exploration and ERCP

Emergency LC has been associated with an increased risk of BDI in those with moderate or severe AC[8] so it is important that surgeons undertaking LC have a construct on how to mitigate the risk of such injuries. Although achieving the critical view of safety has been widely promoted as the key to avoiding BDI, randomised data are lacking, mainly due to the large numbers of patients that would need to be enrolled given the low rate of transectional bile duct injury.[60] Using error analysis methodology key steps have been proposed that if performed will allow the identification of stopping points at which it is unsafe to proceed with trying to achieve the critical view of safety.[61] Instead, when faced with difficult pathology and unclear anatomy it is recommended that consideration be given to calling for help, abandoning the operation or considering subtotal cholecystectomy.[61] Fundus-first cholecystectomy is not recommended as it has been associated with severe vasculo-biliary injuries.[62] Intraoperative cholangiography as a 'preventer' of BDI is a polarising topic, with many surgeons lacking individual equipoise, but profession-wide, considerable clinical equipoise exists. Quality randomised data are lacking due to the large numbers of patients that would be required to adequately power such a trial.[63]

✅ Although population data suggest intraoperative cholangiography may be associated with a reduction in the incidence of BDI, causality cannot be inferred from such data.[63]

A population-based case-control study demonstrated that an intention to perform intraoperative cholangiography was associated with a reduced risk of BDI by 52%.[8]

In an RCT that included patients with mild or moderate AC, routine use of a drain to the sub-hepatic fossa post LC did not reduce risk of postoperative complications (9.6% vs 9.1%, $P = 1.00$).[64]

✅✅ Following LC, postoperative drainage would not appear to be beneficial.

Umbilical port-site infections remain a common complication following LC, particularly with the increasing prevalence of obesity and diabetes. The role of prophylactic antibiotics, retrieval bags and wound toileting have not been studied in the emergency setting. AC (OR 1.69 [1.18–2.42]) but not gallstone pancreatitis has been associated with increased venous thromboembolic events (VTE) post LC, and when combined with other significant risk factors such as age >70 years (OR 2.69 [1.68–4.30]), past history of VTE (OR 50 [27–93]), or >120 minutes operation time (OR 1.66 [1.18–2.35]), thromboprophylaxis should be considered, although it increases the risk of postoperative bleeding (OR 1.72 [1.44–2.05]).[65]

LCBDE has not been widely adopted despite being shown to be equivalent in terms of outcomes to ERCP. Reasons may be multifactorial but are likely to include technical difficulty, need for significant equipment or operating time, and the widespread availability of ERCP. However, for those surgeons wishing to incorporate it into their practice, it is worth considering a recent paper describing a departmental learning curve and technical factors associated with successful transcystic exploration.[66] The authors describe dissecting the cystic duct to within 1 cm of the CBD junction and if necessary extending the cholecystotomy incision along the lateral surface of the cystic duct and onto the common bile duct for 3–5 mm. This increased access to the CBD and allowed extraction of large stones without the need for formally opening the CBD (making primary closure easier). Stones were extracted using wire baskets under vision via a 3–5 mm choledochoscope. Small stones were flushed. No mention was made whether antegrade dilatation of the sphincter was performed to aid distal flushing. If stones were impacted electrohydraulic lithotripsy was employed. From a series of 708 patients, 91% were cleared by transcystic exploration alone (direct 525/644, lateral incision 90/644, lithotripsy

17/644, lateral incision and lithotripsy 12/644), 24 (3%) required LCBDE, 26 (4%) LC only, and 14 (2%) conversion to open surgery.[66] Using CUSUM analysis, the learning curve for the Department, as measured by operative time, was 250 procedures. After the learning curve the median time reduced from 95 (70–130) minutes to 77 (60–111) minutes (P <0.001).[66] However, success rates were equivalent across time periods. A meta-analysis summarising the literature regarding the optimal method of closure and drainage following LCBDE has been published.[67] Primary duct closure without internal or external drainage was associated with fewer complications (OR 0.43 [0.22–0.83], $P = 0.01$) than T-tube drainage, and although biliary specific complications were reduced (11/160 vs 21/173), the difference was not statistically different ($P = 0.09$), perhaps secondary to type II error. Other forms of internal or external biliary drainage did not reduce complication rates as compared to T-tube drainage.

✅✅ Primary closure without biliary drainage is recommended[67] based on a meta-analysis of the literature regarding closure and drainage.

The CBD can be safely closed with a continuous uni-barbed (V-loc, Coviden, USA) running suture to help assist intra-corporeal suturing.[68]

Although ERCP is often performed by gastroenterologists, surgeons should be aware of factors that can mitigate the risk of post ERCP pancreatitis. Correct patient selection is a must, understanding that in the era of EUS and MRCP, ERCP should be restricted to those with therapeutic intent.[69] Patients with suspected sphincter of Oddi dysfunction should be referred to an ERCP-ist familiar with the work-up, performing high-volume ERCP and understanding the current literature with regard to which group of patients will benefit.[69] Technical factors that have been shown to reduce post-ERCP pancreatitis include wire-guided cannulation (OR 0.51 [0.32–0.82] rather than contrast-assisted cannulation.[69] Wire-guided cannulation should be performed gently to avoid side branch perforation of pancreatic ducts.[69] If repeated pancreatic cannulation occurs, the initial wire can be left in situ to straighten the common channel and a second wire used to cannulate the bile duct.[69] Avoiding prolonged attempts at standard cannulation and using pre-cut sphincterotomy or pancreatic sphincterotomy are also recommended.[69] Balloon dilatation of the biliary sphincter can induce pancreatitis, but the incidence can be reduced by longer (2–5 minutes) dilatation rather than short dilatation.[69] A recent systematic review suggests that this may carry the lowest risk for inducing post-ERCP pancreatitis.[70]

✅✅ Prophylactic pancreatic stent placement has been shown to reduce risk of post- ERCP pancreatitis by 60% and should be used in patients deemed to be at high risk of post-ERCP pancreatitis.[69] There is also a strong level of evidence for the use of rectal non-steroidal anti-inflammatory drugs.[69]

✅✅ There are now three randomised controlled trials[71-73] that have shown a reduction in post-ERCP pancreatitis with the use of aggressive hydration with lactated Ringer's in the peri-procedure period (Table 14.4).

It has been associated with 7.7% absolute risk reduction (number needed to treat = 13).[69] Currently the recommended dose is 100 mg rectal indomethacin either before or after the procedure.[69] Importantly, IV or PO formulations have not been shown to be beneficial.[69] It also would appear to have an additive effect to pancreatic stent placement and so the two should be used together.[69]

In the largest of these trials aggressive fluid hydration was also shown to reduce the severity of the pancreatitis ($P = 0.04$) and the effect of reduction was greatest in those at highest risk of post-ERCP pancreatitis (25% vs 9%, $P = 0.04$).[71] The number needed to treat was 18.[71] Important exclusion criteria (other than those deemed at low risk of pancreatitis) in all three trials[71-73] were elderly patients (>70-75 years) and those with significant cardiac, renal or respiratory comorbidity. It is also worth highlighting that none of the patients appeared to receive rectal NSAIDs.[71-73]

Table 14.4 • Randomised trials showing benefit of aggressive hydration with lactated Ringer's solution in preventing ERCP pancreatitis

Variable	Choi et al. 2016[71]		Shaygan-Nejad 2015[73]		Buxbaum 2014[72]	
No.	510		150		62	
Aggressive hydration	10 mL/kg before procedure 3 mL/kg/hr during procedure and continue for 8 hr Bolus 10 mL/kg post procedure		3 mL/kg/hr during and for 8 hr post procedure 20 mL/kg bolus post procedure			
Standard hydration	1.5 mlL/kg/hr during and for 8 hr post procedure					
Rectal NSAID	No		Not stated		No	
	Aggressive	**Standard**	**Aggressive**	**Standard**	**Aggressive**	**Standard**
Outcomes (%)						
Hyper-amylasaemia	7	16	23	44*	23	39
Pain		5		37*	8	22
Pancreatitis	4	10*	5	23*	0	17*

*$P < 0.05$.

Key points

- Acute cholecystitis can be graded by severity based on degree of systemic inflammation and organ dysfunction.
- For patients without organ failure, early laparoscopic cholecystectomy is the treatment of choice while for those patients who are critically ill antibiotics and urgent percutaneous gallbladder drainage is the standard of care.
- Acute cholangitis can be graded by degree of systemic inflammation and requires a combination of antibiotics and urgent biliary decompression.
- The natural history of common bile duct stones is that many will pass spontaneously without symptoms and therefore in a population with a low prevalence (<3%) systematic screening for them may not be cost-effective.

- The management of common bile duct stones is dependent on several factors, including anatomical, presence or absence of the gallbladder, local services and skill sets. ERCP and laparoscopic duct exploration can be considered equivalent treatments.
- Acute pancreatitis requires complex timely decision-making depending on severity and aetiology. Therefore surgical services are encouraged to implement an evidence-based approach and consider optimising clinical workflows to ensure maximal compliance with evidence-based guidelines.

▶ Recommended videos:

- Avoiding bile duct injury – https://tinyurl.com/yc6q7pzy
- Difficult cholecystectomy – https://tinyurl.com/yc7l2t8g
- Laparoscopic transcystic CBD exploration – https://youtu.be/K2O60nPkZGU

🌐 Full references available at **http://expertconsult.inkling.com**

Key references

2. Ansaloni L, Pisano M, Coccolin F, et al. 2016 WSES guidelines on acute calculous cholecystitis. World J Emerg Surg 2016;11:25. PMID: 27307785.
Describes an evidence-based approach to the diagnosis, investigation and management of patients with acute cholecystitis. The authors recommend the use of abdominal US for diagnosis and proceeding to early laparoscopic cholecystectomy unless patient comorbidity is a contraindication to surgery or the patient's symptoms exceed 10 days.

7. Yamashita Y, Takada T, Strasberg SM, et al. TG13 surgical management of acute cholecystitis. J Hepatobiliary Pancreat Sci 2013;20:89–96. PMID: 23307007.
An evidence-based approach examining the evidence for the management of acute cholecystitis. The authors recommend early laparoscopic cholecystectomy. The authors noted the lack of evidence from which to make strong recommendations based on severity of the acute cholecystitis.

24. Giljaca V, Gurusamy KS, Takwoingi Y, et al. Endoscopic ultrasound vs. magnetic resonance cholangiopancreatography for CBD stones. Cochrane Database Syst Rev 2015;2: CD011549.
Both EUS and MRCP have been shown to have a high diagnostic accuracy (summary sensitivities and specificities >0.95) for the detection of CBD stones and can be considered equivalent tests in terms of accuracy. However, the authors qualify this statement that the underlying conclusions were based on studies of poor methodological quality.

33. Miura F, Takada T, Strasberg SM, et al. TG13 flowchart for management of acute cholangitis and cholecystitis. J Hepatobiliary Pancreat Sci 2013;20: 47–54. 23307003.
Describes an algorithm for management of patients with either acute cholangitis or acute cholecystitis. Treatment was stratified by severity. For those with mild, moderate and severe acute cholangitis antibiotics, early biliary drainage and organ support are recommended in summative fashion. For acute cholecystitis early laparoscopic cholecystectomy is recommended except for those with severe acute cholecystitis, in which case organ support and early gallbladder drainage is recommended.

36. Working group IAP/APA acute pancreatitis guidelines. IAP/APA evidence based guidelines for the management of acute pancreatitis. Pancreatology 2013;13: e1–e15. PMID: 24054878.
An extensive evidence-based review of the literature. Using the GRADE system, 21 of the 38 recommendations were rated as strong. The important topics to review in this paper include the evidence around resuscitation and early introduction of oral or enteral nutrition. The use of Ringer's lactate as the initial fluid for resuscitation (GRADE 1B, strong agreement) and using goal-directed therapy (GRADE 1B, weak agreement) is discussed.

42. Dutch Pancreatitis Study Group. Early vs on demand nasoenteric tube feeding in acute pancreatitis. N Engl J Med 2014;371:1983–93. PMID: 25409371.
The aim of this study was to determine if early enteral feeding via a nasoenteric feeding tube would reduce gut-derived infections in patients at high risk of severe acute pancreatitis. There were no differences detected in rates of infection or death in either group. Of note, 69% of the on-demand group tolerated oral diet. The authors concluded that enteral nutrition is only required in those who fail a trial of oral diet.

43. Srimic D, Poropat G, Hauser G, et al. Early nasojejunal feeding vs. nil by mouth in acute pancreatitis: a randomised trial. Pancreatology 2016;16:523–8. PMID: 27107634.
In this RCT patients were randomised on admission to enteral feeding or no nutritional support. A total of 214 patients were enrolled. No differences in the incidence of SIRS, persistent organ failure or mortality were observed between the two groups.

45. Poropat G, Giljaca V, Hauser G, et al. Enteral nutrition formulations for acute pancreatitis. Cochrane Database Syst Rev 2015: CD010605. PMID: 25803695.
This systematic review emphasised the lack of high-quality evidence to support any specific type of enteral feed. The data on immunonutrition were of low quality but a reduction in all-cause mortality was observed. The data on probiotics are contradictory and harm has been reported. It is likely further research will alter our knowledge.

46. Sathiarai E, Murthy S, Mansard MJ, et al. Clinical trial: oral feeding with soft diet compared with liquid diet as initial meal in mild acute pancreatitis. Aliment Pharmacol Ther 2008;28:777–81. PMID: 19145732.
    A randomised trial comparing liquid diet versus a soft diet after mild acute pancreatitis. Allowing patients a soft diet reduced the median hospital stay by 2 days (P <0.001). The authors concluded early feeding with soft diet following mild acute pancreatitis was safe and shortened hospital stay.

47. Moraes JM, Felga GE, Chebi LA, et al. A full solid diet as the initial meal in mild acute pancreatitis is safe and results in shorter length of hospitalisation: results of prospective randomised controlled double blind clinical trial. Pancreas 2013;42:88–91.
    Patients who were offered a full diet consumed more calories earlier and had a shorter length of hospital stay (median reduction of 1.5 days) and did not develop recurrence of abdominal pain.

48. Rajkumar N, Karthikeyan VS, Ali SM, et al. Clear liquid diet vs. soft diet as the initial meal in patients with mild acute pancreatitis: a randomised interventional trial. Nutr Clin Pract 2013;28:365–70. PMID: 23239793.
    Patients who were fed a soft diet as compared to a liquid diet following mild acute pancreatitis tolerated it well and had a mean reduction in length of stay of 2 days as compared to those on a liquid diet.

52. Dutch pancreatitis study group. Same admission vs. interval cholecystectomy for mild gallstone pancreatitis: A multicentre randomised trial. Lancet 2015;386:1261–8. PMID: 26460661.
    In this study 266 patients were randomised. In those undergoing same admission cholecystectomy there was a reduction in the primary endpoint (gallstone-related complications or mortality at 6 months) with a risk ratio (95%CI) of 0.28 (0.12–0.66), P=0.002. Thus same admission cholecystectomy for patients with mild acute pancreatitis is strongly recommended.

67. Yin Z, Xu K, Sun J, et al. Is the end of the T-tube drainage era in laparoscopic choledochotomy for CBD stones coming? Ann Surg 2013;257:54–6. PMID: 23059495.
    A meta-analysis demonstrating that primary closure of the common bile duct following laparoscopic choledochotomy was associated with a reduction in operating time (mean difference 19 mins, P <0.01), reduced biliary specific complications (odds ratio [95%CI] 0.59 [0.38–0.91], P=0.02) and reduction in hospital stay (mean difference 3 days, P <0.01) as compared to those undergoing common bile duct drainage.

69. Elmunzer BJ. Preventing post ERCP pancreatitis. Gastrointest Endoscopy Clin North Am 2015;25:725–36. PMID: 26431600.
    This overview highlights the importance of wire-guided access, the use of rectal NSAIDs and prophylactic pancreatic stents in patients at high risk of post-procedure pancreatitis.

71. Choi JH, Kim HJ, Lee BU, et al. Vigorous periprocedural hydration with lactated Ringer's solution reduces the risk of pancreatitis after retrograde cholangiopancreatography in hospitalized patients. Clin Gastroenterol Hepatol 2017; 15:86–92. PMID: 27311618.
    A randomised trial of 510 patients. Patients who received vigorous IV hydration with lactated Ringer's solution had a reduction in the incidence of post-procedure severe acute pancreatitis (0.4% vs 2%, P=0.40).

72. Buxbaum J, Yan A, Yeh K, et al. Aggressive hydration with lactated Ringer's solution reduces pancreatitis after endoscopic retrograde cholangiopancreatography. Clin Gastroenterol Hepatol 2014;12(2):303–7. PMID: 23920031.
    A randomised pilot study in which none of the patients who received aggressive hydration with lactated Ringer's solution developed post-procedure pancreatitis as compared to 17% of patients who received standard hydration, P=0.016.

73. Shaygan-Nejad A, Masjedizadeh AR, Ghavidel A, et al. Aggressive hydration with lactated Ringer's solution as the prophylactic intervention for postendoscopic retrograde cholangiopancreatography pancreatitis: a randomized controlled double-blind clinical trial. J Res Med Sci 2015;20(9):838–43. PMID: 26759569.
    In patients randomised to aggressive hydration there was reduction in the incidence of post-procedure pancreatitis from 22% to 5%, P=0.002.

15

Acute conditions of the small bowel and appendix

Timothy Forgan
Robert Baigrie

Introduction

Acute disease of the small bowel, from which appendicitis is considered separately, contributes substantially to both the urgent and emergency workload of the abdominal surgeon. There are many causes but disease of any intra-abdominal organ or the peritoneum may involve the small bowel secondarily. The pattern of acute small-bowel disease varies with the age of the patient, some being more common in young people, others in older patients. Its incidence is difficult to estimate but is probably second only to appendicitis as the site of abdominal disease requiring urgent surgical intervention. It primarily manifests itself in one of three ways: obstruction, inflammation (peritonitis) and haemorrhage. These are not mutually exclusive and may coexist in each clinical episode. Treatment may be operative or non-operative, and the timing of surgical intervention is often critical, particularly when bowel ischaemia/infarction is concerned.

Small-bowel obstruction

Although there are many causes of small-bowel obstruction (Box 15.1), the commonest in the developed world is adhesions secondary to previous surgery (approximately 60% of episodes) and malignancy. By comparison, in the developing world the most common cause is hernia. A large retrospective study using Scottish National Health Service data estimated that 5.7% of all hospital admissions following abdominal and pelvic surgery over a 10-year period were directly related to adhesions.[1] While an attempt should be made to diagnose the cause of the obstruction preoperatively (see Chapter 11) to eliminate conditions that might require special treatment, in practice, the cause of the obstruction is often made only at operation. A retrospective study of 102 patients undergoing surgery for adhesive small-bowel obstruction carried out between 1987 and 1992, and followed up for 14 years, reported that a total of 273 further episodes of obstruction occurred, requiring 237 hospital admissions.[2] Nearly half of these resulted in more surgery.

Mechanism

The small bowel responds to obstruction by the onset of vigorous peristalsis. This produces colicky pain, usually in the central abdomen, as the small bowel is of midgut embryological origin. As the obstruction develops, the proximal intestine dilates and fills with fluid, producing systemic hypovolaemia. Further fluid is lost through vomiting, which occurs early if the obstruction is proximal. If the process continues and the blood supply is compromised, infarction and perforation will occur and the pain, initially colicky, will escalate and become continuous. If the blood supply remains intact and the bowel is decompressed by vomiting and nasogastric drainage, peristalsis will stop and the colicky pain will cease, leaving dilated, non-functioning bowel.

Within the lumen
- Gallstone
- Food bolus
- Bezoars
- Parasites (e.g. *Ascaris*)
- Enterolith
- Foreign body

Within the wall
Tumour
- Primary
  - Small-bowel tumour
  - Carcinoma
  - Lymphoma
  - Sarcoma
  - Carcinoma of caecum
- Secondary

Inflammation
- Crohn's disease
- Radiation enteritis
- Postoperative stricture
- Potassium chloride stricture
- Vascultides (e.g. scleroderma)

Outside the wall
Adhesions
- Congenital
- Bands
- Acquired
- Postoperative
- Inflammatory
- Neoplastic
- Chemical (e.g. starch, talc)
- Pharmacological (e.g. practolol)
- Intussusception

Hernia
- Primary
  - Congenital (e.g. diaphragmatic)
  - Acquired (e.g. inguinal, femoral, etc.)
- Secondary
  - Incisional hernia
  - Internal postoperative hernia (e.g. lateral space, mesenteric defect)

Presentation

The typical clinical presentation of small-bowel obstruction is central abdominal colicky pain, vomiting (usually bile-stained), abdominal distension and a reduction or absence of flatus. If the blockage is in the distal ileum, early vomiting may be less of a feature and abdominal distension more obvious.

The vomiting often becomes 'faeculent' as the stagnant small-bowel contents become degraded by bacterial colonisation. Bowel sounds increase and may be audible to the patient. Localised peritonitic pain and tenderness suggests ischaemia and incipient strangulation. In some patients there may be an obvious cause, such as an irreducible hernia. Surgical scars are important clues, as is any history of previous intra-abdominal pathology, and one cause not to forget in the scar-free female abdomen is adhesions from a vaginal hysterectomy.

Although small-bowel obstruction can occur without the development of abdominal pain, the absence of this symptom should be viewed with caution. This is particularly the case in postoperative patients, where small-bowel obstruction and intestinal ileus can be difficult to differentiate.

The history and examination of the patient should be sufficiently thorough to identify small-bowel obstruction and its possible causes, as well as any suspicion of ischaemia or perforation aroused by tenderness and peritoneal irritation. Evaluation of the patient's general state, particularly dehydration and its consequences, will ensure adequate resuscitation prior to any planned surgical treatment.

Initial management

The aim of management is adequate resuscitation, confirmation of the diagnosis and the identification of possible bowel strangulation so that early surgery can be arranged. The absence of strangulation allows a period of decompression and intravenous fluid resuscitation in the hope of spontaneous resolution. However, failure of the obstruction to resolve within 48–72 hours is usually an indication for surgical intervention.

Fluid resuscitation usually requires several litres of normal saline with potassium supplementation or Hartmann's solution (lactated isotonic electrolyte solution) in the first few hours after admission. Patients with a long history are likely to be more severely dehydrated, with an alkalosis and associated hypokalaemia, the former due to loss of hydrogen ions in the vomitus and the latter from renal compensation. Measurement of urinary volume, utilising catheterisation if necessary, is essential and measurement of central venous pressure may be required in the elderly, or patients with coexisting morbidity. Adequate fluid replacement should be given before any surgical intervention is planned and can be given rapidly if required, even in the elderly, provided appropriate monitoring is used (see also Chapter 5).

Although mild obstruction may resolve without a nasogastric tube (NGT), its use in established small-bowel obstruction will reduce vomiting, decompress the bowel and reduce the risk of aspiration. Nasogastric losses should be replaced with additional electrolyte-rich intravenous crystalloid fluids and potassium supplementation if necessary. Adequate analgesia should be given early and will not mask signs of peritonitis, so there is no justification for withholding adequate analgesia while awaiting further clinical assessment[3] (see also Chapter 11). The analgesia requirement should be reviewed regularly, especially in the early stages, as a persistent requirement for increasing amounts may indicate developing strangulation. Anti-thromboembolic prophylaxis should be commenced early and continued until at least discharge from hospital (see Chapter 2).

Investigations

These are aimed at:

1. assessing the general state of the patient;
2. confirming the diagnosis of small-bowel obstruction and possible cause;
3. identifying those patients who need early surgery (those with a high risk of strangulation) and those in whom a non-operative approach is appropriate.

Radiological investigations are discussed in detail in Chapter 11. Contrast-enhanced computed tomography (CT) (**Fig. 15.1**) is increasingly used in the early assessment of patients with small-bowel obstruction, both to identify the underlying cause (particularly malignancy) and to identify features of possible strangulation. CT features of intraperitoneal free fluid, mesenteric oedema and lack of the 'small-bowel faeces sign', in combination with a history of vomiting, have been reported to be highly predictive of requiring operative intervention.[4] A subtle sign on contrast-enhanced CT scanning is hyperaemia of a segment of bowel, which indicates ischaemia. Identifying patients with possible strangulation remains difficult, and where concern persists, early surgery (laparoscopic or open) is advised. The small bowel faeces sign refers to the presence of particulate faeculent material mingled with gas bubbles in the lumen of the small intestine (as seen in the colon on CT). It is believed to be the result of delayed intestinal transit and to be caused by incompletely digested food, bacterial overgrowth, or increased water absorption of the distal small-bowel contents due to obstruction.

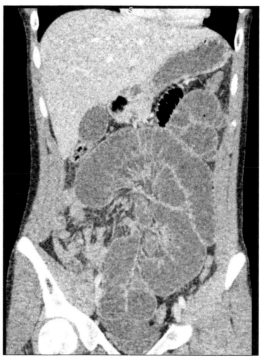

Figure 15.1 • Multislice CT with intravenous contrast demonstrating small-bowel obstruction.

Non-operative management

Intravenous fluids and NGT aspiration are the two components of the first-line 'drip and suck' regimen, particularly when the underlying cause is thought to be adhesions, as spontaneous resolution will occur in the majority. This treatment plan should be abandoned at the first suggestion of underlying strangulation. These patients are good candidates for a Water-Soluble-Contrast-Meal (WSCM), which has both diagnostic and therapeutic properties. The radiological appearance of contrast in the colon within 24 hours from administration predicts resolution in 99% of patients. The use of WSCM, administered either orally or down the NGT, is safe and identifies early those patients who require surgery and those who do not, so reducing hospital stay.[5,6] Although non-operative management can be continued for several days in the absence of any suggestion of strangulation, surgical exploration is generally indicated if the obstruction fails to resolve after 48–72 hours, or the WSCM test fails. It might be worth waiting longer in some patients with known extensive adhesions from multiple previous explorations where surgery is likely to be complex, prolonged and high risk. In this setting, attention should be paid to intravenous nutritional support (see Chapter 6).

✅✅ In the absence of clinical or CT signs of strangulation (free fluid, mesenteric oedema, small-bowel faeces sign, devascularised bowel or hyperaemia), or for patients with partial obstruction, initial non-operative management is appropriate. These patients are good candidates for a trial of orally administered water-soluble contrast medium with both diagnostic and therapeutic purposes. The appearance of water-soluble contrast in the colon on X-ray within 24 hours from administration predicts resolution. The use of contrast is safe and reduces the need for surgery, time to resolution and hospital stay.[5] In the absence of signs of strangulation or peritonitis, non-operative treatment can be prolonged up to 72 hours (Bologna Guidelines for Diagnosis and Management of Adhesive Small Bowel Obstruction).[6]

Surgical management

The particular circumstances of any given patient determine the need for surgical intervention, but some of the commonest features in decision-making are listed in Box 15.2.

Operative principles

Once a decision to operate has been made in the emergency setting, patients should be rapidly resuscitated, their comorbidity optimised (see Chapter 2) and the stomach emptied with a NGT. The wide range of possible surgical procedures should be explained to the patient, including the possibility of a stoma. Antibiotic and antithromboembolic

---

Box 15.2 • Small-bowel obstruction: indications for surgery

Absolute indication (surgery as soon as patient resuscitated)
- Generalised peritonitis
- Visceral perforation
- Irreducible hernia
- Localised peritonitis

Relative indication (surgery within 24 hours)
- Palpable mass lesion
- 'Virgin' abdomen
- Failure to improve (continuing pain, high nasogastric aspirates)

Trial of initial conservative treatment (with further investigations)
- Incomplete obstruction
- Previous surgery
- Advanced malignancy
- Diagnostic doubt (possible ileus)

---

prophylaxis should be administered. In the non-emergency setting, a period of preoperative NGT drainage will serve to decompress the small bowel, facilitating its safer intraoperative handling.

A midline incision has the most utility when the diagnosis is unknown. Too short an incision will result in traumatic manipulation of the dilated loops, and it should be extended sooner rather than later. Where there is a previous midline incision, this should be utilised and extended cranially or caudally so that the peritoneal cavity can be entered through a 'virgin' area. Loops of small bowel may be densely adherent to the back of the old scar and care taken to avoid an inadvertent enterotomy of the attenuated, dilated bowel.

In open surgery, having entered the abdominal cavity, the first step is to identify the point between dilated and collapsed bowel. It is important to demonstrate this transition as it confirms the diagnosis of mechanical obstruction and identifies the obstructing point. The presence of uniformly dilated small bowel, or no definite point of change in diameter of the bowel, suggests that the clinical diagnosis of mechanical obstruction may be incorrect.

The fluid within the bowel makes it heavy and if it is removed from the abdominal cavity, it should be handled and supported carefully, utilising surgical assistants to ensure the mesentery is not damaged or twisted. The large surface area of dilated loops results in considerable insensible fluid loss and if it is anticipated that the viscera will lie outside the abdominal cavity for a significant length of time, it should be placed in a transparent 'bowel' bag or wrapped in moist swabs.

Having identified the point of obstruction, it should be released (**Fig. 15.2**). Although it is not necessary or helpful to divide every last adhesion within the abdomen (as these will inevitably re-form), enough should be divided to confirm that there remains no possible site of obstruction between the duodenojejunal (DJ) flexure and the caecum. It is essential to recognise the patient in whom the clinical diagnosis of mechanical small-bowel obstruction is incorrect, as the presence of adhesions does not in itself confirm the diagnosis.

The small bowel should be resected if it is irreversibly ischaemic, or there is disease or fibrotic narrowing in the bowel at the point of obstruction, and anastomosed if both ends of the bowel are healthy and the patient has no other contraindication from associated comorbidity. If the viability of a segment of bowel is unclear, it should be wrapped in warm moist swabs for several minutes (approximately 15 minutes while you continue with other parts of the operation) and re-examined. Where viability remains in doubt, the segment should be resected, or a planned re-look laparotomy arranged 24–48 hours later.

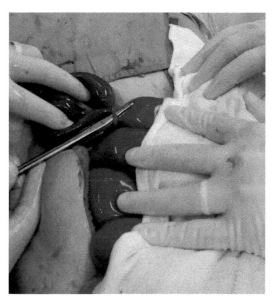

Figure 15.2 • Loop of small bowel obstructed by an adhesive band.
With thanks to Dr Bernie Maree, Consultant Surgeon, Dr Matley and Partners, Cape Town.

Even after removing the obstruction, exteriorisation of the bowel may be indicated if there is generalised disease of the bowel and when there is a high risk of anastomotic dehiscence. In patients who are septic and unwell, stapling off the ends of resected bowel with a planned re-look in 24–48 hours (such as is carried out in the trauma setting, see also Chapter 19), is useful, with subsequent anastomosis performed in more favourable conditions. An ileostomy may be indicated in patients with Crohn's disease as part of their long-term management, and this possibility should be considered and discussed with the patient beforehand.

Laparoscopy

In suitable patients, laparoscopy can be attempted as an alternative to laparotomy using an open access technique. Laparoscopic adhesiolysis, with a low threshold for conversion, may be suitable during a first episode of small-bowel obstruction, particularly when there has been limited previous surgery and a single band is anticipated, for example in a patient with a virgin abdomen or who has had an appendicectomy, oophorectomy or hysterectomy.[6,7] If laparoscopic adhesiolysis is to be attempted, the obstructed bowel must be manipulated with great care to prevent perforation as it is usually thin-walled and distended.

Reducing adhesion formation

There has been considerable research aimed at reducing the development of further adhesions after surgery. Anti-adhesion barriers are compounds that do not actively interfere with inflammation and wound healing. Rather, they act as a spacer that separates injured surfaces of the peritoneum, allowing these surfaces to heal without forming fibrinous attachments, which eventually lead to adhesions. To accomplish this task, such barriers should ideally be inert to the human immune system and be slowly degradable. Anti-adhesion barriers have been demonstrated to reduce adhesion formation and the incidence of subsequent complications.[8] There is evidence that the intraperitoneal administration of icodextrin 4% solution (ADEPT®) at the end of surgery reduces intra-abdominal adhesion formation and the risk of re-obstruction. In a randomised trial the small-bowel obstruction recurrence rate was 2% (2/91) in the icodextrin groups versus 11% (10/90) in the control group after a mean follow-up period of 41.4 months ($P < 0.05$). However, no difference was found in the need for laparotomy.[9] Its use was approved by the US Food and Drug Administration (FDA) in 2013.

Difficult closure

There are some patients in whom, after relief of obstruction, the oedematous bowel makes closure impossible. These patients may have had repeated procedures, and in this setting the use of a low-pressure vacuum-assisted closure dressing may allow delayed closure. Where this is not available, a sterile plastic sheet can be sutured to the wound edges as a temporising measure (Bogota Bag). A 5-litre urology irrigating bag is suitable and invariably available. Further discussions on abdominal sepsis and dehiscence are covered in Chapter 20.

Special conditions

Radiation enteritis

Patients can present with an acute abdomen during radiotherapy due to radiation enteritis or with acute-on-chronic attacks many years later. Patients in the former scenario can present considerable diagnostic difficulties, as they are often neutropenic or suffering other side-effects of their treatment. The possibility of a primary pathology, such as acute appendicitis, arising during the course of radiotherapy must also be borne in mind but, where possible, surgical exploration is best avoided. Laparoscopy may be useful here for both diagnosis and management.

A more common acute presentation is with adhesions due to previous radiotherapy, and these patients normally have obstructive symptoms (**Fig. 15.3**). Again, a prolonged period of non-operative management, even with intravenous nutritional support, may be preferable to surgery.

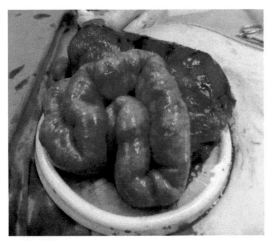

Figure 15.3 • Obstructing loop of irradiated small bowel (closest loop) identified at laparoscopic exploration. Note the pale colour, minimal vascular markings and thickened bowel wall of the irradiated bowel.

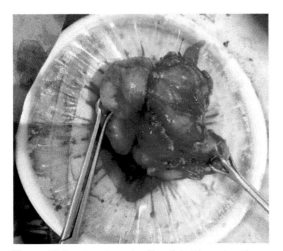

Figure 15.4 • Anastomosis of irradiated (bowel on the left-hand side of the image) to unirradiated small bowel.

These adhesions are often dense and, if the small bowel is injured, there is a significant risk that it might not heal whether it is repaired or anastomosed. If an anastomosis is necessary it is important to adhere to the principle that irradiated bowel should only be anastomosed to non-irraditiated bowel[10] (Fig. 15.4).

Malignant obstruction

Primary tumours of the small bowel are rare but may cause acute small bowel obstruction. The surgical approach will depend on the nature and location of the disease. A more common problem is the patient with advanced intra-abdominal malignancy, with

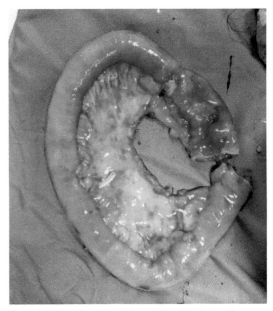

Figure 15.5 • Small-bowel resection for obstructing small-bowel metastases from a previously resected oesophageal adenocarcinoma. Note the stricturing, schirrous nature of the metastasis. Two other smaller metastases are adjacent to the white clips.

or without a past history of surgical treatment for malignancy, who presents with bowel obstruction (Fig. 15.5). If the obstruction fails to settle or rapidly recurs, there is usually time to carry out appropriate investigations to determine the extent of the disease prior to surgery. CT is important in identifying a single area of obstruction, which might be amenable to surgery, as compared to extensive intra-abdominal disease without a single point of obstruction, where surgery has little role to play.

Ascites can be a confusing factor in such a patient and aspiration for cytology to confirm widespread malignancy can be helpful. Clearly, in the presence of advanced and disseminated malignancy, laparotomy should be avoided. However, if the obstruction fails to resolve and the patient is in reasonable condition, surgical bypass may provide relief in some patients, allowing them temporary palliation and to leave hospital. The benefits of surgical bypass in this setting are generally short-lived and this has stimulated increasing expertise among palliative care physicians in the medical management of intestinal obstruction.[11] The principles involve the use of fluid diet, steroids and octreotide, and are aimed at sparing the patient the morbidity and mortality of laparotomy in the terminal phase of their disease. Occasionally the placement of a drainage percutaneous endoscopic gastrostomy (PEG) is possible and appropriate in selected patients to relieve their symptoms of vomiting in the terminal care setting.

Not all patients have obstruction due to their malignant process and have uncomplicated adhesional obstruction. One study of patients who presented with obstruction following previous treatment of intra-abdominal malignancy reported that in one-third of such patients the obstruction was due to a cause other than secondary malignancy.[11] In a Japanese study of 85 patients who had previously undergone surgery for gastric cancer and who were subsequently re-admitted to hospital with intestinal obstruction, the cause was benign adhesions in 20%.[12] This may be a particularly appropriate setting for diagnostic laparoscopy, depending on the extent of the previous surgery.

Abdominal wall hernia

Any hernia can present with intestinal obstruction (**Figs 15.6** and **15.7**), with delayed presentation and gangrene necessitating bowel resection. A Richter's hernia traps only part of the circumference of the bowel wall and the lumen may not be obstructed. Infarction of the trapped segment can still occur, with marked localised tenderness over the hernia site.

Any patient with an acute irreducible hernia should undergo urgent surgery. After bowel resection in the presence of obstruction, with ascites that is often infected, prosthetic mesh should be avoided, especially when there has been gross contamination due to perforation. The incarcerated hernia may reduce spontaneously under general anaesthesia and in this instance it is unlikely that there was strangulation and infarction. However, the bowel

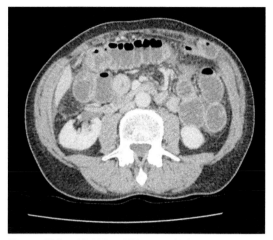

Figure 15.7 • Multislice CT image with intravenous contrast demonstrating small-bowel obstruction secondary to a left-sided Spigelian hernia.

loops should be inspected from within the hernia sac to ensure that a gangrenous loop of bowel or a strictured segment has not dropped back into the abdominal cavity. If it is not possible to inspect the viability of the entire bowel through the hernia sac, laparoscopy may be indicated. A useful approach is to place the laparoscope though the hernia and create a sealed pneumoperitoneum by placing tissue graspers on the defect. Failing this, a standard open laparoscopy through a subumbilical incision cutdown should be used.

A final consideration is the patient with a long history of an uncomplicated hernia who develops acute intestinal obstruction, whereupon the hernia becomes irreducible. The intestinal obstruction raises intra-abdominal pressure, which produces the irreducible hernia, which may be difficult to reduce resulting in its becoming tender. In this setting, a plain abdominal radiograph may demonstrate a dilated colon or the absence of dilated small-bowel loops, suggesting the possibility that the apparently 'incarcerated' hernia is a secondary effect of some other intra-abdominal pathology. In such circumstances a CT is indicated. If the surgeon proceeds and finds the apparently incarcerated hernia easy to release, the wound should be extended to allow exploration, or closed and a laparotomy carried out.

Enterolith obstruction

Enterolith obstruction is rare, the commonest types being gallstones and bezoars.

Gallstone ileus typically occurs in elderly females and follows development of a cholecystoduodenal fistula after cholecystitis with ongoing inflammation. A visible gallstone (if radio-opaque) and gas in the biliary tree are the classic features of a plain

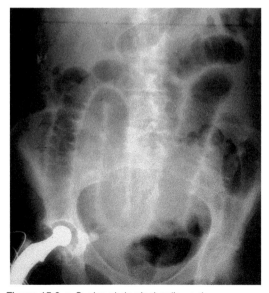

Figure 15.6 • Supine abdominal radiograph demonstrating small-bowel obstruction in a patient with an irreducible femoral hernia.

radiograph. At surgery the stone should be removed via a proximal enterotomy and the proximal intestine palpated to exclude a second stone. The gallbladder should be left alone, as cholecystectomy and duodenal closure can be difficult and dangerous, and are generally unnecessary.

Obstructing bezoars may accumulate in psychiatric patients (hair), or after over-indulging in particular types of food (vegetables and fruit), or those patients without dentures who have swallowed inadequately chewed food. Rarely described, an obstructing bezoar can accumulate in a jejunal diverticulum.

Intussusception

In children, acute presentation is usually to the paediatric department and the main differential diagnosis is gastrointestinal (GI) infection. This is discussed in more detail in Chapter 18. Intussusception in adults is usually caused by tumours of the bowel, which are usually resectable at laparotomy.

Connective tissue disorders

There are several systemic connective tissue disorders that can affect the GI tract and result in a loss of peristaltic power. These patients generally present with chronic symptoms and are usually hard to characterise. Non-operative management of these patients should be pursued whenever possible and a gastroenterologist consulted. In the rare event that this condition progresses to perforation of the bowel, consideration should be given to exteriorisation of the bowel as an ileostomy. Both the ischaemic and healthy bowel should be submitted for histology to attempt to identify the connective tissue disorder. Prolonged postoperative ileus is common and the differentiation of a further episode of mechanical obstruction or continuing ileus presents a diagnostic challenge. The temptation to relook after several days without progress should be resisted. A WSCM should be tried first, and parenteral nutrition and prolonged NGT drainage may be needed. For the surgeon, this is a particularly uneasy and challenging postoperative scenario.

Chronic intestinal pseudo-obstruction

Chronic intestinal pseudo-obstruction (CIPO) is a rare, severe disease characterised by the failure of the intestinal tract to propel its contents, which results in a clinical picture mimicking mechanical obstruction in the absence of any lesion occluding the gut.

Affected individuals are often unable to maintain normal body weight and normal oral nutrition. The severity of the clinical picture, generally characterised by disabling digestive symptoms with intervals of subocclusive episodes, contributes to deterioration of quality of life of the patients.

Furthermore, CIPO often passes unrecognised for a long time, so that patients almost invariably undergo repeated, unhelpful and potentially dangerous surgical procedures. Subtotal colectomy and ileostomy is an approach tried by the optimistic or inexperienced surgeon. It invariably fails and the patient is left with a permanent stoma bag and CIPO of the small intestine.

Management of CIPO remains extremely challenging and often disappointing. There may be a family history and, in severe cases, life expectancy is no more than early adulthood. A greater awareness of the clinical features and natural history of CIPO would help to discourage surgical procedures.[13]

Intestinal obstruction in the early postoperative period

Gastrointestinal ileus or obstruction can occur after any abdominal operation, including gynaecological surgery. The surgeon may also be asked to see patients, often elderly and with comorbidity, who have undergone orthopaedic or cardiac procedures and have apparent bowel obstruction. This group usually have colonic pseudo-obstruction (see Chapters 11 and 16) Each case must be judged on its merits and the differentiation between true postoperative mechanical obstruction and paralytic ileus can be difficult. In patients with a mechanical obstruction appropriate surgical intervention is frequently delayed as a result of this diagnostic dilemma. In these patients, the use of either a WSCM or contrast-enhanced CT is often helpful and should be considered early.[14]

Laparoscopy

In selected patients with small-bowel obstruction, and with appropriate surgical skills, a laparoscopic approach can be attempted using an open access technique. Laparoscopic adhesiolysis may be suitable during an episode of small-bowel obstruction, particularly when there has been limited previous surgery and/or a single band is anticipated, such as might occur in a patient with a virgin abdomen *or* one who has had an appendicectomy, oophorectomy or hysterectomy but no other major abdominal surgery (**Fig. 15.8**). Access to the peritoneal cavity should avoid previous scars and, if away from the midline, be obtained using an open, muscle-splitting approach, with the first trocar inserted in the mid-clavicular line in the left upper quadrant. Most causes of small bowel obstruction are in the lower abdomen and pelvis, so this port site provides an optimal overview of the bowel and lower abdomen when compared with the standard peri-umbilical port, where there may be scar adhesions making access and visibility difficult. This allows early identification of other pathology mandating conversion to open surgery. If laparoscopic surgery

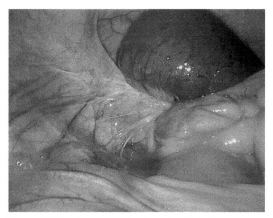

Figure 15.8 • Laparoscopic view of a dilated loop of small bowel proximal to an adhesive band from a gynaecological procedure.
With thanks to Dr Bernie Maree, Consultant Surgeon, Dr Matley and Partners, Cape Town.

is to proceed, further ports can be placed under direct vision in appropriate sites. The availability of a 30-degree camera is essential in order to 'look over' dilated loops of bowel. Successful laparoscopic adhesiolysis allows the patient almost pain-free mobilisation immediately. There is often a need for a few more days in hospital while awaiting a return to normal bowel activity. A low threshold for open conversion should be maintained.[6]

Peritonitis

Small-bowel pathology may present as an acute abdomen, with either localised or generalised peritonitis. This may be as a result of perforation or gangrenous bowel at the end-stage of any condition causing obstruction. This section considers conditions that present primarily with inflammatory signs.

Crohn's disease

Crohn's disease is a chronic relapsing inflammatory disease that can affect any part of the GI tract. A common presentation is inflammation of the terminal ileum and this occasionally presents as an acute abdomen. The small bowel alone is affected in approximately 30% of patients and the small bowel and colon together in 50%.[15]

Where possible, the management of patients with Crohn's disease should be undertaken by a surgeon with a special interest in this condition and the reader is referred to the much more detailed account of this disease in the *Colorectal Surgery* volume of this *Companion to Specialist Surgical Practice* series.[15] Only first principles for managing an acute episode are discussed here.

Presentation

An acute episode of Crohn's ileitis typically presents with abdominal pain, diarrhoea and fever, and this can be the first presentation of the disease in a patient who was previously well. This acute presentation is more likely in young adults; hence it is frequently mistaken for acute appendicitis.

Other clinical presentations occur, although they are less likely to be acute. Resolving Crohn's disease may produce fibrosis in the ileum that can cause obstructive symptoms. These tend to be subacute or chronic, and an acute presentation with small-bowel obstruction is rare.

Entero-enteric or enterocutaneous fistulae occur in Crohn's disease because of the transmural inflammation, sometimes complicated by abscess formation, resulting in local peritonitis.

Investigation

A young patient who presents with right iliac fossa pain, with symptoms that are more insidious than typical appendicitis, should alert a clinical suspicion of Crohn's disease. Inflammatory markers may be markedly elevated (C-reactive protein [CRP], white cell count, platelet count, alkaline phosphatase, erythrocyte sedimentation rate [ESR]), but these are not specific to Crohn's disease. An ultrasound scan may show thickening of the bowel wall or a mass, but contrast-enhanced CT will provide more detailed information and is the preferred investigation in this setting.[16]

Surgery for acute Crohn's disease presenting de novo

If a patient with known Crohn's disease presents with an acute flare-up, or Crohn's disease is diagnosed preoperatively at the first presentation, the patient should be referred to a surgeon with a special interest.[17] The unexpected finding of inflammation of the terminal ileum or caecum at laparoscopy or laparotomy for suspected appendicitis or any other condition, does not necessarily imply Crohn's disease as it can be difficult to differentiate it from infectious (e.g. *Yersinia*) enteritis. Even if it were to be Crohn's ileitis, resection might not be the most appropriate strategy if the dominant symptoms relate to inflammation. In all these scenarios the surgeon should remove the appendix to prevent any future diagnostic dilemma and confusion. No further procedure on the suspected Crohn's disease is required. Further diagnostic investigations are then arranged as appropriate. Only when the patient has obvious small obstruction should the area of inflamed bowel be resected.[18] Stricturoplasty with a full-thickness biopsy is also an option if the stricture is short.

Mesenteric ischaemia

While acute small bowel ischaemia can be caused by a closed loop obstruction, this section reviews mesenteric ischaemia due to embolism or thrombosis, arterial or venous, which may be acute or chronic. Chronic mesenteric ischaemia is also termed 'mesenteric claudication' and is usually caused by a stenosis in the proximal part of the superior mesenteric artery. Patients develop cramp-like abdominal pains after eating, caused by the increased oxygen requirements to the small intestine, which cannot be met by increased blood flow because of the stenosis. The disease is usually associated with atherosclerosis and the investigation of choice is mesenteric angiography (**Fig. 15.9a** and **b**). A specialist vascular surgeon should manage these patients.

This condition is discussed in more detail in the *Vascular and Endovascular Surgery* volume of this *Companion to Specialist Surgical Practice* series and is not discussed further here.

Acute mesenteric ischaemia can affect any part of the GI tract, but is most common in the small bowel and colon. Acute ischaemia to the small bowel will usually produce infarction, whereas ischaemia to the large bowel presents with bloody diarrhoea and abdominal pain, which will usually settle over the course of a few days and is often termed 'ischaemic colitis'. Rarely, delayed strictures may occur.

Thrombosis may occur in the superior mesenteric artery or its branches, usually associated with underlying atherosclerosis. Embolus is often associated with atrial fibrillation, when an atrial thrombus dislodges and lodges in the superior mesenteric artery distribution. Venous thrombosis in the distribution of the superior mesenteric vein is a less common cause of acute small-bowel ischaemia but may be related to increased blood coagulability, portal vein thrombosis, dehydration, infection, compression and vasoconstricting drugs.

Early detection of acute mesenteric ischaemia is difficult (see Chapter 11) and is the primary reason for its high morbidity and mortality. It is more common in the elderly patient who gives a history of vague but worsening abdominal pain, but it is by no means confined to this age group and should be considered in any age group, particularly patients with new onset atrial fibrillation. Further difficulty is added by initial examination findings often being unimpressive, resulting in diagnostic delay.

Where the presentation is a short history with severe pain and tenderness, and there is a high index of suspicion, if possible, early contrast CT should be performed and if a mesenteric thrombus/embolus

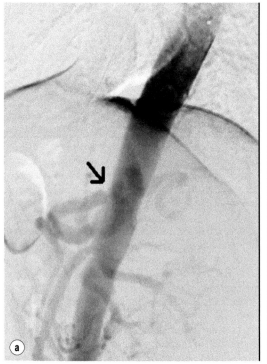 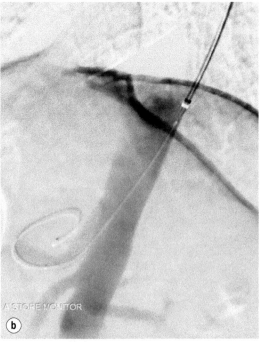

Figure 15.9 • (a) Angiogram demonstrating focal high-grade ostial stenosis of the coeliac artery (*arrow*) in a patient with chronic mesenteric ischaemia. **(b)** The stenotic region has been managed by endovascular stent placement. Images courtesy of Dr Bhavesh Natha, Dr Matley and Partners, Cape Town.

is identified a vascular surgeon should be contacted. The patient should then proceed directly to diagnostic laparoscopy or laparotomy. At surgery a decision must be made as to whether (a) the ischaemic bowel is localised and after resection of frankly gangrenous bowel an adequate length compatible with life will remain; and (b) whether there is an option of vascular reconstruction to salvage the remaining bowel, particularly if it is ischaemic but not yet dead. Exploration of the superior mesenteric artery with removal of an embolus may avoid an extended small-bowel resection and re-vascularise the remaining ischaemic bowel.[19] Bypass for an arterial thrombus with underlying vascular disease is much more complicated and much less likely to be successful and is why a preoperative CT can be helpful for the vascular surgeon to make a decision on what approach may be required, depending on the operative findings.

If surgical resection is carried out, primary anastomosis may be performed, providing the blood supply to both proximal and distal margins is adequate. If embolectomy and vascular reconstruction have been performed, or there is any doubt about the margins, then anastomosis should be deferred. In this situation the safest option is formation of a double-barrelled stoma, or to staple off distal and proximal bowel ends with re-exploration planned within 48 hours. At re-operation an anastomosis may be performed or the proximal limb of bowel exteriorised if anastomosis still appears risky. However, if the patient develops significant postoperative complications, for example cardiac insufficiency, then the planned re-look laparotomy may become life-threatening and untenable. For this reason, in patients with significant cardiac disease, the first option is to be preferred, although management of a high proximal stoma brings with it its own problems of high fluid loss, nutritional supplementation and long-term management. Postoperatively, close attention must be paid to the general condition of the patient to avert or detect any secondary ischaemic event.

Even with prompt intervention, for the majority of patients the affected small intestine is beyond salvage and requires resection. If the whole of the superior mesenteric artery's vasculature has been affected, the majority of the small bowel and part of the proximal colon will often be involved. In this setting the abdomen should simply be closed and no resection performed. These patients should receive intravenous opiates and be kept well sedated, as death will occur shortly afterwards.

✅✅ Overall prognosis is better following acute mesenteric venous infarction as compared to acute mesenteric arterial ischaemia, and survival better following arterial embolism as compared to arterial thrombosis.[20]

Meckel's diverticulum

Meckel's diverticulum is a remnant of the omphalo-mesenteric or vitelline duct. It arises from the anti-mesenteric border of the distal ileum, approximately 60 cm from the iliocaecal valve. It may contain ectopic tissue, usually gastric mucosa, and is estimated to be present in approximately 2% of the population. Meckel's diverticulum may remain asymptomatic throughout life, particularly if it has a broad base and does not contain ectopic gastric mucosa. Occasionally, a band may exist between the diverticulum and the umbilicus, which can cause small-bowel obstruction. This should be treated as for a congenital band adhesion, although resection of the diverticulum, which in this setting is usually elongated and appears pathological, should accompany division of the band. Occasionally, the diverticulum may intussuscept, also causing obstruction. Again, this will require reduction and excision. However reduction is not always possible, in which setting the nature of the lead point will not be obvious, and the entire intussusception mass should be excised. Other common complications of Meckel's diverticulum are haemorrhage and inflammation, when the patient presents with signs and symptoms similar to acute appendicitis. Unless there has been a preoperative CT, this diagnosis is rarely suspected before surgery and the diagnosis is made on the operating table (**Fig. 15.10a**) once a normal appendix has been found. The diverticulum should be excised and the small bowel repaired (**Fig. 15.10b**). Overt, obscure or occult GI bleeding may occur from a Meckel's diverticulum containing ectopic gastric mucosa and the diagnosis is usually established by CT angiogram. The treatment is surgical resection, and this can be done laparoscopically after delivery of the diverticulum through an extended port site incision. If found incidentally at an unrelated operation, an asymptomatic Meckel's diverticulum should not be excised.

Haemorrhage

Disease of the small intestine is an occasional cause of acute GI haemorrhage.[21] There are no specific clinical features that distinguish the small bowel as the source rather than the colon, except that the blood loss may be less 'fresh' and more like melaena. As discussed in Chapter 13, it is important to exclude bleeding from a gastroduodenal source at an early stage by upper GI endoscopy. The commonest causes are vascular malformation, jejunal diverticula, peptic ulceration in a Meckel's diverticulum, and small-bowel tumour. These are all treated by resection. A Dieulafoy lesion presents a particular challenge, as it is frequently not visible

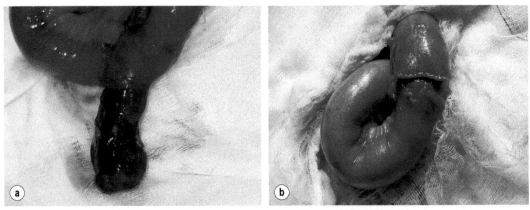

Figure 15.10 • **(a)** Acutely inflamed Meckel's diverticulum identified at laparotomy. **(b)** Operative view after resection of the Meckel diverticulum shown in **(a)**.

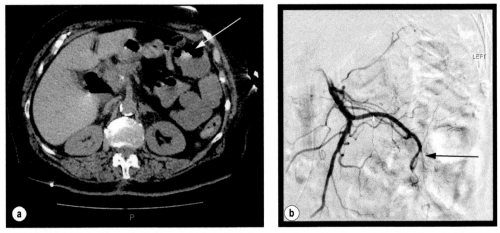

Figure 15.11 • **(a)** CT angiogram with intravenous contrast demonstrating a bleeding point in the jejunum. **(b)** Mesenteric angiogram demonstrating embolisation of the bleeding point shown in **(a)**.

except when it is bleeding and is most common in the stomach. Other vascular malformations, such as haemangiomata, are visible at transillumination. Laparoscopy is not practical in this setting, as the bowel needs to be palpated and illuminated.

Every attempt should be made to identify the site of bleeding before surgery, because at operation a vascular abnormality may produce no external signs. Particularly challenging is bleeding from the biliary tree or distal duodenum beyond the easy reach of the gastroscope. Double balloon and capsule endoscopy have increased the diagnostic yield, the former being both diagnostic and allowing for endoscopic therapies such as Argon plasma coagulation (APC) of vascular malformations. If endoscopic management is unsuccessful the lesion can be tattooed for surgical resection. A limitation of CT angiography results from the mobility and variable anatomical layout of the small bowel, which can make it difficult at laparotomy to

pin-point a radiologically identified bleeding point. CT angiography may identify a bleeding point (**Fig. 15.11a**), following which formal angiography may allow embolisation of the bleeding vessel (**Fig. 15.11b**). It must be remembered that a potential complication of this strategy is bowel ischaemia and a low index of suspicion for bowel ischaemia must be maintained post embolisation.

If the previously mentioned interventions have been unsuccessful and surgery is indicated there are multiple interventions that can help in localisation of the bleeding site, namely: tattoo via double balloon endoscopy, intraoperative endoscopy or, if bleeding appears brisk, segmental soft bowel clamps can be placed throughout the small intestine, resecting the segment that fills up with blood after a period of waiting. Blind resection is often unrewarding and the risks of re-bleeding are high. If no bleeding point can be identified, the surgeon can either close the abdomen and await events, hoping that further bleeding does not occur (and this is often the case), or divide the small bowel around its midpoint, bringing out two stomas. Subsequent bleeding can then be identified to one or other side and endoscopy used to localise it further. These techniques are often heard in surgical discussion, but experience of them is extremely rare. Moreover, emergency surgery is usually not necessary, because ongoing, continuous life-threatening haemorrhage is unusual. This allows investigation of these patients between bleeding episodes.

Appendicitis

Acute appendicitis is the most common intra-abdominal surgical emergency requiring surgery, with an incidence of 7–12% in the population of the USA and Europe. Although frequently described as a childhood illness, the peak incidence is towards 30 years of age. It is slightly more common in males (1.3–1.6:1) but appendicectomy is more common in women because of other mimicking conditions. The reader is referred to Chapter 11 for description of some of the general features and investigation of patients with acute abdominal pain, many of which relate directly to acute appendicitis.

Aetiology and pathology

There are three common aetiological hypotheses for appendicitis, namely: mechanical, infective and hygiene. The *mechanical hypothesis* draws on the fact that appendicitis has a lower incidence in populations with a high-fibre diet, such as in Eastern and Southern Africa. In groups with a low-fibre diet the transit time of stool is slower and thereby, it is proposed, a propensity to form faecoliths.[22] Faecoliths are a specific cause of appendicitis in about one-third of specimens and are composed of fats (coprosterols), inorganic salts (calcium phosphate) and organic residue (vegetable fibres) in a proportion of 50%, 25% and 20%, respectively[23,24] (**Fig. 15.12**). The lumen may also be obstructed by tumours of the caecum or appendix, or by enlargement of lymphoid aggregates within the appendix wall.

The *infective hypothesis* draws on the finding that viruses such as dengue, influenza, Epstein–Barr, rotavirus and cytomegaloviruses, bacteria such as *Campylobacter*, *Brucella* and *Salmonella* as well as parasites like *Entamoeba histolytica*, *Schistosoma mansonii/japonicum* and *Enterobius vermicularis* have been isolated in specimens or indirectly implicated in the pathogenesis of appendicitis. These pathogens are thought to cause appendicitis by invading the lamina propria and initiating oedematous obstruction of the narrow lumen of the appendix.[25,26]

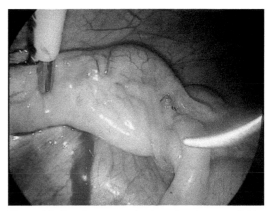

Figure 15.12 • Laparoscopic view of acute appendicitis with a faecolith evident in the proximal third.

The *hygiene hypothesis* stems from the observation that there was an increase in the incidence of appendicitis in Britain from 1895 through 1930 before declining. It was thought that the increase was due to better housing and sanitation. This resulted in a compromised gastrointestinal immune system and an abnormal response to gut pathogens and commensals. Unfortunately none of these hypotheses is completely satisfactory.

The pathology of acute appendicitis is classically described as suppurative, gangrenous or perforated. Typically, there is full-thickness inflammation of the appendix wall. As the disease progresses, adjacent tissues, particularly the omentum, may also become inflamed. Histologically, haemorrhagic ulceration and necrosis in the wall indicate gangrenous appendicitis, and subsequent perforation may be associated with a localised periappendiceal mass/abscess or generalised peritonitis.[24]

Clinical features

The presentation of acute appendicitis varies widely but the classical history and examination findings are described as: central abdominal pain migrating to the right iliac fossa over 4–24 hours; loss of appetite, nausea, sometimes vomiting and fever; diarrhoea is uncommon, but when present should not be confused with gastroenteritis, which is rarely associated with abdominal tenderness (as opposed to pain). In females, the gynaecological history is important, including menses, vaginal discharge or previous endometriosis. On examination, the patient usually exhibits a tachycardia, a low-grade pyrexia and localised peritonitis in the right lower quadrant.

The condition is most difficult to diagnose at the extremes of age: in the very young because of the lack of history and often late presentation; and in the elderly because of a wide list of differential diagnoses and often unimpressive physical signs.

Another factor producing atypical signs is the variation in the position of the appendix. A retrocaecal appendix can give rise to tenderness in the right loin and/or right upper quadrant, whereas a pelvic appendix may be associated with very little abdominal discomfort and a history of diarrhoea, although deep suprapubic pressure and rectal examination may elicit tenderness. Rectal examination tends to be of little value in the diagnosis of acute appendicitis and should rarely be necessary.[27]

Acute appendicitis is one of a dwindling number of conditions where a decision to operate may be based solely on clinical findings. A classic history and the presence of localised right iliac fossa peritonism in a male are highly predictive of acute appendicitis. The risk of morbidity and mortality is significantly increased if the appendix perforates, and to err on the side of over-diagnosing acute appendicitis remains accepted as best surgical practice.

Laparoscopy offers an alternative to what may turn out to be an unnecessary laparotomy and this is especially applicable in women of child-bearing age where a classic history and the presence of peritonism is less reliable than in males. This allows the exclusion of other causes of abdominal pain such as endometriosis, pelvic inflammatory disease and ovarian pathology.

Investigations

The majority of these investigations are discussed at length in Chapter 11 and will not be repeated here except to emphasise the key points. Urinalysis is essential, particularly in women. Although pus cells and microscopic haematuria can occur in appendicitis, their absence may be useful in excluding significant urinary tract disease. The presence of organisms may confirm the diagnosis of urinary tract infection and if in doubt urgent urine microscopy should be requested. Pyelonephrosis or pyonephrosis may be difficult to differentiate clinically from an acutely inflamed retrocaecal appendix and patients with pyuria require urgent investigation of the urinary tract to exclude these diagnoses prior to appendicectomy. Ultrasound may identify gynaecological causes of pain and visualise an inflamed appendix (**Fig. 15.13**), and has a high specificity when positive. However, it cannot reliably be used to exclude appendicitis.

There has been an increasing trend towards using CT (**Fig. 15.14**) in the assessment of patients with acute lower abdominal pain, since its role in acute appendicitis was first reported nearly 20 years ago.[28] A recent meta-analysis concluded that CT utilisation has

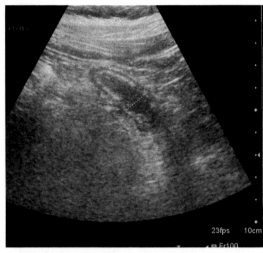

Figure 15.13 • Ultrasound scan demonstrating an acutely inflamed appendix.

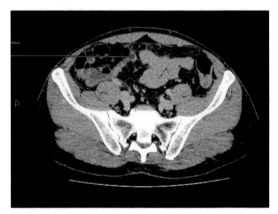

Figure 15.14 • Multislice CT image with intravenous contrast demonstrating an acutely inflamed appendix (*red arrow*).

reduced negative appendicectomy rates, and proposed the routine use of CT in adult patients with suspected appendicitis.[29] However, radiation remains a concern and it seems reasonable to utilise CT only selectively when the diagnosis is in doubt and in elderly patients in whom an underlying colonic neoplasm may be the cause. It remains an appropriate practice to proceed directly to open, or now increasingly, laparoscopic appendicectomy in young males with a high clinical suspicion of appendicitis, and laparoscopy in women of childbearing years. It is reassuring if a preoperative ultrasound demonstrates a pathological looking thickened appendix. However, there should be a low threshold for CT imaging when there is diagnostic doubt, particularly in older patients, and for those in whom the risks of intervention are increased by comorbidity, previous abdominal surgery or morbid obesity.

Differential diagnosis

Just as appendicitis should be considered in any patient with abdominal pain, many other abdominal emergencies must be considered in the differential diagnosis of acute appendicitis. Common conditions presenting in similar fashion include gastroenteritis, mesenteric lymphadenitis, gynaecological diseases, right-sided urinary tract disease and disease of the distal small bowel. Gynaecological disorders are probably the most important group as illustrated by the normal appendicectomy rate being highest in young women. The commonest are acute salpingitis, Mittelschmerz (mid-cycle) pain and complications of ovarian cyst. Torsion, or haemorrhage into an ovarian cyst, usually presents with an acute onset of very severe pain, which may provide a diagnostic clue. To avoid missing a complicated ectopic pregnancy, females of childbearing age should routinely have a pregnancy test (although appendicitis is not uncommon in the first trimester of pregnancy).

The improvement and increased availability of imaging techniques and laparoscopy has provided the opportunity to reduce the stubbornly high proportion of normal appendices removed in the 'open surgery' era, typically up to 20% of patients, and even reaching 29% in women of childbearing age.[30] Although it is clearly advantageous to spare patients unnecessary surgery, the morbidity and mortality of failing to diagnose appendicitis until perforation has occurred is greater than that associated with the removal of a normal appendix. If ultrasound and CT are not readily available, diagnostic laparoscopy is the best option when there is a clinical suspicion of acute appendicitis.

Management

Once acute appendicitis has been diagnosed the options are surgical or non-operative management with antibiotics. Short delays, even up to 24–36 hours in selected patients, are safe and are likely to aid access to imaging and/or laparoscopy, and are not associated with an increased rate of infectious complications. However, where optimal surgical systems allow for expeditious surgery, prompt appendicectomy is advocated.[31] As an example, a patient who is systemically well does not require out-of-hours surgery and can be safely managed with intravenous antibiotics, pending surgery in the morning.[32,33]

Surgical Treatment
Open appendicectomy
The key points for an open appendicectomy are:

1. A transverse muscle splitting incision over McBurney's point.

2. If the appendix is obviously inflamed, it should be removed taking care to make sure the base of the appendix, where it joins the caecum, is properly identified.
3. Local lavage performed and the wound closed.
4. If the appendix is macroscopically normal, examination should be undertaken of the terminal ileum (for at least 60 cm to exclude an inflamed Meckel's diverticulum) and small-bowel mesentery and pelvis, both by palpation and direct visualisation. Any free peritoneal fluid should be collected for subsequent culture. The presence of bile staining indicates proximal bowel perforation, such as perforated peptic ulcer, and faecal fluid indicates colonic perforation. In both instances a full laparotomy is indicated. In the former situation, it is best to close the right iliac fossa incision in preference to an upper midline, but in the latter, some surgeons advocate extending the right iliac fossa incision medially as a muscle-cutting lower abdominal transverse incision. If in doubt, a midline incision is best.

   An alternative technique for evaluating the peritoneal cavity without a laparotomy or wound extension, is to close the appendicectomy wound over a 10-mm laparoscopic port using tissue-grasping forceps or a strong purse-string suture. Laparoscopy can then be undertaken with insertion of more ports as needed to allow manipulation of abdominal organs. If this is difficult, closure of the appendicectomy wound and a standard subumbilical open laparoscopy incision should be performed.
5. It used to be traditional teaching to bury the appendix stump, but laparoscopic appendicectomy has proven that simple ligation of the stump is adequate.[34] If the appendix has perforated at the base, formal repair of the caecal pole is advised. Leaving a long stump should be avoided as this can become ischaemic leading to complications. Similarly, failing to remove all the appendix will result in recurrent symptoms and appendicitis of the remaining stump. The use of surgical drains remains controversial and will ultimately depend on the extent of local contamination and whether or not there was an abscess cavity.
6. All patients should receive prophylactic broad-spectrum antibiotics to reduce wound infection,

which is the commonest complication after appendicectomy.[35,36] A single dose is as effective as three doses for wound prophylaxis. For perforated appendicitis, antibiotics should be continued until signs of sepsis have settled. In complicated appendicitis, provided that there are no ongoing signs of sepsis, postoperative antibiotics should be continued for 3 days.[37] When patients can tolerate diet, completing the course of antibiotics orally will reduce hospital stay without additional complication.[38] Although the risk of deep vein thrombosis is relatively low in young patients, prophylaxis is best administered as a routine, as not all patients will make a swift recovery and early postoperative mobilisation may be delayed. Laparoscopy does not preclude the need for DVT prophylaxis.

✔✔ Prophylactic antibiotics should be administered in all patients undergoing appendicectomy for acute appendicitis in order to reduce the risk of wound infection.[35,36]

Laparoscopic appendicectomy

The advantages of laparoscopic appendicectomy have been extensively studied over the last 20 years, although individual studies have produced conflicting results.[39–41]

As skills in laparoscopic technique have become more widespread, laparoscopic appendicectomy has become increasingly common.[41] It seems reasonable to proceed with laparoscopic appendicectomy for any patient in whom an acutely inflamed appendix is discovered during diagnostic laparoscopy, providing the surgeon has the relevant skills. Obese patients and those of large build, will benefit more from the laparoscopic approach by avoiding the larger wound required at open surgery.

✔✔ A Cochrane database systematic review of 67 studies has confirmed the benefit of the laparoscopic approach in relation to less pain, faster recovery and a lower incidence of wound infections. However, this 2010 review suggested that there is an increase in intra-abdominal abscesses (odds ratio 1.87) in patients undergoing a laparoscopic procedure. These concerns have been discounted by more recent data demonstrating a reduced incidence of abscess and adhesion formation.[39] As a result, the laparoscopic approach is now generally recommended for all patients with suspected appendicitis, with particular advantage in young female, obese and working patients.[40,41]

The key principles for laparoscopic appendicectomy are similar to the open approach with the following additions:

1. The pelvis is much easier to examine and the opportunity to examine it and the rest of the peritoneal cavity should be taken.
2. Thorough lavage is easier but it is important to remove all the effluent. If there has been significant contamination and a large amount of washout has been used, it is advisable to leave a small drain in the pelvis for the first 12 hours or so to allow any residual fluid to drain out after the patient sits up. It can then be removed.
3. While formal ligation and division of the appendix mesentery is standard practice in open appendicectomy this is not necessary in the laparoscopic approach. The appendix can be dissected from its mesentery from tip to base with electro-cautery without formal division of the mesentery. Occasionally larger vessels may require to be clipped, but this is uncommon.

The appendix can be secured with a pre-formed loop ligature or a 15-mm Hem-o-Lok®, which has recently been shown to be both safe and effective[42] (**Fig. 15.15**). The application of an endoscopic stapling device to the appendix and/or meso-appendix is discouraged due to unnecessary associated cost.

It is important to remove the appendix through the abdominal wall without contaminating the soft tissues. Most appendices can be drawn into the 10-mm laparoscopic port, thus eliminating abdominal wall contamination, particularly if the appendix has been dissected off the mesentery. A large, friable or perforated appendix should be handled gently and

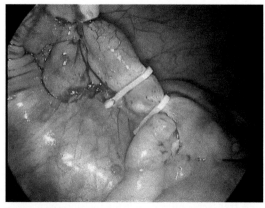

Figure 15.15 • Appendix base secured with Hemolok® at laparoscopic appendicectomy.

removed in a retrieval bag, taking care to remove all debris, including any loose faecolith.

One of the reported complications of laparoscopic appendicectomy is leaving too long a stump and risking recurrent symptoms.[43] Care must therefore be taken to ensure that the entire appendix has been fully mobilised to avoid this complication.

The normal appendix at open surgery

An unexpected normal appendix discovered through a right iliac fossa appendicectomy incision should be removed. While this may be associated with some morbidity, it does avoid future dilemma in patients presenting with recurrent symptoms and a scar that suggests the appendix may have been removed. Postoperative wound infection remains the same as after an open appendicectomy for an inflamed (but non-perforated) appendix. A late complication which also needs to be considered is adhesive small bowel obstruction. In a historical cohort study of 245 400 patients who underwent appendicectomy in Sweden with population-based matched controls, the cumulative risk of surgically treated small-bowel obstruction following open appendicectomy was 1.3% after 30 years compared with 0.21% for non-operated controls.[44]

The normal appendix at laparoscopy

When the appendix is found to be normal and an alternative diagnosis, such as pelvic inflammatory disease or diverticulitis, is identified at laparoscopy, surgical judgement should be used regarding its removal. While removal is usually easy and probably best to perform, this may not be the case if the alternative pathology is complex, such as finding a perforated peptic ulcer, severe diverticulitis or malignancy. As already mentioned above, if suspected Crohn's disease is encountered at either laparoscopy or laparotomy, the appendix should be removed.

In the presence of a visibly normal appendix and no other pathology the arguments in favour of removing the appendix are:

1. There is a small incidence of appendicitis on histological examination of a macroscopically normal appendix.[45] A study evaluating the ability of laparoscopy to discriminate between a normal and an inflamed appendix demonstrated a sensitivity of 92% and a specificity of 85% if an appendix with isolated mucosal inflammation was considered to be inflamed.[46]

2. Removal of the appendix prevents a diagnostic dilemma in the future in a patient who has persistent abdominal symptoms following laparoscopy. The counter argument is the questionable clinical significance of isolated mucosal inflammation in an otherwise normal appendix, and all operations are associated with some risk, however small.

It would seem counter intuitive at laparoscopy to leave an apparently uninflamed appendix when its removal is simple, but the surgical decision-making will vary with the individual clinical setting.

Non-surgical treatment

It is recognised that simple appendicitis can be successfully managed with antibiotics alone in selected patients. This contentious topic has been reviewed in two recent meta-analyses.

The first compared five studies including 1116 patients.[47] Complications were reported in 5% of patients in the antibiotic and 8% in the appendicectomy group. There was a 23% appendicectomy rate within 1 year in the antibiotic group. The study concluded that there should be a change in practice towards shared decision-making around surgery or non-operative treatment in patients with clearly uncomplicated appendicitis.

There are limitations to this meta-analysis, many of which are recognised in the paper. The major morbidity reported in the surgical group is perforation, yet this is part of the disease spectrum of appendicitis and not a complication of surgery. Exclusion of this single complication reduces the complication rate in the surgical group to 9 of 489 patients, or 1.8%. In none of the studies analysed were the complications classified according to severity. There is also evidence of probable selection bias, with slow recruitment in two of the biggest trials, one of which recruited only 20% of all the patients presenting with uncomplicated appendicitis. This raises concerns that the healthier patients were treated with antibiotics. Furthermore only 23% of procedures in the surgical group were performed laparoscopically, which is recognised to have a lower wound infection and adhesion rate than open surgery. A final concern is that the recurrence rate of 23% of appendicitis within 1 year has to be seen as a failure of antibiotic therapy.

The second meta-analysis was of four randomised trials and four cohort studies, including 2551 patients.[48] This study found that 26.5% of patients in the antibiotic group needed appendicectomy within 1 year. The rate of adverse events (3.3% for antibiotic and 1.5% for surgery group) and the incidence of complicated appendicitis was significantly higher in the antibiotic treatment group. Overall, postoperative complications were, however, comparable between the group that underwent immediate surgery and those that had an appendicectomy due to antibiotic failure. The randomised trials analysed showed a significantly longer hospital stay in the antibiotic treatment group. There remains concern as to the longer-term outcomes of the antibiotic-only group in all the studies due to the fact that all trials have so far followed up the patients for only 1 year. The conclusion that is drawn from this second meta-analysis is that although antibiotics may prevent some patients from appendectomy, surgery represents the definitive, one-time-only treatment with a well-known risk profile, whereas the long-term impact of antibiotic treatment on patient quality of life and healthcare costs is unknown.

✔️ While antibiotic treatment will be successful in the short term (up to 1 year), in many patients with uncomplicated appendicitis, the high failure rate (27%) means that laparoscopic appendicectomy remains the authors' treatment of choice in the majority of patients with suspected acute appendicitis. A small subgroup of patients who are well with minimal signs might be considered for antibiotic treatment after full discussion of the risks and benefits, and perhaps taking into account other circumstances.

Treatment of atypical presentation of acute appendicitis

Appendix mass

The natural history of acute appendicitis left untreated is that it will either resolve, become gangrenous and perforate, or become walled off by a mass of omentum and small bowel. The latter prevents inflammation spreading to the abdominal cavity. Such a patient usually presents with a longer history, often a week or more, of right lower quadrant abdominal pain, and appears systemically well but has a tender palpable mass in the right iliac fossa. The differential diagnosis includes Crohn's disease in younger patients and carcinoma of the caecum in older patients. Confirmation is obtained from ultrasound or CT. Appendix mass is best managed non-operatively as the risk of perforation has passed and removal of the appendix at this late stage can be difficult and is associated with a significant complication rate. A 2010 meta-analysis reported that the non-operative treatment of complicated appendicitis (appendix mass or abscess) is associated with a decrease in complications compared to appendicectomy, with a similar duration of hospital stay.[49] In the systemically well patient, non-operative treatment may include percutaneous drainage of any fluid collections.

Following resolution of the symptoms and mass, routine interval appendicectomy (6 weeks to 3 months) was considered essential to prevent recurrent symptoms in the young and to exclude carcinoma in the elderly. However, providing carcinoma can be excluded by other means, such as CT and colonoscopy, routine interval appendicectomy is no longer recommended. In the majority of patients the appendix has been destroyed and in one study only 9% of patients treated non-operatively for an appendix mass subsequently developed recurrent symptoms within 5 months.[50] If symptoms recur then it is reasonable to offer these patients surgery.

✔️✔️ A systematic review has confirmed that non-operative management of an appendix mass will be successful in the majority of patients and recurrence of symptoms is low. As a result, the routine use of interval appendicectomy is no longer justified.[50]

Appendix abscess

In some patients the appendix becomes walled off by omentum but has perforated and an abscess will develop in the periappendiceal region. This may be in the right paracolic gutter, the subcaecal area or the pelvis and can be visualised by either ultrasound or CT (**Fig. 15.16**). Unlike with a simple 'appendix mass', the patient is usually systemically unwell with abdominal tenderness. As for all abscesses, drainage is the best treatment, either under radiological control or surgically. There is no doubt that surgical drainage can be associated with significant complications, not least because tissues and organs adjacent to the abscess will be friable and must be handled with great care. The alternative of radiologically guided drainage (**Fig. 15.17**) has been reported to produce lower complications and equivalent early operation/re-operation rates.[51,52] It would therefore seem reasonable to use the non-operative approach in any patient in whom overt signs of peritonitis are absent. If surgery is required, then the residual necrotic appendix should be

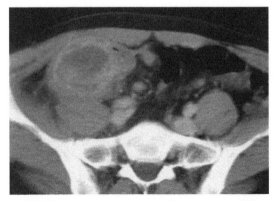

Figure 15.16 • CT demonstrating an appendix abscess.

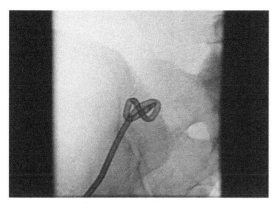

Figure 15.17 • Radiograph of the patient shown in Fig. 15.16, following percutaneous drainage of the appendix abscess, with drain in situ.

identified and resected. In this setting the placement of a drain in the residual cavity is encouraged.

Chronic appendicitis

As noted already, there is certainly a group of patients who suffer from recurrent appendicitis[53] and who benefit from appendicectomy. CT can help assessment in difficult cases, but for many patients laparoscopy is the best investigation, at which the appendix can be removed. A small, randomised trial has reported improvement in chronic recurrent right lower quadrant pain following laparoscopic appendicectomy compared to laparoscopy alone.[54]

Appendicitis in pregnancy

The rate of appendicitis in pregnancy is similar to that in the non-pregnant female population. Suspected appendicitis is the most common indication for surgery for non-obstetric conditions during pregnancy, and occurs in approximately one in 500 pregnancies per year. Appendicitis occurs more frequently in the second trimester than in the first or third.[55] Preoperative diagnosis of acute appendicitis can be difficult in pregnancy, and a low threshold for surgical intervention has traditionally been recommended, as complicated appendicitis is associated with a higher rate of fetal loss and increased maternal morbidity. A systematic review reported a negative appendicectomy rate of 12–24%, higher than in the non-pregnant population, and rates of fetal loss of 3.4%, 12.1% and 7.3% in simple, complicated and negative appendicectomy, respectively.,[55] Recognition of the risk associated with negative appendicectomy[56] has led to the American College of Obstetricians and Gynecologists recommending magnetic resonance imaging (MRI) in patients in whom an ultrasound scan has failed to show acute appendicitis.[57] Where emergency access to such imaging is not possible and

there remains a high suspicion of acute appendicitis, surgery should not be delayed.

Many reports have demonstrated laparoscopic appendicectomy to be a safe and effective procedure during pregnancy. With modification of port positions, the laparoscopic approach has even been reported during the third trimester. The results of a recent systematic review and meta-analysis suggest that laparoscopic appendicectomy in pregnancy results in an almost twofold significantly higher risk of fetal loss compared with open appendicectomy. This was heavily influenced by a single study, which showed a higher risk for laparoscopy, with an odds ratio of 2.3 for fetal loss compared to conventional surgery. After exclusion of this study from the pooled analysis, there was no effect of laparoscopic appendicectomy on fetal loss.[55,56] Currently the Society of American Gastrointestinal and Endoscopic Surgeons continues to recommend laparoscopic appendicectomy as the treatment of choice for pregnant patients regardless of gestation.[58]

A reasonable approach in these patients is to use laparoscopy in the first trimester or when, despite adequate imaging, the diagnosis is in doubt. In later pregnancy open surgery may be preferred when the diagnosis is confirmed, but the approach will depend upon surgeon expertise. In all cases there should be a low threshold for conversion to open surgery if difficulties are encountered. In the third trimester the incision for open appendicectomy may be high in the right upper quadrant and is not a procedure for unsupervised trainee surgeons.

Postoperative complications and outcome

Hospital stay

The duration of hospital stay depends on local resources, policies, the patient's general condition and any coexisting disease. It is now clear that laparoscopic appendicectomy is associated with a more rapid return to normal activities, lower morbidity rate and a shorter hospital stay than conventional surgery.[39-41]

Wound infection

This is the commonest postoperative complication, occurring in around 10–15% of patients following a conventional right iliac fossa incision. In most patients the inflammation is superficial, responding promptly to antibiotics, but in some there will be abscess formation, sometimes requiring surgical intervention. Wound infection is significantly less following laparoscopic appendicectomy.[41]

There is no evidence that wound infiltration with local anaesthetic agents is associated with any increase in the incidence of wound infection.[59,60] After open appendicectomy the skin may be closed with interrupted sutures or a continuous suture and this does not appear to affect wound infection rates. However, in the presence of infection, removal of one or two interrupted sutures may allow irrigation and resolution without complete dehiscence of the wound, which results when a continuous suture is cut to allow access. Some surgeons leave the skin incision open if there has been gross contamination of the wound in perforated appendicitis, with secondary closure a few days later. The subsequent cosmetic result of such a scar is usually satisfactory.

Other septic complications

Pericaecal fluid collections are relatively common and are usually indicated by the presence of abdominal discomfort and a low-grade pyrexia. They can usually be diagnosed by ultrasound, and the initiation of antibiotics with re-laparoscopy and lavage of the right iliac fossa via the previously used port sites results in rapid recovery. An alternative is radiological aspiration. Pelvic abscess is a less common complication that presents with lower abdominal discomfort and swinging pyrexia. The symptoms may be delayed by 10 days or more and a soft tender mass may be palpable on rectal examination, although this is not always the case. Again, ultrasound and often CT is required for diagnosis and, if pus is aspirated, a percutaneous drain should be placed if possible. Occasionally, a pelvic abscess may be difficult to drain percutaneously and in this situation early re-look laparoscopy (in preference to re-look laparotomy) and pelvic washout with drain insertion is usually straightforward and immediately effective. An alternative approach is antibiotics or occasionally drainage of the abscess into the rectum if possible. The decision is influenced by the general condition of the patient. Prolonged use of antibiotics should be avoided and further attempts made for drainage if the collection is not resolving on repeated imaging.

As in any patient who has undergone laparoscopic abdominal surgery, the presence of increased abdominal tenderness or generalised peritonitis in the first 24 hours may indicate an unrecognised iatrogenic injury to the intestine and mandates immediate re-look laparoscopy.

Prognosis

The mortality of appendicitis is associated with the age of the patient and delayed diagnosis (perforated appendix). In a report on 573 244 appendicectomies in the USA from 2006 to 2008 the mortality rate was 0.31%. This was highest in patients with perforated appendicitis.[61] A further consideration is the incidence of subsequent tubal infertility after appendicectomy. Meta-analysis has shown that appendicitis does not affect fertility in women; it does, however, increase the risk of subsequent ectopic pregnancy.[62]

Appendiceal tumours

Neoplasms of the appendix are rare. They are found in approximately 1% of appendicectomy specimens. Neuroendocrine tumours are the most common, comprising 30-80% of all appendiceal neoplasms.[63,64]

Neuroendocrine neoplasm

Appendiceal neuroendocrine neoplasm (NEN) is a relatively frequent subgroup of neuroendocrine neoplasms with an approximate incidence of 0.15–0.6/100 000/year.[64-70] The majority of appendiceal NENs originate from serotonin-producing enterochromaffin cells. The tumours appear to have a neuroectodermal origin and more benign features than other NENs.[65] Appendiceal NEN are prevalent at autopsy and rarely attain clinical significance. Many may perhaps undergo spontaneous involution, since the prevalence is reported as higher in children than in adults.[66]

It follows that appendiceal NEN are often an incidental finding at surgery, and are expected to occur in 3–5 in 1000 appendicectomies.[65,70] Approximately 70% are located in the tip of the appendix, resulting in them seldom occluding the lumen and causing appendicitis.[65,70] Patients with appendiceal NENs are generally younger than those with other NENs, having a mean age of 40 years, with a slight female predominance. The overall metastasis rate is 3.8%, with distant metastases in 0.7%.[66] Early stage NEN have an excellent prognosis, with 5-year survival rates of 95–100% for local disease and 85–100% for regional disease.[64,68,70] This is in contrast with metastatic disease, where 5-year survival is less than 25%.[64,69,70]

✔✔ The majority (approximately 90%) of appendiceal NENs are <1 cm in diameter and have minimal risk of presenting with metastases. These lesions may be cured by simple appendicectomy.[64,66,70] This treatment is also apparently safe for most lesions measuring 1–2 cm, although rare cases in this group have presented with lymph node metastases.[65,70] Right hemicolectomy should be performed for the 1–2 cm NEN with high-risk features, namely: positive or unclear margins, deep meso-appendiceal invasion (>3 mm), high proliferation rate (WHO Grade 2) or angioinvasion. NEN with a diameter >2 cm should likewise be treated with a right hemicolectomy.[70]

Mucinous tumours

Adenomas and low-grade appendiceal mucinous neoplasms typically occur in patients in their sixth decade. The majority of mucinous neoplasms of the appendix are either asymptomatic, present with chronic right iliac fossa pain or a mass. Some patients may present with pain that mimics acute appendicitis.[71–73] Diagnosis is usually made with imaging performed for chronic pain, or occasionally at colonoscopy, where a bulging appendiceal orifice may be recognised (**Fig. 15.18**).

Pseudomyxoma peritonei (PMP) is the consequence of a perforated mucinous tumour of the appendix. This mucinous neoplastic epithelium is gradually seeded throughout the peritoneal cavity.[74,75] PMP is commonly diagnosed by gynaecologists in patients presenting with pelvic discomfort or enlarged ovaries secondarily involved by mucinous tumour deposits. Histological studies of many PMP cases presumed to be due to ovarian mucinous tumour peritoneal spread have been found to be of appendiceal origin.[76,77] The very slow accumulation of mucin means the process of distension and gradual perforation may be minimally symptomatic and occur years before the presentation of PMP.[74,75]

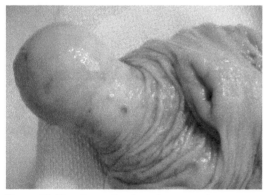

Figure 15.18 • Appendiceal mucinous neoplasm specimen demonstrating bulging appendiceal orifice.

There are three histological entities grouped together as mucinous neoplasms of the appendix: adenoma, low-grade appendiceal mucinous neoplasm (LAMN) and invasive adenocarcinoma.[78] An appendix with an adenoma or LAMN may, on gross examination, appear either unremarkable or dilated with tenacious mucin, although there should be no mucin on the external surface. As the process advances, the wall of an appendix with LAMN frequently becomes fibrotic and hyalinised, and may have extensive calcification creating a 'porcelain appendix'.[73,78] Alternatively, it may become transformed into a fibrotic cyst lined by attenuated neoplastic mucinous epithelium.

Simple appendicectomy is sufficient treatment for adenomas and LAMNS (**Fig. 15.19**), but if the appendix margin is found to be involved at histology then a right hemicolectomy is indicated[73,79] (**Fig. 15.20**). This operation offers no additional benefit over appendicectomy alone for patients with LAMNs that are confined to the appendix.[80,81] Given the possibility of peritoneal recurrence in patients with ruptured tumours, patients with acellular mucin on the appendiceal serosa should have wide excision of the surrounding tissue that has encapsulated the mucin. The peritoneal cavity and omentum should also be copiously washed in an effort to prevent the development of PMP. Some specialist units now offer radical 'peritonealectomy' and high temperature intraperitoneal chemotherapy for patients at high risk of recurrence and referral to one of these units should be considered in such patients.

Adenocarcinoma

In contrast to other appendiceal neoplasms the majority of patients with adenocarcinoma present with a picture of acute appendicitis.[82] Other presentations include a palpable mass, obstruction, gastrointestinal bleeding, or symptoms referable to metastases. Appendiceal adenocarcinomas fall into one of three separate histologic types: (i) the most common is the mucinous type, which produces abundant mucin;

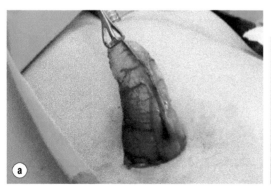
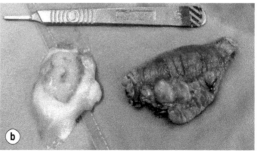

Figure 15.19 • (a) Appendicectomy for mucinous adenoma discovered in pregnant patient with right iliac fossa pain. **(b)** Appendix specimen demonstrating distal dilatation at adenoma site and mucin from within appendiceal lumen.

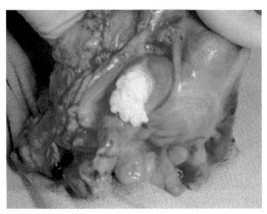

Figure 15.20 • Hemicolectomy for mucinous tumour of appendix involving base of appendix (see Fig. 15.18). Specimen opened to demonstrate appendiceal mucin.

(ii) the less common intestinal or colonic type closely mimics adenocarcinomas found in the colon; and (iii) the least common is signet ring cell adenocarcinoma, which is associated with a poor prognosis.[83]

Although controversial, invasive adenocarcinoma of the appendix on histology warrants a subsequent right hemicolectomy both to achieve complete tumour resection and to adequately stage the tumour by examining the right colic lymph nodes.[84-87] Most studies have shown that right hemicolectomy offers improved 5-year survival rates relative to appendicectomy alone; however, the prognosis of appendiceal carcinoma is worse than for adenocarcinoma of the colon.[84,85,87] See also the *Colorectal Surgery* volume of the *Companion to Specialist Practice* series.

Key points

- The commonest emergency conditions affecting the small bowel are obstruction, haemorrhage and ischaemia.
- Early management requires adequate clinical and radiological assessment, which might include contrast radiology and CT (see also Chapter 11).
- Surgery for acute appendicitis is superior to antibiotics alone because of the latter's high recurrence rate.
- Laparoscopic appendicectomy results in less pain, fewer wound complications and faster return to normal activities than open appendicectomy.
- A non-operative approach is indicated in the majority of patients with appendix mass or abscess, with radiological drainage as required. Subsequent interval appendicectomy is only indicated in those patients with recurrent symptoms. Care must be taken to ensure that underlying diseases other than appendicitis have been excluded (e.g. caecal carcinoma and Crohn's disease), which usually requires CT and colonoscopy.

Acknowledgement

The 5th edition of this chapter was written by Peter Lamb. We have retained much of the information, revising and updating it as appropriate. We acknowledge the excellence of his work.

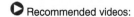 Recommended videos:

- Laparoscopy of ischaemic bowel –https://youtu.be/wyohLCbFTV0
- Laparoscopic adhesiolysis – https://youtu.be/BKo0mAoog6M
- Open appendectomy – https://youtu.be/8OK-_4Wx3QY
- Laparoscopic appendicectomy – https://youtu.be/GfmicbfAeD0
- Laparoscopic appendicectomy in a pregnant patient – https://youtu.be/mvVOWLh6_vE
- Other useful videos from the authors can be viewed on https://www.youtube.com/channel/UCLSczWba4suPd-j6CAD615Q

Full references available at **http://expertconsult. inkling.com**

Key references

20. Schoots IG, Koffeman DA, Levi M, et al. Systematic review of survival after acute mesenteric ischaemia according to disease aetiology. Br J Surg 2004;91:17–27. PMID: 14716789.

   Data from 45 observational studies including 3692 patients were reviewed. Prognosis after acute mesenteric venous thrombosis is better than for arterial ischaemia, and that for arterial embolism is better than that for arterial thrombosis.

35. Andersen BR, Kallehave FL, Andersen HK. Antibiotics versus placebo for prevention of postoperative infection after appendicectomy: update of Cochrane Database Systematic Review

2003;(2). Cochrane Database Syst Rev 2005;3: CD001439. PMID: 16034862.

This systematic review confirmed the advantage of prophylactic antibiotics in reducing wound infection following appendicectomy.

36. SIGN guideline 104. Antibiotic prophylaxis in surgery. Scottish Intercollegiate Guideline Network; April 2014. www.sign.ac.uk.

This guideline demonstrated that prophylactic antibiotics during appendicectomy reduced wound infection with an odds ratio of 0.33 and the number needed to treat to prevent one wound infection being 11.

39. Masoomi H, Mills S, Dolich MO, et al. Comparison of outcomes of laparoscopic versus open appendectomy in adults: data from the nationwide inpatient sample (NIS), 2006–2008. J Gastrointest Surg 2011;15:2226–31. PMID: 21725700.

This nationwide review confirms the decrease in infective morbidity from laparoscopic appendicectomy.

40. Sauerland S, Jaschinski T, Neugebauer EA. Laparoscopic versus open surgery for suspected appendicitis. Cochrane Database Syst Rev 2010;(10) CD001546. PMID: 20927725.

This Cochrane review recommends laparoscopic appendicectomy for the obese, women of childbearing age and working individuals.

42. Lucchi A, Berti P, Grassia M, et al. Laparoscopic appendectomy: Hem-o-lok versus Endoloop in stump closure. Updates Surg 2016. PMID: 28013455.

Randomised trial demonstrating no difference between Endoloop and Hem-oLok in closure of the appendix stump during laparoscopic appendicectomy, but Hem-o-Lok costs less and is easier to use. See also https://www.sages.org/meetings/annual-meeting/abstracts-archive/application-of-hem-o-lok-clip-in-basic-laparoscopic-procedures-a-single-center-experience-on-856-cases-and-review-of-data-from-food-and-drug-administration/; .

48. Harnoss JC, Zelienka I, Probst P, et al. Antibiotics versus surgical therapy for uncomplicated appendicitis: systematic review and meta-analysis of controlled trials (PROSPERO 2015:CRD42015016882). Ann Surg 2017;265(5):889–900. PMID: 27759621.

Meta-analysis of 8 trials, reporting 1 year appendicitis recurrence rate of 26.5%. Found increased rate of adverse events and complicated appendicitis in the antibiotic only group. Recommends surgery as the treatment for acute, uncomplicated appendicitis.

50. Deakin DE, Ahmed I. Interval appendicectomy after resolution of adult inflammatory appendix mass – is it necessary? Surgeon 2007;5(1):45–50. PMID: 17313128.

A systematic review confirming that non-operative management will be successful in the majority of patients and recurrence of symptoms is low.

70. Pape UF, Niederle B, Costa F, et al. Consensus guidelines for neuroendocrine neoplasms of the appendix (excluding goblet cell carcinomas). Neuroendocrinology 2016;103(2):144–52. PMID: 26730583.

ENET consensus guideline.

16

Colonic emergencies

Scott R. Kelley
David W. Larson

Introduction

Colonic emergencies result from obstruction, inflammation/infection, perforation, haemorrhage, or ischaemia. Herein we discuss aetiology, pathogenesis, presentation and management. Emergency compared to elective colon surgery is associated with a two- to threefold increase in mortality, hence interventions to convert an emergency into an elective operation should be considered when safe to do so. In addition to a thorough history and physical examination, patients must be resuscitated and optimised as far as practicable prior to proceeding to the operating room. Multidisciplinary approaches to patient care and thorough radiographic and colonoscopic evaluation are often extremely beneficial for planning and treating this complex population. When possible patients should be preoperatively evaluated, educated and site-marked by stoma therapists. If facilities are inadequate, transfer to a referral centre should be considered.

Colonic obstruction

Colonic obstruction can occur secondary to multiple causes (Table 16.1) and can be partial or complete, intrinsic or extrinsic, and adynamic or mechanical. The most common causes are neoplasia, diverticulitis and volvulus. Treatment for obstruction is dependent on the location, cause, patient presentation and goals of care.

A distal colonic obstruction in the presence of a competent ileocaecal valve hindering retrograde flow of enteric content, or colonic volvulus, will result in a closed loop obstruction. Antegrade flow of enteric content and bacterial overgrowth progressively increase intraluminal pressure, which is followed by venous occlusion, intramural hypoperfusion, arterial occlusion, thrombosis, ischaemia, necrosis and perforation. Consequently a closed loop obstruction mandates expedited care.

Mild obstruction (stenosis) typically presents with cramping abdominal pain and constipation. Imaging may reveal an area of luminal stenosis. Endoscopic advancement through the stricture is often not possible. Colon proximal to the stricture is not dilated and surgery can be planned in an elective fashion. Severe obstruction presents with proximal bowel dilatation, pronounced abdominal distension, absolute constipation (failure to pass flatus or stool) and varying degrees of tenderness, which in combination with signs of systemic toxicity (elevated heart rate, leukocytosis) necessitate emergency surgery.

Neoplastic obstruction

Approximately 20% of patients with colon cancer will present with an obstruction, with the majority being elderly. Nearly 30% will have hepatic metastasis at the time of surgery. Obstruction secondary to colon cancer often presents with a constellation of symptoms including abdominal distension, alteration in bowel habits, weight loss, change in stool calibre and/or consistency, nausea, emesis, obstipation and absence of flatus. Symptoms usually develop slowly and typically reflect the site of obstruction. Right-sided masses typically cause obstructive symptoms (abdominal cramping, pain) whereas left-sided

Table 16.1 • Causes of colonic obstruction

Neoplasm
Volvulus
Diverticulitis
Pseudo-obstruction
Hernia
Stricture
Faecal impaction
Inflammatory
Intussusception
Endometriosis
Adhesions
Ischaemia

cancers are more commonly associated with a change in stool calibre, consistency and alteration in bowel habits.

Initial management includes bowel rest, analgesia, resuscitation and correction of laboratory abnormalities. Nasogastric tubes do not decompress the colon and are not necessary unless the patient is experiencing nausea/emesis. Plain abdominal radiographs will identify large bowel dilatation and if the ileocaecal valve is incompetent small intestine distension may also be noted. Computed tomographic (CT) imaging informs surgical planning and provides staging information which may be key in defining goals of care, and should be obtained unless immediate operative intervention cannot be delayed. If CT is not available, a water-soluble contrast enema will identify the level of obstruction and can be useful in distinguishing pseudo-obstruction (Ogilvie's syndrome) from causes of mechanical obstruction. Endoscopy may be both diagnostic and therapeutic.

Intervention: colonic stents

Colonic self-expandable metal stents (SEMS) may be used as a bridge to surgery for those with partial obstruction or for palliation in patients with inoperable disease.[1] Although technical success is greater than 90%, complications include stent migration (12%), obstruction/occlusion (7%) and perforation (4%).[2] Perforations are more common with intraluminal stents left in place for a prolonged period of time, stents crossing acute angles and in patients receiving bevacizumab.[3-4] Non-palliative stenting ('bridge to surgery') provides the opportunity to decompress the distended proximal colon, medically optimise patients in preparation for surgery, complete a preoperative colonoscopy, and pursue a single-stage operation using a minimally invasive approach. However, clinically silent microperforations associated with stents have been documented at the time of surgery,

raising concerns regarding oncological outcomes. Small and colleagues at the Mayo Clinic identified five risk factors associated with complications from self-expandable colonic stents, which included male gender, complete colonic occlusion, balloon dilatation prior to stent placement, mid-stent diameter less than 22 mm, and placement by an interventionalist not familiar with pancreaticobiliary procedures.[3] The first randomised prospective study comparing open surgery to SEMS followed by a minimally invasive resection (endolaparoscopic) for left-sided colon cancer was reported in 2009. No stent-related complications were reported, technical and clinical success for stenting was 83%, and only 38% underwent a single-stage operation in the open compared to 67% in the endolaparoscopic arm. All in the stent arm underwent ostomy reversal and six in the open group were left with a permanent stoma.[5] Pirlet and colleagues in a French multicentre prospective randomised controlled trial compared the outcomes of emergency surgery to SEMS as a bridge for surgery. The primary outcome was the need for a stoma (temporary or permanent) for any reason. The secondary endpoints were mortality, morbidity and length of hospital stay. The study was closed early secondary to stent-related perforations. Among the 60 patients accrued, 17 in the open group versus 13 in the SEMS group were left with a stoma.[6] The multi-institutional Dutch Stent-In Study Group evaluated colonic stenting as a bridge to elective surgery versus emergency surgery, with the primary outcome of mean global health status during a 6-month follow-up. The study was closed early secondary to increased morbidity in the SEMS group, and specifically six perforations in the SEMS versus none in the operative arm. They concluded colonic stenting has no decisive clinical advantages to emergency surgery.[7] Compared to proceeding directly to surgery, endoluminal stents for obstruction in non-palliative circumstances have not been shown in a Cochrane systematic review to confer an advantage in regards to morbidity and mortality.[8] The American Society of Gastrointestinal Endoscopy (ASGE) and European Society of Gastrointestinal Endoscopy (ESGE) currently only recommend self-expanding metal stents for patients who are poor surgical candidates who need medical optimisation.[1]

✓✓ According to the European Society of Gastrointestinal Endoscopy (ESGE) and American Society of Gastrointestinal Endoscopy (ASGE):
1. Prophylactic colonic stent placement is not recommended. Colonic stenting should be reserved for patients with clinical symptoms and imaging evidence of malignant large-bowel obstruction, without signs of perforation.

2. Colonic self-expandable metal stent (SEMS) placement as a bridge to elective surgery is not recommended as a standard treatment of symptomatic left-sided malignant colonic obstruction.

3. SEMS placement is recommended as the preferred treatment for palliation of malignant colonic obstruction, except in patients treated or considered for treatment with anti-angiogenic drugs (e.g. bevacizumab).[1]

Intervention: operative

Resectable disease can be pursued in an oncological fashion in single or multiple stages. Choice of operative approach is multifactorial and dictated by surgeon experience, clinical condition of the patient and operative factors (tissue quality, contamination, synchronous cancer, proximal dilatation). For those not in extremis a single stage primary anastomosis with or without a protective diverting ostomy can be pursued. Morbidity and mortality have been shown to be equivalent between single and multi-staged procedures in appropriate candidates.[9] Laparoscopic approaches have typically been avoided secondary to lack of visualisation, risk of iatrogenic perforation and increased time to perform the procedure, although in the hands of skilled laparoscopic surgeons these are not absolute contraindications.

Some form of intraoperative colonic decompression is usually required to facilitate handling of the distended colon and visualisation of the intracoelomic cavity. Techniques to decompress through a laparotomy incision include needle aspiration, suction, lavage and endoscopic. However, on-table lavage of faeces has not been noted to decrease anastomotic complications.[10]

For needle decompression a purse-string suture using a small needle is placed through the tenia of an accessible portion of dilated colon. A large angiocath (14-gauge or larger) is placed through the middle of the purse-string and the needle is removed leaving the soft flexible catheter sheath in the lumen of colon (**Fig. 16.1**). The sheath is then connected to suction. Needle decompression works well to decompress gas,

though is too small to decompress stool and blood. If unable to decompress adequately, a pool tip suction catheter can be placed through the same defect after making a small colotomy (**Fig. 16.2**). Once adequate decompression is obtained the catheter can be removed and the purse-string suture secured.

More thorough lavage can be carried out after placing a large diameter catheter with multiple distal holes connected to a Y-connector through the ileocaecal valve into the right colon. One limb of the Y-connector is connected to irrigation and the other to suction (**Fig. 16.3**). If the catheter becomes clogged it can be readily irrigated. After decompression is achieved the catheter can be removed and the purse-string secured, or pushed into the ascending colon and removed with the specimen for a right colectomy. Closed systems for retrograde colonic lavage are also available.

Evaluation for synchronous tumours, liver metastasis, local invasion and the presence of peritoneal carcinomatosis should be carried out. A curative resection, including en bloc resection of surrounding involved structures, is pursued when possible. Metastasis does not preclude resection and re-establishment of

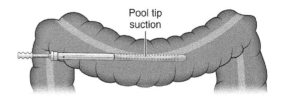

Figure 16.2 • Pool suction decompression of colon. Used with permission of Mayo Foundation for Medical Education and Research, all rights reserved.

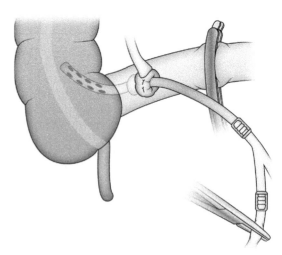

Figure 16.3 • Catheter lavage and decompression of colon. Used with permission of Mayo Foundation for Medical Education and Research, all rights reserved.

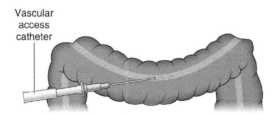

Figure 16.1 • Needle decompression of colon. Used with permission of Mayo Foundation for Medical Education and Research, all rights reserved.

intestinal continuity. For palliation during surgery a decompressive ostomy is the preferred approach in those with unresectable disease who are operative candidates. If creation of an ostomy is not possible an intestinal bypass procedure can be considered. In rare instances a loop ostomy can be performed under local anaesthesia for palliation in decompensated patients unable to tolerate general anaesthesia.

Diverticular

In Westernised countries, diverticular disease affects around 40% by age 60 and 60% by age 80, and the diagnosis appears to be rising.[11] Acute diverticulitis occurs in 10–25%, and of those 20–25% experience a complicated form (perforation, abscess, stricture, fistula). Recurrent episodes of diverticulitis can result in fibrosis of the colon wall, stricturing and obstructive symptoms. Approximately 10% of colonic obstructions result from diverticular strictures.

Initial management and imaging is as noted above. For obstruction presenting with a concomitant abscess, active inflammation, or phlegmon a trial of conservative treatment including antibiotics, with or without interventional radiology-guided procedures, may allow the obstruction to resolve as inflammation improves.

Urgent/emergency surgery is rarely performed for colonic strictures secondary to diverticular disease and only in cases of complete obstruction. Partial obstruction solely related to stricturing is pursued in an elective fashion. Self-expandable metal stents can be used as a bridge to surgery allowing for decompression of the distended proximal colon, provide the opportunity to medically optimise patients, complete a preoperative colonoscopy and pursue a single-stage surgery. Few studies describe SEMS for diverticular strictures and most are single institution experiences.[12–13] Small and colleagues described the use of stents in 23 patients, of whom 16 were associated with diverticular disease. Complications included perforation (4), migration (2) and re-obstruction (2), and 87% of the time occurred 7 days after placement. An emergency procedure was converted to an elective surgery for 84%, although the authors recommended that resection should be attempted within 7 days of SEMS placement.[13] Utilising self-expandable metal stents for diverticular strictures is unproven at this time.

Operative approaches include open or minimally invasive segmental resection, with or without a protective diverting ostomy, and Hartmann's procedure. It is important to note that in many cases it may not be possible to distinguish diverticular stricture from malignancy preoperatively, in which case resection should follow oncological principles given that malignancy is more frequent. As noted

above, the choice of operation and need for ostomy is dependent on the condition of the patient, tissues and the experience of the surgeon. Procedures for decompressing the colon apply as described above.

Sigmoid volvulus

Sigmoid volvulus is for the most part an acquired condition and encompasses 60–80% of all colonic volvulus. In Westernised countries it is most commonly associated with the elderly, debilitated, neurological conditions, those institutionalised or taking psychiatric medications, and laxative abuse. Males and females are equally affected. Although the aetiology is unknown, it is thought to be secondary to constipation and colonic lengthening. Sigmoid volvulus in younger age groups is more common in non-Westernised countries. Worldwide, sigmoid volvulus is the most common cause of bowel obstruction during pregnancy. Congenital anomalies such as Hirschsprung's disease, gut malrotation and parasitic disease caused by *Trypanosomi cruzi* (Chagas disease) are also associated with sigmoid volvulus. Volvulus of the sigmoid colon can occur in either a clockwise or counter-clockwise orientation as the colon elongates and rotates on a narrow pedicled mesenteric base.

Although a few patients describe symptoms of recurrent distension followed by spontaneous detorsion resulting in explosive large-volume bowel movements, the vast majority present as an emergency with abdominal pain, distension and absolute constipation. Diagnosis can be made most of the time with an abdominal X-ray revealing a dilated colon in the shape of a 'coffee bean' or 'omega loop' with its apex pointing toward the right upper quadrant, though only present radiographically in 50–80% (**Fig. 16.4**).[14] A water-soluble contrast enema

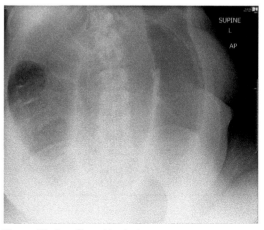

Figure 16. 4 • Sigmoid volvulus.

reveals a 'bird's beak' appearance in the rectosigmoid region, which is secondary to narrowing at the level of the torsion. CT has become the imaging modality of choice and in addition to a dilated loop of colon often reveals a characteristic 'whirl sign' whereby the mesentery twists around the vasculature.

Fluid and electrolyte abnormalities, common in patients with sigmoid volvulus, need to be corrected. For patients without perforation or peritonitis, rigid or flexible sigmoidoscopy with minimal air insufflation is performed to detort the volvulus and decompress the proximal colon. Flexible endoscopy allows for direct visual inspection of the colonic mucosa and in those with suspicion of necrosis detorsion should not be attempted and surgery should be pursued. Detorsion alone results in recurrence in the majority of cases. A rectal tube may be placed to decrease the chance of immediate re-volvulisation while the patient is optimised for colonic resection, preferably during the same hospitalisation. Evaluating patients in the United States Veterans Affairs Medical System, Grossmann et al. noted mortality of 24% for emergency surgery versus 6% for those able to be treated in an elective fashion following endoscopic decompression.[15] A single-centre experience of 952 patients over a 46-year period noted morbidity and mortality for emergency surgery was 35% and 16% compared to 12.5% and 0% for elective.[16] If the patient has not had a recent colonoscopy, and if feasible, a full mechanical bowel preparation and endoscopic colonic evaluation should be pursued prior to proceeding to the operating room. In addition to higher rates of recurrence, non-operative management has been shown to be associated with higher mortality rates in those without prohibitive operative risks.[17]

✓✓ A single-centre experience of 952 patients over a 46-year period noted morbidity and mortality for emergency surgery was 35% and 16% compared to 12.5% and 0% for elective. The principal strategy in the treatment for sigmoid volvulus is early non-surgical detorsion followed by elective surgery in uncomplicated patients, while emergency surgical treatment is performed for patients with bowel gangrene, perforation, or peritonitis, other difficulties with diagnosis, unsuccessful non-surgical detorsion, and early recurrence.[16]

Emergency surgery is pursued for perforation, peritonitis, ischaemia, or the inability to endoscopically reduce the volvulus. Unless prohibited at the time of surgery (haemodynamic instability, intraperitoneal contamination, etc.) a segmental resection and primary anastomosis should be pursued. In those with uncomplicated sigmoid volvulus morbidity and mortality have not been shown to differ between primary anastomosis and Hartmann's procedure. Faecal decompression with on-table lavage carries

the added risk of spillage and contamination and has not been noted to decrease anastomotic complications. If the volvulus is ischaemic, resection should be pursued without reducing the volvulus to decrease the chance of systemically disseminating toxins. Previously described fixation and plasty procedures (sigmoidopexy, mesenteric fixation, mesosigmoidoplasty, etc.) are associated with high rates of recurrence and should be avoided.

Caecal volvulus

Caecal volvulus comprises around 15–30% of all colonic volvulus and is more common in those with prior abdominal surgery, women, younger age groups, pregnancy and constipation. Volvulisation most commonly occurs in a clockwise orientation when there is a lack of retroperitoneal fixation and includes the ascending colon and terminal ileum, rather than just the caecum.

Patients often present with sudden onset of abdominal pain, distension, nausea and emesis. Spontaneous detorsion of the volvulus is uncommon. Abdominal X-ray may reveal a large dilated loop of intestine in the shape of a 'coffee bean' or 'comma' extending across the abdomen to the left upper quadrant (**Fig. 16.5**).[14] CT has become the imaging modality of choice and in addition to a dilated loop of colon often reveals a characteristic 'whirl sign' where the mesentery twists around the vasculature (**Fig. 16.6**).

Endoscopic decompression should not be attempted and definitive management requires operative intervention. Once resuscitated, and unless prohibited at the time of surgery (haemodynamic instability, severe intraperitoneal contamination, etc.) a segmental resection of the hypermobile segment and primary ileocolonic anastomosis should

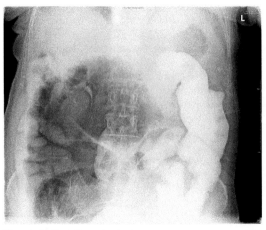

Figure 16.5 • Caecal volvulus.

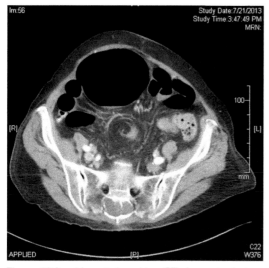

Figure 16.6 • Mesenteric swirl on CT of caecal volvulus.

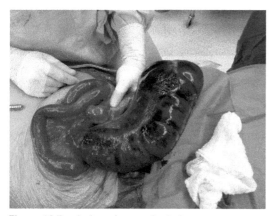

Figure 16.7 • Ischaemic caecal volvulus.

be pursued. If the volvulus is ischaemic, resection should be undertaken without reducing the volvulus to decrease the chance of systemic dissemination of toxins (**Fig. 16.7**).[18]

Other surgical procedures described for caecal volvulus include caecostomy and caecopexy. Both are associated with recurrence rates as high as 25% and mortality as high as 33%. Caecostomy is associated with inadequate decompression, clogged tubing, abdominal wall infection, persistent fistulisation, perforation and peritonitis. Unless surgical resection is contraindicated caecostomy and caecopexy should be avoided.

Caecal bascule

Caecal bascule is a type of caecal volvulus that results from the caecum folding anteriorly onto itself without mesenteric twisting. Patients often present with intermittent and recurrent obstructive symptoms making diagnosis difficult. CT is the most useful imaging modality. Management and operative intervention is the same as for caecal volvulus.

Acute colonic pseudo-obstruction

Acute colonic pseudo-obstruction, also referred to as Ogilvie's syndrome, results in non-mechanical distension of the colon and is primarily a problem of transiently absent colonic motility. It is most commonly associated with elderly, frail, institutionalised patients but also occurs in hospitalised patients after orthopaedic, gynaecologic and abdominal surgeries as well as those with cardiac and infectious aetiologies. It is has been postulated that parasympathetic inhibition likely plays a key role, though the pathophysiology is unknown.

The clinical presentation is characterised by marked abdominal distension, discomfort, nausea, emesis and constipation. Pain on examination is typically less than expected. Abdominal X-rays reveal significant dilatation of the entire large intestine (**Fig. 16.8**). Mechanical obstruction of the left colon should be ruled out radiographically with a water-soluble contrast enema or CT scan with rectal contrast, which will reveal free flow of contrast through the colon without a point of obstruction. Perforation is rare but caecal diameter greater than 12 cm is associated with higher rates of spontaneous perforation and mortality doubles with an increase from 12 to 14 cm. Ischaemia and perforation are associated with mortality greater than 40%.[19]

Non-operative supportive care (bowel rest, resuscitation, correction of electrolyte abnormalities) is pursued in the absence of perforation or suspected ischaemia. Suspected precipitating illnesses such as urinary tract infections should be sought and treated.

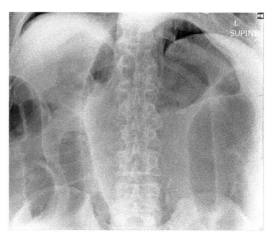

Figure 16.8 • Acute colonic pseudo-obstruction.

Nasogastric tubes do not decompress the colon and are not necessary unless the patient is experiencing nausea/emesis with small intestine and gastric distension. Medications that inhibit gastrointestinal transit (opiates/narcotics, antidepressants, antipsychotics, calcium channel blockers, antidiarrhoeal agents, anticholinergics) should be discontinued. Medications shown to worsen pseudo-obstruction, such as laxatives and enemas, should also be avoided. In most cases colonic pseudo-obstruction will resolve spontaneously, though failure to resolve after 6 days is more commonly associated with perforation.

The use of neostigmine, a reversible acetylcholinesterase inhibitor, may be considered in selected patients as first-line therapy.[20] However, serious side-effects including bradycardia, bronchospasm, hypotension and asystole effectively exclude most patients with the condition in UK practice.

Endoscopic decompression helps to ease the discomfort of severe colonic distension. Perforation, peritonitis and ischaemia are all contraindications to proceeding. Mechanical bowel preparation and enemas should be avoided. Advancement to the caecum is often difficult to achieve and not necessary. A long colonic decompressive tube positioned at the hepatic flexure can be placed to gravity or low wall suction to help sustain decompression (**Fig. 16.9**). To maintain patency the tube should be flushed every 4–6 hours. Once the pseudo-obstruction resolves, the decompression tube can be removed. It is not uncommon for patients to undergo multiple colonoscopic decompressions (15–30%) before a sustained response is achieved.[21]

Subcutaneous methylnaltrexone, a peripheral mu-opioid antagonist, can be used in patients receiving chronic opioid therapy, though supporting data are lacking.[22] Low-dose daily polyethylene glycol (PEG) solution has been shown to be effective in preventing recurrence of acute pseudo-obstruction.[23] Blocking sympathetic outflow with epidural anaesthesia has been shown to improve pseudo-obstruction in small series.

> ✅ Administration of polyethylene glycol (PEG) in patients with Ogilvie's syndrome after initial resolution of colonic dilatation may increase the sustained response rate after initial therapeutic intervention.[23]

When all non-operative measures have failed to resolve acute colonic pseudo-obstruction, surgical intervention may be considered. However, the inordinately high risk secondary to underlying frailty and comorbidities in this patient population effectively rules out surgery for most.[24] Decompressive ostomies do not prevent recurrence of pseudo-obstruction, increase long-term morbidity and are inadvisable.

Poor surgical candidates can be considered for percutaneous tube caecostomy to vent the colon if they cannot tolerate surgery, fail medical management and endoscopic decompression, and are without perforation, peritonitis or ischaemia.[25] Only case reports and small series have documented the success of tube caecostomy, which can be performed endoscopically, under radiological guidance, or laparoscopically. Issues with the procedure include inadequate decompression, clogged tubing, retraction, dislodgement, skin erosion, abdominal wall infection, leakage, fistulisation, perforation and peritonitis. Morbidity is noted to be around 50% and mortality 20–30%.

Inflammation/infection

Toxic colitis/megacolon

Toxic megacolon may occur as the initial manifestation of acute colonic inflammation or an acute exacerbation of chronic colitis. It is characterised by acute colitis, ≥6 cm non-obstructive segmental or complete dilatation of the colon, and signs of systemic toxicity (Table 16.2). Although multiple rare causes have been described in the literature (Table 16.3), it is most commonly associated with inflammatory bowel disease (ulcerative colitis, Crohn's, indeterminate colitis) and pseudomembranous (*Clostridium difficile*) colitis. The pathophysiology is thought to be secondary to local inflammatory mediators inhibiting smooth muscle tone causing colonic dysmotility and toxic dilatation.

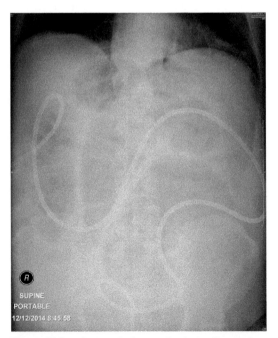

SUPINE
PORTABLE
12/12/2014 8:45:58

Figure 16.9 • Acute colonic pseudo-obstruction post endoscopic decompression.

Table 16.2 • Toxic megacolon diagnostic criteria

Radiographic evidence of colonic dilatation
  Classic finding of more than 6 cm in the transverse colon
Any 3 of the following:
  Fever (>38°C/101.5°F)
  Tachycardia (>120 beats/min)
  Leukocytosis (>10.5×10^3/μL)
  Anaemia (<60% of normal)
Any 1 of the following:
  Dehydration
  Altered mental status
  Electrolyte imbalances
  Hypotension

Adapted from Jalan KN, Sircus W, Card WI, et al. An experience of ulcerative colitis. I. Toxic dilation in 55 cases. Gastroenterology 1969;57(1):68–82.

Table 16.3 • Causes of toxic megacolon

Inflammatory bowel disease
Infectious colitides
  Clostridium difficile
  Salmonella typhi
  Shigella
  Campylobacter jejuni
  Yersinia enterocolitica
  Entamoeba histolytica
  Cryptosporidium
  Cytomegalovirus
Chronic obstructive pulmonary disease
Diabetes
Immunosuppression
Kidney failure
Chemotherapeutic drugs
Kaposi's sarcoma
Colonoscopic overdistension
Cystic fibrosis

Patients often present critically ill (fever, tachycardia, leukocytosis) with abdominal distension and tenderness, tympany and diarrhoea. A high index of suspicion is essential since symptoms may be non-specific or masked by medications (steroids, immunosuppressants, narcotics/opioids) or other factors (elderly, debilitated). Opiates/narcotics, antidepressants, antidiarrhoeal agents, anticholinergics, hypokalaemia and barium enemas are known to induce and exacerbate the condition. Systemic toxicity differentiates patients with toxic megacolon from those with colonic dilatation due to other processes.

In confirmed inflammatory bowel disease, aggressive medical therapy for a period of 5–7 days can be continued if clinically stable and no deterioration is appreciated. This must be pursued cautiously, ideally with collaborative decision-making by gastroenterologists and surgeons. However, toxic megacolon is a late sign, and surgery should be aggressively pursued in the face of deterioration or a lack of measurable improvement within 24–72 hours given the devastating consequences of colonic perforation: mortality rates leap as high as 20% in cases of colonic perforation in comparison to 4% without.[26]

Aggressive resuscitation and correction of electrolyte derangements should be pursued with the goal of reversing physiological defects and the toxic state. Patients should be closely monitored with serial examinations and resuscitated in a critical/intensive care unit. Serial abdominal X-rays can track the progression of colonic distension, though the diameter of the colon is not as important as the patient's overall clinical picture. Abdominal and pelvic computed tomography may help determine aetiology and evaluate for pneumatosis, subclinical perforation and abscesses. Medications that slow colonic motility and function must be avoided. For significant gastrointestinal bleeding and anaemia, transfusion may be necessary.

Treatment of severe/fulminant colitis secondary to inflammatory bowel disease includes the initiation of high-dose intravenous corticosteroids. Upwards of 20–40% will fail to respond and treatment beyond 7 days adds no benefit in those without a response. Increased rates of colonic perforation have not been documented with high-dose steroids. Other medical regimens showing some success in small studies, though unproven at this time, include oral 5-ASA compounds, topical regimens, ciclosporin and immunomodulators. Empiric broad-spectrum antibiotics, although routinely administered, have not shown benefit in those lacking infection.

Patients presenting with toxic megacolon without a history of inflammatory bowel disease should be empirically treated for *C. difficile* colitis until proven otherwise. *C. difficile* colitis has been associated with an increasing prevalence (3%) of toxic megacolon since 2000, which is attributable to a more virulent strain (BI/NAP1/027) with less responsiveness to standard therapies and higher rates of relapse. These patients are more likely to present with an ileus and therapy should not be delayed since failure to make an early diagnosis will result in worse outcomes.

Limited lower endoscopy with minimal air insufflation by an experienced endoscopist may be helpful in obtaining biopsies, evaluating for pseudomembranes, and therapeutically decompressing the colon. Pseudomembranes are seen in nearly 90% of patients with *C. difficile* colitis (**Fig. 16.10**), though rectosigmoid sparing is present in up to 20–30%. Continuously diseased mucosa with deep ulcerations

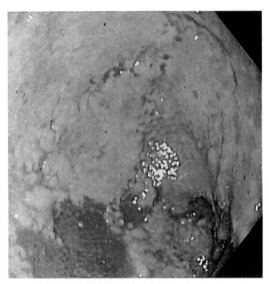

Figure 16.10 • *Clostridium difficile* colitis – pseudomembranous colitis.

and extensive mucosal pseudopolyps may indicate severe ulcerative colitis, whereas intervening normal mucosa, rake ulcers and aphthous ulcers are more suggestive of Crohn's disease.

Indications for emergency surgery include diffuse peritonitis, pneumoperitoneum, uncontrolled sepsis and major haemorrhage. Urgent surgery is pursued in those with increasing abdominal pain and/or colonic distension, progressive physiological deterioration, a lack of objective improvement within 24–72 hours and sustained transfusion requirements. Early surgical intervention should be pursued for patients who are immunocompromised, severely debilitated, malnourished, or have multiple comorbidities.

Treatment for severe complicated *C. difficile* colitis (WBC >15×10⁶/L, Cr >1.5 mg/dL, hypotension, shock, ileus, megacolon) includes vancomycin 500 mg by mouth every 6 hours and metronidazole 500 mg by mouth or intravenously every 8 hours. For those unable to tolerate oral intake medications can be administered through a nasogastric tube. Fidaxomicin has not been proven to be more beneficial than vancomycin in cases of complicated *C. difficile* colitis. Patients with an ileus may have vancomycin introduced through a retention enema (500 mg/100 mL normal saline) every 6 hours, or directly instilled colonoscopically since adequate intracolonic concentrations of vancomycin may not be achieved with oral administration.

Refractory *C. difficile* infection can be treated with faecal microbiota transplantation. Small studies have show benefit in treating patients with acute colitis and toxic megacolon with an efficacy rate of >90%. There is no clear consensus regarding the most appropriate method of delivery (upper endoscopy, nasoenteric tube, colonoscopically, enema), preparation, donated volume, or volume instilled. Some advocate faecal transplant if no improvement with aggressive pharmacotherapy is noted within 48 hours, and more than one transplant may be required to obtain maximal benefit.[27]

Management of toxic megacolon associated with colitides other than *C. difficile* or IBD should follow the same general principles while focusing treatment on the underlying aetiology.

The surgical approach for toxic megacolon, whether performed as an emergency or urgently, most commonly involves an open total or subtotal colectomy with creation of a Brooke ileostomy with preservation of the rectum for a potential future restoration of intestinal continuity. If the rectosigmoid stump is too friable or oedematous to close a sigmoid mucous fistula or subcutaneously exteriorised proximal rectosigmoid stump is an option (**Fig. 16.11**). Laparoscopic-assisted approaches are feasible and not a contraindication in the hands of a skilled laparoscopic surgeon. A proctocolectomy with end Brooke ileostomy is very rarely performed and typically only in cases of life-threatening rectal haemorrhage, severe disease preventing creation of a Hartmann pouch or mucous fistula, rectal perforation, or when re-establishment of continuity or a restorative procedure will not be considered in the future. Re-establishment of intestinal continuity (ileocolonic/rectal anastomosis) or a restorative procedure (ileal pouch anal anastomosis) is not recommended at the time of resection in these patients, as the combination of severe systemic illness, impaired nutrition and high-dose immunosuppression makes anastomotic failure highly likely. Reconstructive options should

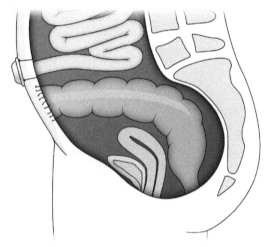

Figure 16.11 • End ileostomy with subcutaneously extracorporealised rectosigmoid stump.

be deferred until the patient has recovered from colectomy (at least 3 months).

Patients with severe complicated *C. difficile* colitis can be treated with creation of a diverting loop ileostomy followed by colonic lavage with polyethylene glycol, vancomycin and metronidazole, though robust literature is lacking for this procedure. Neal and colleagues at the University of Pittsburg demonstrated lower mortality (19 vs 50%) and higher rates of colonic preservation (39 of 42 patients). However, any deterioration or lack of improvement following lavage necessitates proceeding with a colectomy.[28]

Neutropenic enterocolitis

Neutropenic enterocolitis, also known as typhlitis, is associated with inflammation and thickening of any portion of the intestine, though most commonly the caecum and terminal ileum. The pathophysiology is unclear and typically seen in patients receiving chemotherapy for neoplastic diseases, but also documented in transplant recipients and those with aplastic anaemia.

Patients present with abdominal pain, diarrhoea with or without haematochezia, nausea, emesis and pyrexia. Neutropenia is a common finding and often resolves as the patient improves. CT is the imaging modality of choice. Most can be treated non-operatively with intravenous fluids, bowel rest and broad-spectrum antibiotics. Emergency surgery is pursued for perforation and peritonitis and urgent surgery for a lack of improvement with supportive measures.

Perforation

Complicated colonic diverticulitis

Complicated colonic diverticular disease affects 20–25% of those diagnosed with diverticulitis and is associated with abscess formation (15%), stricture (10%), fistulas (<5%) and perforation (1.5%).[29] Emergency surgery is rarely indicated for stenosis/partial obstruction or fistula, unlike complete obstruction and perforation. Diverticulitis associated with abscess formation (Hinchey I and II) is commonly managed conservatively with bowel rest, broad-spectrum antibiotics and interventional-guided percutaneous drainage. Purulent (Hinchey III) and faeculent (Hinchey IV) peritonitis usually requires urgent/emergency surgical intervention.

Patients with Hinchey III and IV diverticulitis present with systemic signs of sepsis, focal or generalised peritonitis, nausea, pyrexia, rebound tenderness and guarding. Some with purulent peritonitis improve with supportive measures and can be managed non-operatively. Computed tomography is the imaging modality of choice. Initial management includes resuscitation and administration of broad-spectrum antibiotics covering anaerobic and Gram-negative bacteria. Careful clinical observation is required in these patients: some improve markedly in the first 24 hours, but any sign of systemic deterioration requires prompt surgical intervention.

After evacuation of faecal matter and/or purulence the abdomen is irrigated with 6–10 L of warm saline solution. Although of unproven benefit, antibiotic irrigation (gentamicin, polymyxin, etc.) has not been shown to be harmful. Following resection of the diseased sigmoid colon, Hartmann's procedure or primary anastomosis, with or without diversion, may be pursued. Most presenting with Hinchey IV disease undergo a Hartmann's procedure, which removes the septic focus, but future re-establishment of intestinal continuity necessitates a second major operation with resultant morbidity and mortality. Up to 30% of patients never have their end colostomy reversed.[30] In the appropriate population a primary anastomosis with or without diversion may be pursued. Relative contraindications to creating a primary anastomosis include haemodynamic instability, vascular compromise, severe protein calorie malnutrition, anaemia, bowel oedema, connective tissue disorders and immunosuppression. Primary diversion with a loop ileostomy or colostomy is inadvisable as it leaves the source of sepsis in situ.

Touting low morbidity and mortality, small series have proposed laparoscopic lavage as an alternative to resection in selected patients with purulent peritonitis, though a large number of those studies included patients with Hinchey II disease.[31–32] The studies are heterogeneous, describing different volumes of irrigation, solutions and placement of drains. In order to help define the utility of laparoscopic lavage large randomised controlled trials have been conducted recently. The Ladies trial was a multicentre (Belgium, Italy, Netherlands) study composed of two arms (LOLA and DIVA) that terminated at 33% of the planned sample size secondary to increased morbidity and mortality in the lavage group. The LaparOscopic LAvage (LOLA) arm compared lavage to Hartmann's procedure and sigmoidectomy with primary anastomosis with or without protective diversion in a 2:1:1 randomisation. Out of 90 patients, 47 were randomised to the lavage group, 21 to a Hartmann's procedure and 22 underwent primary anastomosis. The trial found lavage was not superior to sigmoidectomy for perforated purulent diverticulitis at 12 months.[33] The DIVerticulitis arm (DIVA) compared sigmoidectomy with or without anastomosis, though the results are still pending. The multicentre (Sweden and Norway) randomised Scandinavian Diverticulitis (SCANDIV) trial compared lavage to Hartmann's procedure and noted inferior outcomes in the lavage group. Although the SCANDIV trial included all Hinchey stages, the lavage group experienced more severe complications, higher morbidity and higher rates of reoperation.[34] The multicentre DIverticulitis LAparoscopic LAvage (DILALA) trial compared laparoscopic lavage to Hartmann's procedure for Hinchey III diverticulitis and randomised 39 patients to lavage and 36 to the Hartmann's arm. Data within 30 days of surgery and mortality within 90 days revealed that lavage was feasible and safe in the short term, though 12 month results are still pending.[35] The randomised controlled Laparoscopic Lavage for Acute Non-faeculant Diverticulitis (LapLAND) trial by Winter and colleagues from St Vincent's University Hospital, Ireland concluded in December 2015, and the results are still pending.

✅✅ The LaparOscopic LAvage (LOLA) and the Scandinavian Diverticulitis (SCANDIV) randomised controlled trials both noted laparoscopic lavage vs primary resection did not reduce severe postoperative complications and concluded a lack of support for laparoscopic lavage of perforated diverticulitis.[33-34]

Stercoral

Hard inspissated stool (stercus) impacted in the rectum or rectosigmoid region can result in ischaemic necrosis, ulceration and perforation. The true incidence of stercoral perforation is unknown with only around 100 cases reported in the literature. The median age of presentation has been noted to be 60 with an equally reported incidence in men and women. Secondary to increased age, debility and comorbidities stercoral perforation is associated with mortality rates close to 50%. Factors noted to be associated with stercoral ulceration and perforation include chronic constipation, debility, megacolon, scleroderma, hypercalcaemia, renal failure and renal transplantation. Medications associated with stercoral perforation include opioids/narcotics, antacids, calcium channel blockers and antidepressants. Maurer and colleagues from the University of Berne, Switzerland noted the incidence of stercoral perforation of the colon is likely underestimated secondary to a lack of defined diagnostic criteria.[36] As a result they proposed the criteria should include: (1) round or ovoid colonic antimesenteric perforation exceeding 1 cm in diameter; (2) faecalomas present within the colon and protruding through the perforation site or lying within the abdominal cavity; (3) microscopic evidence of pressure necrosis or ulcer and chronic inflammatory reaction around the perforation site; and (4) exclusion of other pathological causes of perforation.

Presenting symptoms may include marked abdominal distension, discomfort, peritonitis, nausea, emesis and obstipation. Aggressive resuscitation and correction of electrolyte derangements is carried out in preparation for surgery. Radiological imaging is non-specific and rarely identifies stercoral perforation. Serpell and Nicholls from St Thomas' Hospital, London, UK noted only 11% were correctly diagnosed prior to surgery.

Management of patients with stercoral perforation is surgical and the diseased segment must be resected. At the time of surgery multiple ulcers and perforations may be encountered and the entire colon is often filled with inspissated stool. The decision to proceed with resection and stoma versus resection and anastomosis is for the discretion of the surgeon.

Colonoscopic

Perforation during colonoscopy is a rare event occurring in less than 1/1000 procedures with rates in large studies noted to be between 0.012 and 0.016%.[37-38] Higher rates are associated with biopsy, polypectomy and diseased colons (IBD, diverticular). Mechanisms thought to result in perforation include: (1) mechanical as a result of direct trauma from the scope; (2) barotrauma; and (3) procedural-related (biopsies, polypectomies, use of energy, dilatation, placement of endoluminal stents, etc.). The most common site of perforation is the sigmoid colon, likely secondary to its narrow and tortuous nature. The ascending colon and caecum are most susceptible to barotrauma.

Symptoms include marked abdominal distension, discomfort, peritonitis, nausea, emesis, diarrhoea and constipation. The diagnosis of perforation is not always obvious at the time of colonoscopy and upwards of 50% have delayed presentation.

Initial management includes bowel rest, resuscitation and correction of laboratory abnormalities. Nasogastric tubes do not decompress the colon and are not necessary unless the patient is experiencing nausea/emesis. Flat and upright abdominal radiographs will identify free air. Computed tomography with contrast or a water-soluble enema can be used to confirm the diagnosis.

Management depends on both the procedure performed and presentation of the patient. If clinically stable, non-operative management with bowel rest, resuscitation and broad spectrum IV antibiotics can be pursued. Peritonitis, deterioration, or a lack of measurable improvement necessitates surgery or procedural intervention. Placement of endoclips to manage perforations is showing promise in small studies. Trecca and colleagues presented their own experience in addition to reviewing the literature and found in 78 reported cases clips were successful in controlling perforations 69–93% of the time.[39] Large defects and peritoneal contamination will require operative intervention whether open or laparoscopic. Depending on the initial colonoscopic procedure performed, segmental resection and anastomosis, primary repair of the colonic defect and resection and creation of a stoma are all options.

✅✅ Trecca and colleagues' review of the literature and personal experience noted in 78 cases colonoscopically placed endoclips were successful in controlling perforations in 69–93% of cases.[39]

Anastomotic leak/dehiscence

Rates of colonic anastomotic leaks following resection depend on the reporting criteria utilised and have been documented to be as high as 20%, especially for very low anastomoses. Bruce and colleagues from the University of Aberdeen, UK reviewed 97 anastomotic leak studies and noted 56 different definitions for what constituted a leak. Multiple patient and procedural factors are associated with increased risk of anastomotic leaks (Table 16.4). Mortality rates ranging from 10% to 22% have been documented in association with leaks. Morbidity (long hospitalisation, multiple interventional procedures, wounds, hernias, additional

Table 16.4 • Risk factors for anastomotic leak

Operative factors
Blood loss
Poor surgical technique
Anastomotic tension
Anastomotic blood supply
Length of surgery
Preoperative mechanical bowel preparation
Left colon/Low anastomosis
Failure to intraoperatively leak test left/low anastomoses
Patient factors
Immunocompromised
Diabetes
Protein calorie malnutrition
Anaemia
Tobacco use
COPD
Obesity
Male
Alcohol abuse
Prior radiation
Emergency surgery
Disease (connective tissue disorders, IBD, diverticular)
Prior abdominal surgery

surgical procedures, infection, bowel obstructions, stoma issues, impaired bowel function, DVT/PE, etc.) is significantly increased. Time of diagnosis probably reflects how avidly the complication is sought by the surgeon. Leaks are usually diagnosed during the same inpatient admission but have also been documented beyond 30 days. Patients with an early leak (within 1 week of surgery) often present with relatively subtle signs of sepsis; frank peritonitis is uncommon.

Prompt diagnosis and treatment are imperative to decrease the sequelae of sepsis and prevent mortality. Peritonitis and haemodynamic instability necessitate operative intervention and few if any imaging studies are necessary in this population. The difficulty lies in patients presenting with vague (poor appetite, generally not feeling well, etc.) and minimal symptoms, and few clinical signs. There is no one pathognomonic testing modality for identifying an anastomotic leak. As shown by Erb, Hyman and Osler at the University of Vermont,[40] just as many patients without leaks, as those with, experience postoperative tachycardia, tachypnea, leukocytosis, hypotension and pyrexia. CT and contrast studies are the imaging modalities of choice although radiological findings can be equivocal and falsely negative, thus necessitating a high index of suspicion. Flat and upright abdominal films can reveal gas under the diaphragm, but are of debatable significance in the immediate postoperative period. Localised extraluminal pockets of free air can be seen on CT up to 26 days after surgery, and frank free air up to 9 days. Only air associated with a loculated fluid collection has been shown to be more prevalent in those with an anastomotic leak.[41] Equally, the absence of pneumoperitoneum should not discourage one from pursuing further investigations to evaluate the integrity of the anastomosis.

In addition to the timing of presentation management also depends on patient and anastomotic factors. Leaks later than 7–10 days make surgical intervention more difficult and indicate higher risk secondary to the desmoplastic peritoneal reaction. For those presenting with peritonitis and haemodynamic instability aggressive resuscitation and correction of laboratory derangements is pursued while planning for emergency surgery.

Peritonitis, deteriorating sepsis, or a lack of measurable improvement necessitates surgical intervention. The peritoneal cavity is thoroughly lavaged followed by evaluation of the anastomotic defect, tissue integrity and surrounding structures. Historically the treatment of choice was resection with creation of a stoma and possibly mucous fistula, and is still a safe option. The reader should take careful note of comments in Chapter 20 regarding ill-advised attempts to repair anastomotic leaks in the presence of sepsis as a leading cause of complex intra-abdominal sepsis and intestinal fistulation.

In clinically stable patients it is possible to salvage anastomotic leaks by non-operative means with good outcome. Highly selected patients with small contained leaks, whether proximally diverted or not, can be treated conservatively with close observation, bowel rest, parenteral nutrition, broad-spectrum antibiotics and percutaneous interventional guided procedures. Future restoration of intestinal continuity is difficult for distal leaks and a diverting loop stoma and (transanal) drainage of the area can preserve anastomotic continuity for small leaks.

Other modalities described in the literature for treating low anastomotic leaks include endoscopic (clip, covered stent) and vacuum-assisted devices, though to date these lack robust supporting evidence.

Haemorrhage

The colon accounts for approximately 20% of all cases of acute gastrointestinal haemorrhage. Sources, in decreasing frequency, include diverticular disease, neoplastic/polyp, inflammatory bowel disease, ischaemic, angioectasias, post polypectomy and post surgery. The elderly are more commonly affected. For the majority, bleeding stops spontaneously and emergency surgery is rarely required. Urgent investigation and control is necessary for unremitting bleeding. Higher rates of bleeding are associated with diverticular disease and vascular ectasias.

Management of colonic haemorrhage depends on the source and includes medical, endoscopic, angiographic, and surgical approaches. Depending on the patient's haemodynamic status colonoscopy, radionuclide imaging, selective mesenteric angiography, and CT angiography can all be utilised to identify the source of bleeding. Selective angiography and colonoscopy have the advantage of being both diagnostic and therapeutic.

Once an upper gastrointestinal source is excluded, colonoscopy may be pursued if the patient is haemodynamically stable. Studies have documented high caecal intubation rates and diagnostic accuracy for emergency colonoscopies performed without bowel preparation, though most describe finding sources associated with lower rates of bleeding (ischaemia, inflammatory bowel disease, neoplastic/polyp) that did not require intervention.[42] For haemodynamically stable patients mechanical bowel preparation should be administered to enhance visualisation of mucosal abnormalities. Treatment of localised sources of bleeding (diverticular, angiodysplastic, polyp) includes injection with epinephrine, coagulation, placement of an endoclip, and polypectomy. India ink tattoo should be placed at the site of bleeding to help localise the site in the event repeat endoscopic procedures are required. Risks of sedation and perforation must be taken into consideration when pursuing colonoscopy.

For those who cannot tolerate an endoscopic procedure, or colonoscopic localisation was not possible, imaging modalities are pursued. Radionucleotide imaging with a patient's own red blood cells labelled with technetium 99 m (^{99m}Tc-RBC) can identify rates of bleeding as low as 0.1 mL/min.[43] Technetium 99 m remains active for up to 48 hours and reimaging can be pursued for intermittent or recurrent bleeding. A negative scan provides evidence there is no active bleeding, and a blush is indicative of bleeding. Disadvantages to ^{99m}Tc-RBC scanning include the time required to perform the test (several hours), high false localisation rate (25%) and inability to identify the source (25–60%). Patients with haemodynamic instability are not good candidates for radionucleotide imaging.

CT angiography (CTA) has largely supplanted ^{99m}Tc-RBC scanning by providing the benefit of fast image acquisition, reformatted three-dimensional vascular reconstruction, localisation of the site of bleeding and higher resolution imaging. CTA can detect bleeding as low as 0.3 mL/min and when active bleeding is present can localise the region 91–92% of the time.[44] Patients with haemodynamic instability, renal insufficiency and allergy to contrast dye are not candidates for the test.

Selective mesenteric angiography can detect bleeding rates as low as 0.5 mL/min. Unless imaging has already localised the bleeding to a particular region, the superior mesenteric artery is typically visualised first followed by the inferior mesenteric artery. CTA is commonly performed prior to mesenteric angiography. When mesenteric angiography is performed <150 minuets following a positive CTA the likelihood of identifying an active source of bleeding is 2.89 times higher,[45] and if within 90 minutes, 8.56 times higher.[46] As shown by Jacovides and colleagues from the University of Pennsylvania, with the precise localisation on CTA the cumulative contrast load with mesenteric and CT angiography is no different than mesenteric angiography following ^{99m}Tc-RBC scanning. Sensitivity for identifying a bleeding source ranges from 40–95%. For intermittent presentations, provocative measures (administration of heparin, vasodilators, thrombolytics, or a combination) utilised to induce bleeding to help identify the source have been described in small studies, with diagnostic yields ranging from 29% to 38%. Caution must be taken secondary to the risks of intracranial and uncontrolled haemorrhage. When bleeding is identified, transcatheter therapeutic intervention is pursued. Superselective embolisation of small vessels through microcatheters with microcoils, gelfoam, or polyvinyl alcohol is now the preferred procedure. Cessation of active arterial bleeding is as high as 50–75%, with rebleeding rates of only 22–24%.[47,48] Embolisation of larger vessels is no longer performed secondary to high rates of transmural ischaemia, perforation and stricture formation. Risks of mesenteric angiography include vascular injury, thromboembolic events, contrast-induced renal insufficiency/failure and pseudoaneurysm formation.

> ✅✅ Two retrospective studies evaluating the timing of selective mesenteric angiography following a positive CT angiography revealed an increase in the probability of detecting the source of bleeding, with a 2.89 times higher likelihood if performed within 150 minutes and 8.56 times higher if within 90 minutes.[45–46]

Indications for emergency/urgent surgery include transfusion requirements greater than 6 units during resuscitation, ongoing or recurrent haemorrhage unresponsive to non-operative approaches, and persistent haemodynamic instability. An increase in mortality is directly correlated with the units of blood transfused. It has been documented that those requiring more than 10 units of blood experience mortality as high as 27% versus 7% for those requiring less than 10. Transfusion of 4 or more units of packed red blood cells in the first 24 hours of resuscitation is associated with a 50% operative rate. Every effort should be made to localise the source of bleeding prior to proceeding to the operating room. Segmental resection of a localised area of bleeding carries a mortality rate less than 10% versus 10–30% for a total abdominal colectomy. If the source of bleeding cannot be localised, a thorough exploratory evaluation of the entire intestine is performed. On-table intestinal endoscopy by an experienced endoscopist can be utilised to help localise the source. If unable to localise, a total abdominal colectomy is performed when small intestinal sources have been excluded. An ileosigmoid or ileorectal anastomosis, with or without protective diversion, may be considered in haemodynamically stable patients.

Ischaemia

Colon ischaemia, also known as ischaemic colitis, results from reduced colonic perfusion and is the most common type of mesenteric ischaemia. There are multiple causes (Table 16.5). Ischaemia occurs secondary to a lack of sufficient flow to maintain colonocyte metabolic activity, which results in hypoxia. The most common causes are non-occlusive disease, arterial embolic or thrombotic occlusion, and mesenteric vein thrombosis. The superior and inferior mesenteric arteries supply the colon through certain regions, referred to as watershed areas, which receive only collateral circulation. These low flow vulnerable areas include the caecum, splenic flexure (Griffith's point) and the rectosigmoid region (Sudek's point). The most common area of inconsistent collateral

Table 16.5 • Causes of colon ischaemia

Physiological
Hypotension
Hypovolaemic
Haemorrhage
Cardiovascular
Heart failure
Atherosclerosis
Hypercoagulable
Factor V Leiden
Protein C and S deficiency
Prothrombin G2010A mutation
Antiphospholipid syndrome (Lupus anticoagulant)
Antithrombin III deficiency
Polycythaemia vera
Disseminated intravascular coagulation (DIC)
Heparin-induced thrombocytopenia and thrombosis (HITT)
Tobacco (acquired)
Drugs
Vasopressors
Oral contraceptives
Cocaine
Diuretics
Antiarrhythmics
Antihypertensives
Surgery/procedural
Cardiac
Aortic
Autoimmune disease
Systemic lupus erythematosus
Other
Haemodialysis
Embolic/thrombotic
Long distance running
Trauma (blunt or penetrating)
Connective tissue disorders
Mechanical bowel obstruction

circulation is Griffith's point. Although all areas of the colon can be affected by non-occlusive disease, the watershed areas are the most prominent. Arterial embolic or thrombotic occlusion and mesenteric vein thrombosis more commonly affect the proximal colon. Colon ischaemia predominantly affects those over 65 years of age, is more common in women, and is estimated to be responsible for 16 out of every 100 000 hospital admissions.[49] Most cases will not require surgical intervention. Emergency surgery is associated with a mortality rate as high as 50%, and highest for right-sided ischaemia. Baseline mortality ranges from 4–12%. Mortality in renal transplant recipients has been documented as high as 70%.

Signs and symptoms are often non-specific, depend on the duration and extent of ischaemia, and can include abdominal pain, distension, haematochezia, an urgent desire to defaecate, nausea, emesis, pyrexia, diarrhoea, constipation, renal failure and sepsis. Any patient presenting with abdominal pain and bloody diarrhoea should be evaluated for colonic ischaemia. Markers of ischaemia such as acidosis and elevated lactate, lactate dehydrogenase, amylase and alkaline phosphatase are often absent until late in the course of severe disease. Computed tomography is the imaging modality of choice and will reveal segmental bowel wall thickening and mesocolic oedema and stranding. Pneumatosis and portal venous gas suggests transmural ischaemia or infarction and mandates urgent surgical intervention.[50] Since the vast majority of colon ischaemia is secondary to non-occlusive disease (95%) vascular imaging studies are typically not necessary unless acute mesenteric ischaemia is suspected, such as pain out of proportion on examination with a lack of haematochezia. Diagnosis with flexible endoscopy is the gold standard and allows for direct visualisation of the ischaemic segment, which can range from submucosal oedema to full-thickness necrosis (Table 16.6), and the ability to obtain biopsies (**Fig. 16.12**). To decrease the risk of perforation endoscopy is typically preformed with minimal air insufflation, in an unprepped bowel, and not advanced proximal to the area of ischaemia. Biopsies of gangrenous areas are avoided. A single inflammatory band of erythema with erosion along the lateral axis of the colon, referred to as the 'single-stripe sign', is highly specific for colon ischaemia. Abdominal X-rays and barium enemas can reveal thumb-printing, a sign of submucosal oedema, though it is non-specific and can be found in multiple inflammatory and infectious colitides.

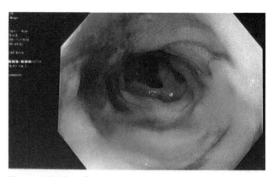

Figure 16.12 • Colonic ischaemia.

✔✔ A meta-analysis of three prospective and three retrospective studies revealed contrast-enhanced multidetector CT correctly identifies the diagnosis of primary acute mesenteric ischaemia with high pooled sensitivity (93.3%) and specificity (95.9%), thus supporting its use as a first-line imaging modality.[50]

Once the diagnosis of colon ischaemia is made a cause is sought and appropriately treated. Mild disease is noted to be segmental, not isolated to the right colon, and lacking poor prognostic factors observed in moderate disease. Moderate disease includes any three of the following: tachycardia, abdominal pain without rectal bleeding, hypotension, male sex, blood urea nitrogen level greater than 20 mg/dL, serum sodium less than 136 mEq/L, white blood cell count greater than 15×10^9/L, haemoglobin less than 12 g/dL, or colonoscopically identified ulceration. Severe disease is defined as more than three of the moderate disease criteria or peritoneal signs, pneumatosis or portal venous gas with CT imaging, gangrene on colonoscopy, and pancolonic or isolated right colon ischaemia on CT or endoscopy.[51] For those presenting with full-thickness necrosis and gangrene, peritonitis, pneumoperitoneum, and haemodynamic instability surgery is immediately pursued. Mild and moderate colon ischaemia is treated supportively with bowel rest, resuscitation, correction of laboratory abnormalities, and treatment of the underlying cause of ischaemia. Over 80% respond and avoid surgical intervention. Administration of broad-spectrum empiric antibiotics to decrease the sequel of bacterial translocation may be entertained, despite a lack of robust data to support doing so. Nasogastric tubes do not decompress the colon and are not necessary unless the patient is experiencing nausea/emesis. Peritonitis, deterioration, or a lack of measurable improvement necessitates surgery intervention.

During surgery any portion of the colon affected by ischaemia, necrosis and perforation is widely resected

Table 16.6 • Endoscopic colon ischaemia findings

Mild ischaemic colitis
Pale-appearing mucosa
Mucosal oedema
Petechial haemorrhages
Ulcerations

Moderate ischaemic colitis
Dusky-appearing mucosa
Submucosal haemorrhage
Haemorrhagic ulcerations

Severe ischaemic colitis
Frank necrosis
Circumferential involvement

and an ileostomy or colostomy created. Taking into consideration the risk of progression of ischaemia, physiological derangements that led to surgery, and tenuous blood flow, a primary anastomosis is not advised. Extensive or patchy involvement can be treated with a temporary abdominal closure and second-look laparotomy to determine the need for further resection.

Key points

- The most common causes of colonic obstruction are neoplasia, diverticulitis and volvulus. Treatment for obstruction is dependent on the location, cause, patient presentation and goals of care.
- The American Society of Gastrointestinal Endoscopy (ASGE) and European Society of Gastrointestinal Endoscopy (ESGE) currently recommend self-expanding metal stents only for patients who are poor surgical candidates who need medical optimisation.
- CT has become the imaging modality of choice for volvulus. In addition to a dilated loop of colon a characteristic 'whirl sign', whereby the mesentery twists around the vasculature, is typically seen. Detorsion alone results in recurrence in the majority of cases. Colonic resection should preferably be pursued during the same hospitalisation.
- Acute colonic pseudo-obstruction requires non-operative supportive care (bowel rest, resuscitation, correction of electrolyte abnormalities) is pursued in the absence of perforation or suspected ischaemia. The use of neostigmine may be considered in selected patients as first-line therapy. Endoscopic decompression can help ease the discomfort of severe colonic distension. When all non-operative measures have failed to resolve acute colonic pseudo-obstruction surgical intervention may be considered. However, the inordinantly high risk secondary to underlying frailty and comorbidities in this patient population precludes pursuing surgery for most.
- Toxic colitis is characterised by acute colitis, ≥6 cm non-obstructive segmental or complete dilatation of the colon and signs of systemic toxicity, and is most commonly associated with inflammatory bowel disease and pseudomembranous (*Clostridium difficile*) colitis.
- Early surgical intervention should be pursued for patients who are immunocompromised, severely debilitated, malnourished, or have multiple comorbidities. Urgent surgery is pursued in those with increasing abdominal pain and/or colonic distension, progressive physiological deterioration, a lack of objective improvement within 24–72 hours, and sustained transfusion requirements. Indications for emergency surgery include diffuse peritonitis, pneumoperitoneum, uncontrolled sepsis and major haemorrhage.
- Diverticulitis associated with abscess formation (Hinchey I and II) is commonly managed conservatively with bowel rest, broad-spectrum antibiotics and interventional-guided percutaneous drainage. Purulent (Hinchey III) and faeculent (Hinchey IV) peritonitis usually requires urgent/emergency surgical intervention.
- Management of colonoscopic perforation depends on both the procedure performed and presentation of the patient. If clinically stable, non-operative management with bowel rest, resuscitation and broad-spectrum IV antibiotics can be pursued. Peritonitis, deterioration, or a lack of measurable improvement necessitates surgery or procedural intervention.
- In clinically stable patients it is possible to salvage anastomotic leaks by non-operative means with good outcome. Highly selected patients with small contained leaks, whether diverted or not, can be treated conservatively with close observation, bowel rest, parenteral nutrition, broad-spectrum antibiotics and percutaneous interventional guided procedures. Peritonitis, deteriorating sepsis, or a lack of measurable improvement necessitates surgical intervention.
- CT angiography (CTA) has largely supplanted ^{99m}Tc-RBC scanning by providing the benefit of fast image acquisition, reformatted three-dimensional vascular reconstruction, localisation of the site of bleeding, and higher resolution imaging. CTA can detect bleeding as low as 0.3 mL/min and when active bleeding is present can localise the region 91–92% of the time.

- Mesenteric angiography with superselective embolisation of small vessels through microcatheters with microcoils, gelfoam, or polyvinyl alcohol will result in cessation of active arterial bleeding 50–100% of the time with rebleeding rates of only 22–24%.
- Indications for emergency/urgent surgery include transfusion requirements greater than 6 units during resuscitation, ongoing or recurrent haemorrhage unresponsive to non-operative approaches, and persistent haemodynamic instability.
- In acute colonic ischaemia computed tomography is the imaging modality of choice and will reveal segmental bowel wall thickening and mesocolic oedema and stranding. Pneumatosis and portal venous gas suggest transmural ischaemia or infarction and mandate urgent surgical intervention.
- Diagnosis with flexible endoscopy is the gold standard and allows for direct visualisation of the ischaemic segment and the ability to obtain biopsies.
- Mild and moderate colon ischaemia is treated supportively with bowel rest, resuscitation, correction of laboratory abnormalities, and treatment of the underlying cause of ischaemia, and over 80% respond and avoid surgical intervention.

⊕ Full references available at **http://expertconsult. inkling.com**

Key references

8. Sagar J. Colorectal stents for the management of malignant colonic obstructions. Cochrane Database Syst Rev 2011;(11):CD007378. PMID: 22071835.

A meta-analysis of five randomised trials including 207 patients (102 colorectal stent and 105 emergency surgery) revealed the use of colonic stents in malignant colorectal obstruction seems to have no advantage over emergency surgery. There was no statistically significant difference in the 30-day mortality between two groups, with both being 2.3%. The stent-related perforation was 5.88%, and migration and obstruction rates both 2.13%. The complication rate was 39.22% in the stent and 45.71% in the emergency surgery group.

16. Atamanalp SS. Treatment of sigmoid volvulus: a single-center experience of 952 patients over 46.5 years. Tech Coloproctol 2013;17(5):561–9. PMID: 23636444.

A single-centre experience of 952 patients over a 46-year period noted morbidity and mortality for emergency surgery was 35% and 16% compared to 12.5% and 0% for elective. The principal strategy in the treatment for sigmoid volvulus is early non-surgical detorsion followed by elective surgery in uncomplicated patients, while emergency surgical treatment is performed for patients with bowel gangrene, perforation, or peritonitis, other difficulties with diagnosis, unsuccessful non-surgical detorsion and early recurrence.

20. Valle RG, Godoy FL. Neostigmine for acute colonic pseudo-obstruction: a meta-analysis. Ann Med Surg (Lond) 2014;3(3):60–4. PMID: 25568788.

A meta-analysis of four randomised trials including 127 patients (65 in the neostigmine group and 62 in the control group) revealed neostigmine is a safe and effective option for patients with acute colonic pseudo-obstruction (ACPO) who failed to respond to conservative management. ACPO resolved in 89.2% treated with one dose of neostigmine versus 14.8 in the control group.

33. Vennix S, Musters GD, Mulder IM, et al. Laparoscopic peritoneal lavage or sigmoidectomy for perforated diverticulitis with purulent peritonitis: a multicentre, parallel-group, randomised, open-label trial. Lancet 2015;386(10000):1269–77. PMID: 26209030.

A multicentre, parallel-group, randomised, open-label trial in 34 teaching hospitals and eight academic hospitals in Belgium, Italy, and the Netherlands (the LOLA arm) compared laparoscopic lavage with sigmoidectomy and concluded lavage is not superior to sigmoidectomy for the treatment of purulent perforated diverticulitis. The study was terminated early secondary to an increased event rate in the lavage group. The primary endpoint occurred in 30 (67%) of 45 patients in the lavage group and 25 (60%) of 42 patients in the sigmoidectomy group (odds ratio 1·28, 95% CI 0.54–3.03, P=0·58). By 12 months, four patients had died after lavage and six patients had died after sigmoidectomy (P=0·43).

34. Schultz JK, Yaqub S, Wallon C, et al. Laparoscopic lavage vs primary resection for acute perforated diverticulitis: the SCANDIV randomized clinical trial. JAMA 2015;314(13):1364–75. PMID: 26441181.

A multicentre, randomised clinical superiority trial from 21 centres in Sweden and Norway compared the outcomes from laparoscopic lavage (n=101) with those for colon resection (n=98) for perforated diverticulitis. Among patients with likely perforated diverticulitis and undergoing emergency surgery, the use of laparoscopic lavage vs primary resection did not reduce severe postoperative complications and led to worse outcomes in secondary endpoints. Their findings did not support laparoscopic lavage for treatment of perforated diverticulitis. Mortality at 90 days did not significantly differ between the laparoscopic lavage group (14 patients [13.9%]) and the resection group (11 patients [11.5%]; difference, 2.4% [95% CI, (7.2–11.9%]; $P = 0.67$). The reoperation rate was significantly higher in the lavage group (15 of 74 patients [20.3%]) than in the resection group (4 of 70 patients [5.7%]; difference, 14.6% [95% CI, 3.5–25.6%]; $P = 0.01$) for patients who did not have faecal peritonitis.

35. Angenete E, Thornell A, Burcharth J, et al. Laparoscopic lavage is feasible and safe for the treatment of perforated diverticulitis with purulent peritonitis: the first results from the randomized controlled trial DILALA. Ann Surg 2016;263(1):117–22. PMID: 25489672.

A multicentre prospective, randomised, controlled trial comparing laparoscopic lavage and open Hartmann procedure was conducted in nine surgical departments in Sweden and Denmark. A total of 83 patients were randomised (39 in the lavage and 36 in the Hartmann group). Follow-up at 12 months revealed morbidity and mortality after laparoscopic lavage did not differ when compared with the Hartmann procedure. Long-term data are still pending.

37. Rathgaber SW, Wick TM. Colonoscopy completion and complication rates in a community gastroenterology practice. Gastrointest Endosc 2006;64(4):556–62. PMID: 16996349.

A single-centre study evaluating colonoscopic complications was conducted prospectively and results reviewed retrospectively. A total of 12407 consecutive patients were evaluated. Two perforations occurred (0.016%).

38. Shi X, Shan Y, Yu E, et al. Lower rate of colonoscopic perforation: 110785 patients of colonoscopy performed by colorectal surgeons in a large teaching hospital in China. Surg Endosc 2014;28(8):2309–16. PMID: 24566747.

A retrospective single-centre study evaluating colonoscopic complications was conducted. A total of 110785 consecutive patients were evaluated. Two perforations occurred (0.016%). A total of 14 incidents (0.012%) of perforation were reported (7 males and 7 females), of which 9 cases occurred during diagnostic colonoscopy (0.01%) and 5 after therapeutic colonoscopy (3 polypectomy cases, 1 endoscopic mucosal resection, and 1 endoscopic mucosal dissection).

45. Tan KK, Shore T, Strong DH, et al. Factors predictive for a positive invasive mesenteric angiogram following a positive CT angiogram in patients with acute lower gastrointestinal haemorrhage. Int J Colorectal Dis 2013;28(12):1715–9. PMID: 23836115.

Of 30 patients with non-diverticular aetiologies of lower gastrointestinal bleeding, a selective mesenteric angiography within 150 minutes of a positive CT angiography was 2.89 times more likely to identify the source of bleeding.

46. Koh FH, Soong J, Lieske B, et al. Does the timing of an invasive mesenteric angiography following a positive CT mesenteric angiography make a difference? Int J Colorectal Dis 2015;30(1):57–61. PMID: 25367183.

Of 48 mesenteric angiographies for lower gastrointestinal bleeding a selective mesenteric angiography within 90 minutes of a positive CT angiography was 8.56 times more likely to identify the source of bleeding.

50. Menke J. Diagnostic accuracy of multidetector CT in acute mesenteric ischemia: systematic review and meta-analysis. Radiology 2010;256(1):93–101. PMID: 20574087.

A meta-analysis of three prospective and three retrospective studies revealed contrast-enhanced multidetector CT correctly identifies the diagnosis of primary acute mesenteric ischaemia with high pooled sensitivity (93.3%) and specificity (95.9%), thus supporting its use as a first-line imaging modality.

17

Anorectal emergencies

Sarah A. Goodbrand
B. James Mander

Introduction

Acute anorectal pathology constitutes a significant proportion of the general surgeon's workload. The problems encountered range from the acute pain of thrombosed haemorrhoids and perianal sepsis to the management of anorectal bleeding, trauma and irreducible rectal prolapse. Effective management depends upon sound knowledge of anorectal anatomy, accurate classification of the pathology and timely intervention to ensure minimal disruption to normal function.

Anorectal anatomy

The anal canal is a 3- to 4-cm-long tube running downwards and backwards from the anorectal angle to the anus. It is divided in half by the dentate line, which demarcates hindgut-derived columnar epithelium above and stratified squamous epithelium that merges at the anus with the perianal skin below. Above the dentate line is the anal transitional zone, lined by cuboidal epithelium for 1–2 cm. The hindgut sensory innervation is supplied by autonomic hypogastric nerves, sensitive only to stretch. Anoderm below the dentate line is innervated from the somatic inferior rectal nerves, making it sensitive to pain, pressure and temperature. However, the dentate line is not a reliable boundary between somatic and autonomic sensation; pain can certainly be felt within the anal transitional zone, which explains why some patients experience severe and immediate pain after rubber band ligation of haemorrhoids despite

the band being applied apparently well above the dentate line.

The anorectal sphincter complex can be thought of as a gut tube within a funnel of muscle essential for the maintenance of normal continence. The inner muscle layer is the involuntary internal sphincter, a thickened continuation of the circular muscle of the rectum. Outside this is the funnel of the voluntary external sphincter, formed from striated muscle, continuous at its superior edge with the levator plate. Between these two muscle layers is the intersphincteric space, which contains mucous-secreting anal glands. These glands drain through the internal sphincter via their respective Crypts of Morgani at the level of the dentate line.

Three submucosal anal cushions comprising fibroelastic tissue and arteriovenous anastomoses are found within the anal canal, usually at the 3, 7 and 11 o'clock positions. They normally appose to form a tight seal within the canal, which helps to maintain continence, but in some patients they may enlarge to form troublesome symptomatic haemorrhoids.

Anorectal abscesses

Anorectal abscesses, defined as sepsis within the soft tissues that surround the anus, are among the commonest surgical emergencies, with operative treatment being required in about 1 in 5000 of the population in the UK annually.[1] They occur predominantly in adults, frequently in the third and fourth decades of life, with a male preponderance. An anorectal abscess is thought to originate within the intersphincteric space, due to obstruction and suppuration of the anal crypt glands (the cryptoglandular theory). Ninety per cent of anorectal abscesses arise as a result of this process and are termed primary anorectal abscesses. The resultant primary infection will produce an intersphincteric abscess which can spread, in a vertical, horizontal or circumferential direction, along several anatomical planes to collect in a number of potential anorectal spaces: perianal, intersphincteric, pelvi-rectal (ischiorectal, or post anal) or supralevator. Circumferential spread results in a horseshoe abscess (see **Fig. 17.1**). The relative frequency with which abscesses occur in the various anatomical locations is shown in Table 17.1.[2]

Both aerobic and anaerobic bacteria are responsible for the abscess formation, with the predominant anaerobic bacteria being *Bacteriodes* spp., *Peptostreptococcus* and *Clostridium*; the most commonly isolated aerobic and facultative bacteria are *Staphylococcus aureus*, *Streptococcus*, *Enterobacteriaceae* and *Enterococcus*.[3–5]

Suppurating skin infections, including carbuncles, furuncles and infected apocrine glands, can also cause primary abscesses. The responsible bacterium in these cases is almost invariably staphylococcus and as these abscesses do not communicate with the anal canal they are not associated with fistula formation.[6]

Secondary abscesses are much less common, accounting for just 10% of presentations.[7] They are a manifestation of distinct underlying disease processes, with Crohn's disease, colorectal neoplasia, diabetes mellitus, AIDS and tuberculosis all being potential causes. They can also occur as a complication of anorectal surgery or as a consequence of trauma.

Clinical features

Anorectal abscesses present with signs and symptoms of acute inflammation, with pain being the most common symptom. On examination a perianal abscess can usually be seen as a red, tender, fluctuant swelling near the anal verge; however, ischiorectal abscesses often present as a less distinct brawny swelling on one side of the anus and intersphincteric abscesses usually cannot be seen externally at all. Although this last type of abscess can be felt through the anal wall as a smooth, tender collection, digital rectal examination is usually excruciatingly painful. This diagnosis should therefore be suspected in patients with severe anal pain and fever. Satisfactory examination is usually only possible under general anaesthesia. In a few patients (particularly those who are immune-compromised or with diabetes mellitus) the perianal sepsis can be associated with cellulitis, which can progress to life-threatening necrotising infection if not treated promptly.[8]

All patients presenting with anorectal sepsis or pain should have an examination of the anorectum, including proctosigmoidoscopy. It is our opinion that this can usually only be performed satisfactorily under general anaesthesia. As the diagnosis is usually obvious, few people would routinely recommend preoperative imaging (although some advocate its use, arguing that by identifying cavities and fistulas there is a reduction in the incidence of recurrence[9]).

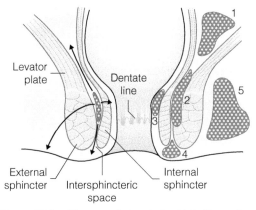

Figure 17.1 • The spread of anal gland infection and common sites of anorectal sepsis. Infection of the anal gland within the intersphincteric space can spread in a variety of directions (see left side of diagram), resulting in abscess in a number of classical sites: 1, supralevator; 2, intersphincteric; 3, submucosal; 4, perianal; 5, ischiorectal. Note also the possibility of circumferential extension of sepsis ('horseshoeing') in the intersphincteric, ischiorectal and supralevator planes.

Table 17.1 • Location of anorectal sepsis by anatomical site

Anatomical site	Number	Percentage
Perianal abscess	437	42.7
Ischiorectal	233	22.8
Intersphincteric	219	21.4
Supralevator	75	7.3
Submucosal	59	5.8

Data from Ramanujam PS, Prasad MI, Abcarian H, et al. Perianal abscesses and fistulae: a study of 1023 patients. Dis Colon Rectum 1984;27:593–7. With kind permission from Wolters Kluwer Health.

Radiological imaging

Diagnostic radiology is seldom required to image uncomplicated anorectal sepsis. Its role in the management of acute anorectal sepsis is for

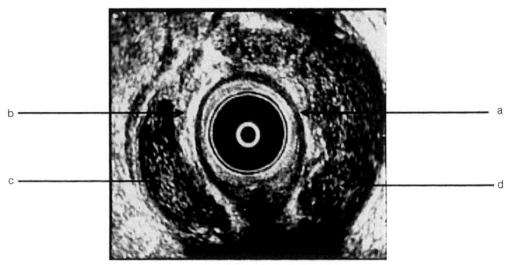

b — a

c — d

Figure 17.2 • Endoanal ultrasound examination carried out on a patient under general anaesthesia. This patient presented with severe anal pain and perianal induration but without any specific area of fluctuance. The ultrasound demonstrates an extensive ischiorectal abscess cavity **(c,d)** extending around the anal canal (**a**, internal sphincter; **b**, external sphincter).
With thanks to Mr Mike Hulme-Moir, previous Clinical Fellow in Colorectal Surgery, Royal Infirmary, Edinburgh.

investigating complex fistula disease in Crohn's disease or patients with supralevator sepsis to differentiate an intrapelvic source from extension of an intersphincteric or ischiorectal abscess. Imaging is also useful if the diagnosis is unclear, if there is non-resolution of symptoms after operative intervention or in cases of recurrent sepsis. Magnetic resonance imaging (MRI) is a sensitive and specific modality for identifying anorectal abscesses and associated fistula tracts and in UK practice is the technique of choice.[10,11]

Endoanal ultrasound has also been shown to be an accurate method of determining the origin of the sepsis and delineating the fistula anatomy (**Fig. 17.2**). In experienced hands it has been shown to be as accurate as MRI.[12,13]

Treatment

Undrained pus is remarkably destructive and hence sepsis must be drained promptly, whilst minimising iatrogenic damage to the sphincter complex and preventing recurrence. In most patients this involves external drainage via a curvilinear (not radial) incision at the lateral edge of the abscess cavity. This should not be placed too laterally as it will make subsequent fistula management more challenging for those patients who develop a fistula. Adequate drainage should result in prompt resolution of the patient's symptoms; if not, a repeat examination under anaesthetic (EUA) or MRI is recommended to ensure that all sepsis has been completely drained.

Historically, it was suggested that thoroughly 'deroofing' the abscess cavity with a wide cruciate incision was beneficial but this does little other than giving the patient a larger wound that will take longer to heal.[14] Similarly, a short-lived enthusiasm for primary wound closure after incision has been abandoned as studies have shown that it offers little immediate benefit in terms of time to wound healing and probably increases the chance of recurrent sepsis.[15]

If the abscess cavity is very large, an alternative to making a huge incision is to insert a de Pezzer or Malecot catheter via a smaller skin incision. One study showed that using such treatment meant hospital stay (1.4 vs 4.5 days) and the need for community dressings was shorter, with no disadvantages seen at long-term follow-up.[16]

Antibiotics should be used only as an adjunct to surgical treatment in immune-compromised patients, or when there is evidence of florid cellulitis or suspicion of necrotising infection.

It is the opinion of the authors that all anorectal abscesses should be drained under general anaesthetic, although in some centres perianal abscess drainage is commonly executed under local anaesthesia. Performing perianal abscess drainage under general anaesthetic allows a comprehensive examination and drainage to be undertaken, and prevents a significant proportion of re-operations. A large retrospective case study of 500 patients treated for perianal abscess at the Mayo Clinic was reported in 2001 and revealed a 7.6% re-operation rate.[17] The reasons for re-operation included incomplete drainage of the abscess cavity at the first operation, missed abscesses (most often posterior collections) and postoperative bleeding. There was no association reported between patient variables (such as age, immune suppression or diabetes) and so it might be concluded that surgical error contributed to these findings, emphasising the need for a thorough primary examination.

Technical tips

The management of specific abscesses is shown diagrammatically in **Fig. 17.3**. Simple perianal

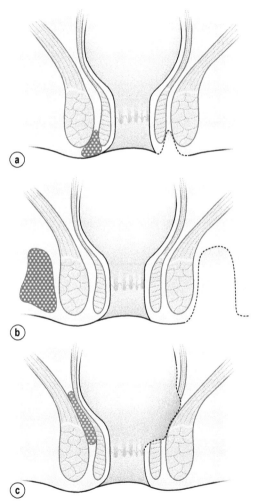

(a)

(b)

(c)

Figure 17.3 • Management of specific abscesses.
(a) Perianal abscess is treated by excision of a small disc of skin and curettage of the cavity. **(b)** Ischiorectal abscess may require excision of a substantial amount of tissue to facilitate drainage. The alternative is to introduce a drainage catheter through a small stab incision.
(c) Intersphincteric abscess is treated by excision of the mucosa and internal sphincter overlying the abscess. Such an abscess should not be drained through the perineal skin or a high fistula will result.

abscesses should be drained externally and the cavity gently curetted (Fig. 17.3a). With ischiorectal abscesses, the cavity is often large (Fig. 17.3b), and should be incised as near to the anal verge as possible in order to minimize the distance to the external opening of any subsequent fistula. A large horseshoe abscess in the ischiorectal space is better drained through multiple short incisions than one large circumferential incision. As mentioned earlier, the size of the drainage wound can be minimised if a drainage catheter is used. Intersphincteric abscesses are more challenging and require drainage into the anorectum, which requires excision of part of the internal sphincter (Fig. 17.3c). Submucosal abscesses, although rare, are drained into the anal canal. Supralevator abscesses pose a unique challenge compared to the drainage of other anorectal abscesses. They develop in a space above levator ani, lateral to the rectum. Drainage transrectally is associated with high recurrence rates,[18] whilst concomitant drainage through the ischiorectal fossa results in high fistula-in-ano, which can be difficult to manage.[14] It is therefore recommended that such abscesses be approached radiologically or via an open transabdominal approach. In true pelvic abscesses unrelated to spread from the anal glands, drainage can be achieved into the rectum or vagina. If the abscess is related to pelvic pathology, the primary disease process will need to be resected along with drainage of the pus to prevent recurrence.

Routine bacteriological swabs at the time of abscess drainage do not predict fistula or recurrence rates, and are therefore unnecessary and costly.[19,20]

Internal packing of anorectal abscess cavities is commonly practised within the UK. However, a 2016 Cochrane review concluded that there is a paucity of high-quality evidence to confirm whether packing influences time to healing, recurrence or fistula rates.[21] A recent UK multicentre observational study (2016) demonstrated significant levels of pain, resource utilisation and expense associated with internal packing.[22] In our opinion, packing should therefore be omitted as it serves only to cause discomfort, inconvenience and cost, with no clear clinical advantage.[21,22]

✓ Perianal abscesses are best incised under general anaesthesia with the cavity left open. Routine bacteriology swabs do not alter management and are unnecessary. There is no evidence that packing the abscess cavity is clinically beneficial.[21,22]

Fistula-in-ano

Perianal abscesses are associated with anal fistulas in about 60% of patients from the outset;[23,24] but only 27-37% of these persist after the acute inflammation has resolved.[22-26] Fistula-in-ano increases the likelihood of recurrent anorectal sepsis, a non-healing wound or persistent discharge, and thus the requirement for repeat interventions. For these reasons, many surgeons consider fistula treatment at the primary drainage procedure. However, identifying a fistula when acute inflammation is present can be difficult, especially for the less experienced surgeon. The probing of fistula tracts within friable, oedematous tissue can also lead to the creation of false fistula tracts which can be difficult to manage, and may cause disproportionate damage to the anal sphincter complex and thus continence.

✔✔ The majority of anorectal abscesses are adequately treated with incision and drainage alone and if a fistula tract is not obvious, it should not be sought.[24,25]

So should synchronous fistulotomy ever be performed? A Cochrane review of six randomised control studies from five different centres from 1987 to 2003 looked at concomitant fistula surgery at the time of abscess drainage in terms of recurrence, need for further surgery and postoperative incontinence.[27] However, as would be expected, the eligibility criteria and treatments offered varied considerably between the trials, making definitive recommendations difficult. Three studies also reported fistula rates of 83–90%,[26,28,29] which is higher than would be expected, raising questions about whether iatrogenic tracks may have been created.

The majority of the studies included in the review dealt only with the surgical treatment of low fistulas. In one of these, patients were randomized *after* the initial abscess drainage, with fistulotomy performed as a second procedure on day 3 of the acute admission.[28] Most studies excluded those with recurrent anorectal sepsis, previous surgery and inflammatory bowel disease (IBD).[27]

All the studies showed that recurrence was less likely after fistula surgery (risk ratio 0.07–0.24), although follow-up times varied. Only two studies looked at short-term incontinence, with one (which included only low fistulas, $n = 52$) reporting no clinical incontinence in either group despite anal manometry revealing a transient reduction in the anal resting pressure in the fistulotomy group (76.3 mmHg vs 91.1 mmHg), which had disappeared by week 12. Squeeze pressures were unaffected.[29] The other group (which included high trans-sphincteric and suprasphincteric fistulas treated with cutting setons) reported transient incontinence of flatus in 3/100 of controls and 15/100 of the intervention group. In patients who underwent drainage alone this had entirely resolved by 6 months; however, in the fistula surgery group, 6% were still having problems after 1 year.[24]

Long-term continence rates were documented in five studies and were normal in four of them following simple drainage alone at 1 year or later. Of the studies performing low fistulotomy, incontinence of flatus was 0/24,[30] 8/20[28] and 0/24.[29] A study that included high fistulas reported 2% incidence of incontinence for flatus and 4% for liquid.[24] In another study, fistulectomy and partial internal sphincterectomy was performed and reported flatus/liquid incontinence in 6/32 of controls and 13/34 of the intervention group, with four and one patients from each group, respectively, lost to follow-up.[31] All these data combined to give a risk ratio of 2.64 for long-term altered continence following synchronous fistulotomy.[27]

The overall conclusions of the Cochrane meta-analysis were that synchronous fistulotomy is appropriate for low, uncomplicated fistula tracts. It should not be performed for high fistulas or anterior fistulas in women. It should also be avoided for groups where the risk of incontinence is high (e.g. those who have undergone previous anorectal surgery or have IBD).[27]

✔✔ Synchronous fistulotomy can be performed at the time of abscess drainage for low, uncomplicated fistula tracts to reduce the risk of abscess recurrence and further operations without compromising continence.[27]

Management of secondary perianal sepsis

Malignant disease

These abscesses should be drained like any other anorectal abscess, but definitive treatment will require appropriate management of the malignant lesion. The presence of anorectal sepsis in this context, however, indicates advanced disease either from direct tumour infiltration or perforation, which has implications for further treatment. Consideration should be given to a defunctioning stoma at the time of sepsis drainage in this subset of patients.

Inflammatory bowel disease

All abscesses in patients with IBD should be drained promptly and setons inserted into any fistulous tracts as necessary. Management in patients with ulcerative colitis follows the principles outlined above, but the presence of anorectal sepsis and fistulas in IBD should always raise the possibility of the correct diagnosis being Crohn's disease. MRI is often helpful in demonstrating fistula tracts. Recurrent disease is often very hard to treat and an expert opinion should be sought.

Necrotising infection

Necrotising infection of the perianal tissues is characterized by the rapid progression of synergistic sepsis along fascial planes. The presentation is of a toxic patient with severe perianal pain, though often there may be very little to find on superficial perineal examination at initial presentation. Predisposing factors include poor health, diabetes and immunosuppression.[32] The condition carries a high mortality (up to 80%)[32] and requires urgent drainage and radical debridement of all involved tissue. A defunctioning stoma may be required to facilitate wound management and several repeat examinations under anaesthetic are often necessary to ensure that only healthy tissue remains. Tissue should be sent for urgent microbiological analysis and antimicrobial advice sought to cover both aerobic and anaerobic organisms.

Anorectal sepsis in neutropenic patients

The classical features of abscess formation may be absent in neutropenic patients with perianal sepsis. The management of this subset of patients is poorly defined. The largest published study compared operative versus non-operative management and demonstrated comparable mortality.[33] Patients with pathognomonic features of an abscess should be managed operatively, whilst those without should be managed with antibiotics and careful serial clinical examination.[34]

Anorectal sepsis in HIV patients

Improved outcomes in HIV patients presenting with anorectal sepsis tend to reflects optimisation of antiretroviral medical treatment. Wound healing does, however, remain a problem and is correlated with the CD4 count.[32] The best management of HIV patients with anorectal sepsis is identification of specific pathogens, involvement of HIV specialists, liberal drainage and fistulotomies for simple and low fistulas. Invasive procedures should ideally be avoided whenever the $CD4^+$ lymphocyte count is less than 50 cells/μL.[32]

Pilonidal abscess

Pilonidal sinus disease is an acquired condition that typically occurs in the midline of the natal cleft. The resultant primary skin pits allow debris and loose hairs to penetrate and generate a chronic foreign body reaction in epithelial tracts, which can become acutely infected forming an abscess or cause chronic blood-stained discharge.

Risk factors for pilonidal sinus disease include male gender (twice as many men are affected), hirsutism, obesity, a deep natal cleft and lifestyle factors, particularly prolonged sitting.[35,36] It is rarely seen in patients over 45 years and therefore alternative diagnosis or a secondary cause should be sought in older patients.

The causative organism, as with many skin infections, is often *Staphylococcus* but mixed anaerobes may be cultured.[37]

In the emergency setting the objective of treatment is simply to drain the abscess to relieve acute symptoms and prevent spreading sepsis. The optimal technique of draining a pilonidal abscess is via a longitudinal lateral incision.[38] Primary drainage alone has a recurrence rate of approximately 50%.[39]

Excision of the whole sinus tract at the same time as abscess drainage has been attempted but has been associated with recurrence rates of up to 60%.[37] It is therefore advisable to drain the primary abscess only as the initial wound will be much smaller.

A study from Israel assessed 58 patients with acute pilonidal abscess: 29 patients were treated with incision and drainage, the other 29 with wide excision (without closure). The risk of recurrent pilonidal suppuration was similar in the two groups, although those who underwent excision had a longer time off work.[39]

It is therefore recommended that excision of the sinus tract is not undertaken synchronously.[40] It is the authors' usual practice to offer formal excision only after the second presentation with a pilonidal abscess and this is always performed as a separate procedure after the acute sepsis has settled.

Novel techniques for pilonidal abscess drainage are evolving. A UK centre has recently reported their initial experience of Endoscopic Pilonidal Abscess Treatment (EPAT) in 19 patients, showing complete wound healing for all patients within 6 weeks, with 21% requiring definitive surgery for pilonidal disease in the longer term.[41] Longer-term results for this technique are awaited.

✅ Fifty per cent of all pilonidal abscesses will be cured with incision and drainage alone.[39] Definitive surgery should be reserved for those who have recurrent disease and be performed in the elective setting.[37,40]

Acute anal fissure

An anal fissure is a superficial ulcer in the anoderm distal to the dentate line. Anal fissure is common, with an incidence of 1 in 350 people, with acute fissures being significantly more prevalent than chronic anal fissures.[42] It can occur at any age but is uncommon in the elderly, and thus if an elderly patient presents with symptoms suggestive of a fissure, serious underlying pathology such as a low rectal or anal cancer must be excluded. Anal fissures can be primary or secondary depending on whether there is a clear causative factor. The pathophysiology of an anal fissure is local trauma, which leads to internal anal sphincter (IAS) spasm, increased resting anal pressure, reduced blood flow and finally ischaemia.[43,44] Most patients will present via the outpatient clinic but some attend emergently, because of severe pain on defecation, or with a complication of the anal fissure such as bleeding, anorectal fistula, abscess or faecal impaction. The distinction between acute and chronic anal fissures is somewhat arbitrary; an acute fissure is likely if the patient has had symptoms for less than 4 weeks. It is usually a simple diagnosis to make on visual inspection; an acute fissure will present as a small fresh laceration, most commonly in the posterior midline (6 o'clock) position. A chronic anal fissure has additional features, including partially healed edges, visible IAS fibres in its base, hypertrophied anal papilla and sometimes a sentinel tag.

The initial treatment of an acute anal fissure is a combination of conservative measures, which includes stool softeners, sitz baths and analgesia. Fifty per cent of acute anal fissures will heal with such measures within 2 weeks.[45]

For those patients with symptoms >2 weeks, topical agents (for 6–8 weeks to allow for re-epithelialisation), which include smooth muscle relaxants such as glycerine trinitrate (GTN)[46] or diltiazem can be used.[47] They are correlated with excellent short-term results, leading to the healing of 90% of acute fissures without the need for surgery.[48] However, the long-term outlook is less encouraging, with one meta-analysis showing recurrence rates of up to 50%.[49]

In a Cochrane Review of 15 RCTs that looked at GTN versus placebo, GTN was found to be significantly better than placebo in healing anal fissures (49% v. 37%, $P < 0.004$). There was no significant difference in efficacy when comparing calcium channel blockers with GTN, although the included studies were clinically heterogeneous. The Cochrane review also found botulinum toxin type A injection was no better at healing anal fissure than placebo or local lidocaine, and no better or worse than topical GTN or a calcium channel blocker. The use of Botox has been assessed mainly for chronic anal fissure, although an Egyptian randomised control trial demonstrated good results when used for acute fissures.[50]

Lateral internal sphincterotomy (LIS) is much more successful than chemical methods at reducing recurrence rates (approximately 2%), and although some studies have raised concerns about disturbance of continence, it has been shown that a well-planned procedure in selected patients has very little effect on continence.[51,52] However, it has no place in the acute setting and should be reserved for patients with chronic symptoms.

In those with atypical or intractable symptoms EUA should be performed to exclude occult sepsis or an alternative aetiology. If a fissure is confirmed at EUA it is the opinion of the authors that local anaesthetic and Botox should be infiltrated under the fissure and into the IAS, respectively, to provide symptomatic relief.

✓✓ Most anal fissures will heal with conservative treatment.[46,48] However, a EUA should be performed for those with severe unremitting symptoms. Definitive surgery should be reserved for those with recurrent or non-healing disease.[49,51]

Haemorrhoids

Symptoms relating to haemorrhoidal disease occur in approximately 5% of the population. Haemorrhoids occur because of abnormal transformation within the vascular, muscular and connective tissue condensations within the anal canal termed the 'anal cushions'. Degeneration of the muscular and fibrous components of these cushions leads to a reduction in the muscle-to-fibre ratio. They can be classified according to their anatomic location relative to the dentate line. Internal haemorrhoids arise from the endoderm and are thus covered by columnar epithelium. External haemorrhoids arise below the dentate line and therefore from the ectoderm and are covered by squamous epithelium. They are innervated by cutaneous nerves from the sacral plexus via the pudendal nerve, and are sensitive to pain.

Most haemorrhoids are asymptomatic or cause minor symptoms only. Patients with complicated haemorrhoidal disease may present as an emergency with anorectal haemorrhage or acute prolapse and thrombosis.

Thrombosed haemorrhoids

Thrombosed haemorrhoids occur either as an acutely thrombosed external haemorrhoid (often used interchangeably with perianal varix/haematoma) or thrombosed or strangulated internal haemorrhoids. They can be differentiated by the presence of anoderm overlying a thrombosed external haemorrhoid, which will also usually present as a single 'lump' at the anal margin. Internal haemorrhoids can prolapse chronically but become thrombosed when the tissue becomes fixed outside the sphincter, impeding venous return. Spontaneous thrombosis of the inferior haemorrhoid plexus is the precipitating event in external haemorrhoid thrombosis. There is usually a history of straining and constipation with the onset of acute pain thereafter.

Although acute haemorrhoidal prolapse/thrombosis is immensely painful it tends to resolve spontaneously within 4–5 days. The mainstays of non-surgical management are good analgesia, laxatives and topical treatments such as nifedipine.[53] The main argument for not undertaking emergency haemorrhoidectomy for acutely thrombosed haemorrhoids is firstly that it is painful for about the same amount of time as for natural healing, and secondly the benefits of surgery lessen as the condition resolves. Recent reviews suggest that patients who present after 72 hours of symptoms are best served by non-operative treatment, while those who present before this time may benefit from conventional haemorrhoidectomy.[54,55] However, the only prospective randomised controlled study comparing operative and non-operative treatment showed that non-operative treatment was associated with shorter hospital stay and less anal sphincter damage.[56]

There is a relative paucity of published literature pertaining to the longer-term consequences of conservative management and the need for subsequent haemorrhoidectomy. A small study from St Mark's Hospital suggested that there is a high incidence of persistent symptoms and requirement for haemorrhoidectomy (54.7%) in these patients.[57]

Definitive emergency surgical treatment can be difficult, but many retrospective and case-controlled studies suggest outcomes when experienced surgeons perform emergency haemorrhoidectomy are similar to outcomes from elective haemorrhoidectomy (Table 17.2).[58] If surgery is to be undertaken, several studies have shown that stapled anopexy (PPH) in the acute setting is associated with shorter hospital stays, reduced pain and earlier return to work compared to conventional open haemorrhoidectomy.[59–61]

✅✅ Thrombosed haemorrhoids should be treated by conservative management, particularly if presentation is more than 72 hours after onset of symptoms.[54–56] If surgery is to be undertaken a stapled haemorrhoidectomy is associated with improved short-term outcomes (e.g. pain) compared to open haemorrhoidectomy.[59–61]

Anorectal haemorrhage

Rectal bleeding is a common reason for emergency hospital admission. In the majority of cases (>90%) it will cease without intervention. In a major UK audit of lower gastrointestinal (GI) bleeding, haemorrhage from a benign anorectal source accounted for 17% of the cohort,[62] and included haemorrhoids, proctitis, rectal varices, rectal prolapse, anal fissures, solitary rectal ulcer syndrome and anal ulceration. Performing basic investigations such as digital rectal examination, proctoscopy and rigid sigmoidoscopy during the index admission will readily identify an anorectal source of lower GI bleeding.[62,63]

Anorectal trauma

Anal sphincter injuries

Anal sphincter injuries can be divided into obstetric and non-obstetric injuries; the latter include direct anal sphincter disruption and iatrogenic damage during other anorectal procedures.

Obstetric anal sphincter injuries

Between 4 and 6.6% of all vaginal births are complicated by perineal or pelvic floor trauma, and

Table 17.2 • Results from comparative study on emergency and elective haemorrhoidectomy

	Elective surgery (n = 500)	Emergency surgery (n = 204)	P value
Haemorrhage	27 (5.4)	10 (4.9)	NS
Blood transfusion	10[2]	4[2]	NS
Anal stenosis	15[3]	12 (5.9)	NS
Disturbance of continence	26 (5.2)	9 (4.4)	NS
Sepsis	0	0	NS
Recurrence	38 (7.6)	14 (6.8)	NS

Numbers in parentheses are percentages. NS, non-significant.
Data from Eu KW, Seow Choen F, Goh HS. Comparison of emergency and elective haemorrhoidectomy. Br J Surg 1994;81:308–10. © British Journal of Surgery Society Ltd. Reproduced with permission. Permission is granted by John Wiley & Sons Ltd on behalf of the BJSS Ltd.

can occur as a result of vaginal delivery or as an extension to an episiotomy leading to damage of the anal mucosa and/or the anal sphincter complex.[64-68] The severity of sphincter injury can be graded by the degree of disruption of both the internal (IAS) and external anal sphincter (EAS). Third-degree tears include complete or partial disruption of the sphincter complex, whilst fourth-degree tears refer to damage of the anal mucosa with complete division of the sphincter complex.

Many obstetric sphincter injuries are not diagnosed in the immediate postpartum period (rates of 26–87% missed injury have been reported[68,69]) and are the commonest cause of anal incontinence in the longer term.

The repair of recognised sphincter injuries can be delayed for 8–12 hours with no impact on continence.[70] The type of repair (end-to-end approximation or overlapping technique) was evaluated in a 2013 Cochrane review, which found no specific advantage of different techniques.[71] The overlapping technique requires more extensive mobilisation of the EAS and is therefore only possible for injuries that involve more than 50% of the EAS.[68] Suture-related morbidity is equivalent for PDS or vicryl.[72] Separate repair of the IAS is recommended, as women with an IAS defect on endoanal ultrasound have higher long-term incontinence rates.[68]

The overall outcomes for primary repair are poor, with overall rates of faecal incontinence ranging from 6 to 53% depending on duration of follow-up.[68]

Non-obstetric trauma

Isolated injuries of the sphincter complex are unusual and are normally associated with concomitant injuries to adjacent viscera. The management of such injuries should therefore be directed towards correctly identifying disrupted anatomy and prioritising management. Early treatment is aimed at debridement of all non-viable tissue and faecal diversion, deferring reconstructive surgery.

Rectal injuries

Injury sustained to the intraperitoneal rectum can sometimes be primarily repaired but if there is significant contamination, major tissue loss, devascularisation or nearby open fractures, resection and formation of a stoma should be preferred.[73] Damage to the extraperitoneal rectum can also be repaired primarily but again proximal diversion may be needed if injuries are extensive.[74] Sigmoidoscopy should always be performed if blood is seen in the rectal lumen or if an extraperitoneal haematoma is seen adjacent to the rectum at laparotomy. Radiological tests incorporating rectal contrast may also be useful.

Foreign bodies

Rectally inserted foreign objects and the innovative techniques used to remove them are extensively reported in medical literature. A review of these case reports suggests that in many cases removal is possible under conscious sedation, either digitally for low objects or bimanually for those above the rectosigmoid junction.[75] Endoscopic extraction with or without fluoroscopic guidance may be worth attempting. However, the authors' experience is that general anaesthesia is invariably preferable for transanal retrieval of objects of significant size and making an adequate assessment for tissue injury. If transanal extraction measures fail, or there is radiographic evidence of perforation, laparotomy is required. It is recommended that all patients undergo sigmoidoscopy after extraction to ensure no damage to the rectal mucosa has been sustained.

Irreducible rectal prolapse

Irreducible rectal prolapse presents mainly in elderly patients and is likely to become a more frequent reason for emergency admission in today's ageing population. Firstly, it is essential to distinguish a full-thickness external prolapse from a mucosal prolapse: they are differentiated by the presence of concentric rings of mucosa and a prolapse containing the muscle layers of the rectal wall, rather than mucosa alone. Secondly, it must be ascertained whether the prolapse is ischaemic. In the absence of ischaemia conservative measures can be undertaken. To reduce the oedema sugar can be applied and manual reduction attempted thereafter with sedation or general anaesthesia, with definitive surgery deferred to a later stage. In the presence of ischaemia, surgical management is the only option. There are no large series to support a surgical procedure of choice and either a perineal rectosigmoidectomy or laparotomy with resection may be appropriate; the choice is usually dictated primarily by the general fitness/comorbidity of the patient.[76]

Key points

- Anorectal sepsis should be managed by prompt drainage following sound anatomical principles.
- Synchronous fistulotomy can be undertaken with care in low, uncomplicated fistulas but should be avoided in those at high risk of incontinence or when the fistula is not easily distinguished.
- Acute pilonidal abscesses should be treated with off-midline incision and drainage alone.
- Abscess cavities should not be packed following drainage.
- Anal fissures should be managed pharmacologically, with surgery reserved for those that fail to heal.
- Acute thrombosed haemorrhoids should be managed non-operatively. Emergency haemorrhoidectomy is recommended only if carried out within 72 hours of symptom onset and by an appropriately skilled surgeon.
- Management of anorectal trauma and retained foreign bodies should be determined by the site of injury and the anorectum should always be re-examined by sigmoidoscopy following removal.

Full references available at **http://expertconsult. inkling.com**

Key references

24. Oliver I, Lacueva FJ. Vincente Perez, et al. Randomised clinical trial comparing simple drainage of anorectal abscess with and without fistula track treatment. Int J Colorectal Dis 2003;18(2):107–10. PMID: 12548410.

A prospective, randomised trial of 200 consecutive patients showed recurrence reduced from 29% to 5% in patients in whom definitive treatment of the fistula track was attempted rather than simple drainage. However, due to the higher risk of incontinence these recommendations were limited to those with low fistulas.

25. Read DR, Abcarian H. A prospective study of 474 patients with anorectal abscess. Dis Colon Rectum 1979;22:566–8. PMID: 527452.

A large prospective study showing good results for primary fistulotomy along with drainage.

27. Malik AI, Nelson RL, Tou S. Incision and drainage of perianal abscess with or without treatment of anal fistula. Cochrane Database Syst Rev 2010;7:CD006827. PMID: 20614450.

A review of the current evidence for concurrent fistulotomy at the time of incision and drainage of an acute abscess, showing good results for fistulotomy in low, uncomplicated disease.

46. Lund JN, Scholefield JH. A randomised, prospective, double-blind, placebo-controlled trial of glyceryl-trinitrate ointment in treatment of anal fissure. Lancet 1997;349(9044):11–4. PMID: 8988115.

This study of 80 consecutive patients demonstrated rapid relief of symptoms and after 8 weeks of ongoing treatment 68% demonstrated fissure healing compared to 8% in the placebo group.

48. Frezza EE, Sandei F, Leoni G, et al. Conservative and surgical treatment in acute and chronic anal fissure: a study on 308 patients. Int J Colorectal Dis 1992;7(4):188–91. PMID: 1293238.

A large study concluding that the condition is self-limiting in the vast majority of patients.

49. Nelson R. Non surgical therapy for anal fissure. Cochrane Database Syst Rev 2006;4:CD003431. PMID: 17054170.

A review of 53 randomised controlled trials comparing medical and surgical therapy for anal fissure showed some advantage to topical treatments over placebo for acute fissure symptoms but that surgery was by far the best solution for chronic fissure problems.

51. Brown CJ, Dubreuil D, Santoro L, et al. Lateral internal sphincterotomy is superior to topical nitroglycerin for healing chronic anal fissure and does not compromise long-term fecal continence: six-year follow-up of a multicenter, randomized, controlled trial. Dis Colon Rectum 2007;50(4):442–8. PMID: 17297553.

A study of 82 patients with chronic anal fissure randomised to GTN treatment or LIS showed better long-term patient satisfaction in the surgical group with no significant compromise to continence.

54. Rivadeneira DE, Steele SR, Ternent C, et al. Practice parameters for the management of hemorrhoids (revised 2010). Dis Colon Rectum 2011;54:1059–64. PMID: 21825884.

Guidelines issued by the American Society of Colorectal Surgeons reflecting the predominantly office-based practice in North America for these conditions.

56. Allan A, Samad AJ, Mellon A, et al. Prospective randomised study of urgent haemorrhoidectomy compared with non-operative treatment in the management of prolapsed thrombosed internal haemorrhoids. Colorectal Dis 2006;8(1):41–5. PMID: 16519637.

This study of 50 patients found that conservative treatment was associated with shorter admission duration and less anal sphincter damage as assessed by endoanal ultrasound, with no difference in the number of symptomatic patients at 24-month follow-up.

58. Eu KW, Seow-Choen F, Goh HS. Comparison of emergency and elective haemorrhoidectomy. Br J Surg 1994;81(2):308–10. PMID: 8156371.
This single centre non-randomised study of >700 patients concluded that results of Milligan–Morgan haemorrhoidectomy for elective and emergency presentations were comparable; however, enthusiasts for acute intervention should note that the emergency group developed anal stricture in 6.9% and altered continence in 4.4%.

59. Wong JC, Chung CC, Yau KK, et al. Stapled technique for acute thrombosed hemorrhoids: a randomized, controlled trial with long-term results. Dis Colon Rectum 2008;51(4):397–403. PMID: 18097723.
This study compared open and stapled haemorrhoidectomy in patients with acute thrombosed haemorrhoids and found reduced pain, faster return to work and greater satisfaction in the stapled haemorrhoidectomy group.

62. http://hospital.blood.co.uk/media/28411/national-comparative-audit-of-lower-gastrointestinal-bleeding-and-the-use-of-blood-light.pdf.
A major UK snapshot audit of management and transfusion practice in lower GI haemorrhage demonstrating variation in management and over-use of blood products.

18

Paediatric surgical emergencies

Dafydd A. Davies
Jacob C. Langer

Introduction

While paediatric surgery has increasingly become the domain of the subspecialist paediatric surgeon, adult general surgeons are still often faced with the challenges of assessing and managing children with surgical emergencies. The unique differences between adults and children must be taken into account when addressing every aspect of surgical management, including assessment, diagnosis, resuscitation and operative interventions. Children face a different spectrum of conditions, have different physiological responses to trauma, illness and surgical stress, and have different psychosocial needs.

This chapter will address the common abdominal paediatric surgical emergencies encountered by general surgeons. These will be categorised according to age: (i) neonates (up to 44 weeks post-gestational age), (ii) infants (1 month to 2 years of age) and (iii) children (2 years of age and older).

Neonatal period

Prenatal diagnosis

Routine prenatal ultrasonography has become the standard of care in many parts of the industrialised world, and has resulted in the detection of many congenital anomalies before birth. Common detectable anomalies relevant to the general surgeon include: abdominal wall defects, congenital diaphragmatic hernia, intestinal obstruction and intra-abdominal masses.

Whenever possible these patients should be referred for prenatal consultation with obstetrics, neonatology and paediatric general surgery. In most cases, delivery should occur at a hospital with a neonatal intensive care unit and paediatric surgical service. If this is not possible they should be immediately transferred following delivery and resuscitation.

Intestinal obstruction

Intestinal obstruction is the most common abdominal emergency in the neonatal period, and is usually due to a congenital, developmental or genetic anomaly.

Assessment

Assessing neonatal patients for obstruction requires a thorough history, including the nature of any vomiting and the presence or absence of abdominal distension. Since neonates are unable to verbalise, surgeons must gather as many clues as possible from the prenatal, perinatal and family historical details (Table 18.1).

Examination of neonates with suspected intestinal obstruction should start with vital signs and an assessment of the level of resuscitation required. Certain forms of obstruction can cause severe dehydration or sepsis, which will need to be addressed early. Dysmorphic features may give clues to syndromes in which obstruction is common. The abdominal examination should make note of discolouration, distension and signs of peritoneal inflammation such as guarding and rigidity. It is important to look for an incarcerated inguinal hernia as the cause of obstruction (see later). A thorough

Table 18.1 • Important considerations in the neonatal history

Prenatal history	Previous pregnancies (complications and outcomes)
	Maternal gestational illnesses (e.g. gestational diabetes, pregnancy-induced hypertension)
	Screening ultrasonoography (dates and findings)
	Other prenatal investigations and outcomes (e.g. maternal alpha-fetoprotein/BetaHCG/oestrogen levels, chorionic villous sampling, amniocentesis)
Perinatal history	Weeks of gestation
	Induced or spontaneous labour
	Complications of delivery
	APGAR scores
Neonatal history	Complications
	Infections
	Feeding history (initiation, type, rate achieved)
	Passage of meconium in the first 24 hours of life
	Other anomalies identified
Family history	Maternal and paternal health
	Previous congenital anomalies
	Cystic fibrosis
	Consanguinity

evaluation of the perineum must also be performed to ensure normal location and patency of the anus.

Routine blood work including electrolytes and complete blood count are helpful in assessing the level of dehydration as well as helping to determine if electrolyte disturbances or sepsis are contributing to the presentation. It should be kept in mind that serum creatinine in the newborn reflects the mother's levels, and may not be helpful in assessing the neonate's renal function.

Abdominal radiography should be the initial imaging modality for neonates with possible intestinal obstruction. Typically, infants with duodenal obstruction have a 'double-bubble' appearance (**Fig. 18.1**), whereas those with distal intestinal obstruction will have multiple dilated bowel loops. It is impossible to differentiate distal small-bowel obstruction from colonic obstruction based on the plain abdominal radiograph in neonates, as the haustral markings seen in adults are not visible in this age group.

A contrast study is often required to definitively diagnose the aetiology of intestinal obstruction. If malrotation is suspected, an urgent upper gastrointestinal contrast study should be performed first. Once this has been excluded, a contrast enema can be done to exclude distal pathology if this is indicated. For those infants with distal obstruction on plain radiograph, a contrast enema will help to differentiate the three most common causes of distal obstruction: meconium ileus, jejuno-ileal atresia and Hirschsprung disease (**Fig. 18.2**). Water-soluble

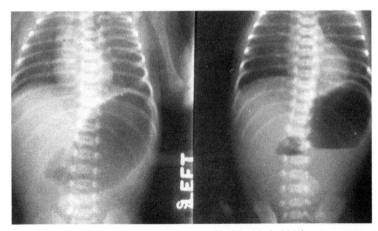

Figure 18.1 • Abdominal radiograph of an infant showing the typical 'double-bubble' appearance resulting from duodenal obstruction.

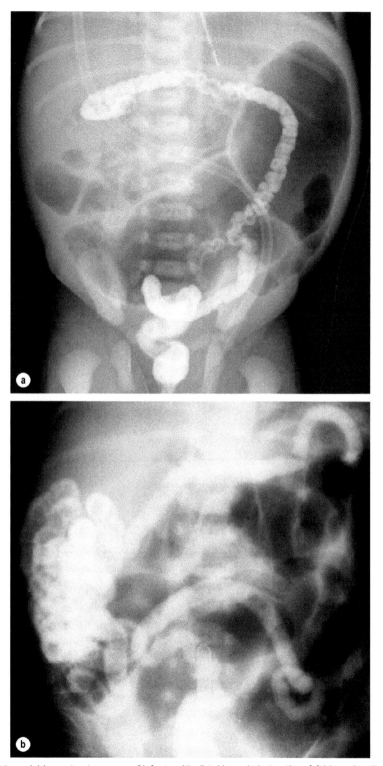

Figure 18.2 • Water-soluble contrast enemas of infants with distal bowel obstruction. **(a)** Meconium ileus, showing a microcolon, dilated proximal small bowel and a soap-bubble appearance in the right lower quadrant. **(b)** Ileal atresia, showing a microcolon, contrast entering the distal small bowel but dilated proximal small bowel without contrast.

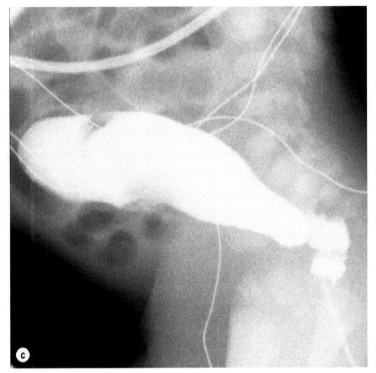

Figure 18.2 • cont'd (c) Hirschsprung disease: lateral film showing a contracted distal rectum with dilated bowel proximally.

contrast should always be used instead of barium, to avoid the possibility of barium leaking into the abdominal cavity should a perforation occur, and also because water-soluble contrast is more effective in relieving the obstruction in cases of meconium obstruction.

Neonates with suspected intestinal obstruction should be transferred in a temperature-controlled transport isolette to a specialised paediatric surgical unit for evaluation and definitive management. Resuscitation should begin as soon as the patient is assessed and should continue during transport. Nasogastric decompression with a large-calibre nasogastric tube (size 8-10 French) is important to improve ventilation, monitor resuscitation and limit bowel distension and subsequent ischaemia.

Specific forms of intestinal obstruction

Oesophageal atresia

This anomaly is characterised by a gap in the oesophagus, resulting in a blind-ending proximal pouch. In 90% of cases, the distal oesophagus is connected to the back of the trachea as a tracheo-oesophageal fistula. Oesophageal atresia is usually first suspected when the baby has difficulty swallowing saliva and may have coughing or respiratory distress during the first feed.[1] Intubation may be needed if ventilation or respiration are significantly impaired. The diagnosis is confirmed by inability to pass a 10–12 French nasogastric tube. This tube should be left in the proximal oesophageal pouch and placed on continuous suction to reduce aspiration of secretions. Operative repair should only be performed by an experienced paediatric surgeon and involves division of the fistula and end-to-end anastomosis of the proximal and distal oesophagus. Associated cardiac anomalies are common with this condition and should be ruled out prior to the baby receiving a general anaesthetic.

Meconium ileus

Cystic fibrosis (CF) is the most common autosomal recessive disorder in Caucasian children.[2] The disease alters the regulation of chloride transport in epithelial cells resulting in a variety of clinical manifestations. Ten to fifteen per cent of children born with CF will develop meconium ileus, in which the meconium becomes sticky and causes intraluminal obstruction. This can further lead to complications of volvulus, atresia or perforation. In addition, meconium ileus may occasionally occur in children without CF. A diagnostic work-up, including both sweat chloride determination and genetic studies, must be done on all children with meconium ileus.

Abdominal radiograph may show distal intestinal obstruction with a bubbly appearance in the right lower quadrant due to gas mixing with the viscous meconium (**Fig. 18.2a**).[2] There may also be intraperitoneal calcification if in-utero perforation has occurred.

Following resuscitation and nasogastric decompression, a water-soluble contrast enema will reveal a microcolon (small calibre) and multiple meconium plugs in the terminal ileum (**Fig. 18.2a**). In approximately 50% of cases the contrast enema will relieve the obstruction. If progress is made, but the infant remains obstructed after the initial enema and is otherwise stable, the procedure can be repeated. If the contrast enema is unsuccessful in relieving the obstruction and/or no further progress has been made, a laparotomy must be done. If there is no volvulus or perforation, enterotomies are made and mechanical washout is performed. Complications of volvulus, acquired atresia or perforation are managed by intestinal resection with or without a stoma, depending on the condition of the bowel and of the patient.

Intestinal atresia/stenosis

Atresia and stenosis can occur at any point in the alimentary canal. The two prominent aetiological theories are failure of recanalisation of the intestine during fetal development, or an ischaemic event in utero.[3] Early resuscitative measures should be initiated and confirmatory diagnosis can usually be made with either upper or lower gastrointestinal contrast studies. The presence of a 'double-bubble' sign on abdominal radiograph is considered diagnostic for duodenal atresia (**Fig. 18.1**), although this finding associated with distal gas may also be due to stenosis, duodenal web, or malrotation. Trisomy 21 is present in one-third of children with duodenal atresia. Patients with distal atresia will typically have multiple dilated loops of bowel on the plain abdominal radiograph. Although a diagnosis of proximal obstruction can be confidently made based on plain radiography, those with distal obstruction should always undergo water-soluble contrast enema to differentiate atresia from meconium ileus or Hirschsprung disease (**Fig. 18.2a–c**).

Since most infants with intestinal atresia are stable once decompressed and resuscitated, we recommend transfer of such neonates to a facility with paediatric surgical expertise. Most of these anomalies are treated with a primary anastomosis. If there is significant dilatation of the proximal segment, tapering enteroplasty should be done, as the dilated bowel tends not to have effective peristalsis.

Hirschsprung disease

Hirschsprung disease (HD) is a congenital disorder characterised by lack of ganglion cells in the distal bowel. This results in failure of peristalsis and functional obstruction. The 'transition zone' is usually located in the rectosigmoid, but HD can affect the entire colon and in rare occurrences the small bowel. HD most often presents in the neonatal period with distal bowel obstruction and failure to pass meconium in the first 24 hours of life. Patients can present later in life with a history of severe constipation. Early identification and management are important to prevent complications of HD such as enterocolitis and nutritional problems.

Water-soluble contrast enema has a sensitivity and specificity of 70% and 83%, respectively, and may therefore be normal, particularly in the newborn.[4] The gold standard for the diagnosis of HD is rectal biopsy, either by a suction technique at the bedside, or full-thickness biopsy.

Initial management, after resuscitation and nasogastric decompression, includes digital rectal stimulation and/or rectal irrigations (10 mL/kg normal saline).

✅ Although the historical teaching for Hirschsprung disease was routine diverting colostomy followed by a 'pull-through' operation several months later, the current standard of care is primary reconstructive surgery without a routine colostomy in most patients.[5]

Preliminary levelling colostomy should be reserved for infants presenting with severe enterocolitis, colonic perforation or failure to decompress with rectal stimulations and irrigations.

There are a number of options for surgical correction of HD, including the Swenson, Soave and Duhamel procedures. In recent years, laparoscopic and transanal approaches have been described, which have decreased morbidity and shortened hospital stay. These operations should all be performed by an experienced paediatric surgeon.

Anorectal malformations

Anorectal malformations can be divided into low and high anomalies. Low anomalies are characterised by rectoperineal or rectovestibular fistulas in female patients. Most males with high malformations have a fistula from the rectum to the bladder neck or urethra. Females with high anomalies usually have a single channel (cloaca) formed by coalescence of the urethra, vagina and rectum. Less commonly, there may be rectal atresia without a fistula, and some infants present with an anal membrane or anal stenosis.

Infants with these malformations usually present in the first day of life with distal bowel obstruction. Low malformations in girls with large fistulas can permit adequate evacuation of stool, and are occasionally missed. Careful examination of the perineum of all newborns for anal patency and position is important. Many of these patients will suffer from associated anomalies that need to be investigated prior to proceeding with anatomical repair of the anorectal malformation.

The next consideration is to determine if the defect is amenable to primary repair or whether faecal flow should be diverted with a colostomy followed by delayed secondary anatomical repair. Children with a rectoperineal fistula can usually be managed with a local procedure from below, without a colostomy. Children with high anomalies are usually managed with a preliminary colostomy. The use of a colostomy in females with a rectovestibular fistula is controversial. The colostomy can be made using either the transverse or the sigmoid colon, and can be a loop or divided stoma. The authors agree with Pena's recommendation for a divided colostomy in the proximal sigmoid colon.[6] Predictors for poor long-term continence in these patients include a rectourinary fistula to the bladder neck or prostatic urethra, tethering of the spinal cord and the presence of an absent or hypoplastic sacrum. Depending on the nature of the anomaly, repair can be carried out using a posterior sagittal approach, a laparoscopic approach, or a combination of posterior and abdominal approaches. Technical expertise is crucial to success, and these procedures should only be performed by experienced paediatric surgeons.

Malrotation

The process of normal rotation and fixation occurs between the 6th and 10th week of development. If no rotation occurs, the patient is left in a position of non-rotation, which has a wide-based mesentery and does not require correction. Classic malrotation occurs when the process is interrupted part way through, leaving the caecum and the duodenal-jejunal junction (ligament of Treitz) close to each other (**Fig. 18.3**). Because this arrangement results in a narrow-based mesentery, the bowel is prone to midgut volvulus around the superior mesenteric vessels, which may lead to intestinal ischaemia. Malrotation with midgut volvulus is one of the true paediatric surgical emergencies. Failure to recognise this condition early can be catastrophic, leading to loss of large portions of bowel and subsequent short-bowel syndrome or death.

Rotation abnormalities are most often asymptomatic. While volvulus can occur at any time, it is most common in the first week of life.[7] The most common presentation of malrotation is bilious vomiting, which may occur for two reasons: midgut volvulus with kinking of the duodenum, or compression of the duodenum by Ladd's bands. Peritonitis and shock from midgut volvulus are late symptoms and are associated with a worse prognosis. Every attempt should be made to diagnose and correct malrotation before this occurs.[8] For this reason, every infant who presents with bilious vomiting should be considered to have malrotation with midgut volvulus until proven otherwise.

Any patient with suspected malrotation and volvulus needs urgent imaging and surgical consultation. Abdominal radiograph is often

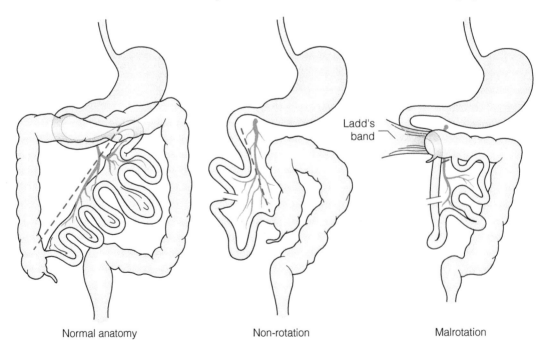

Ladd's band

Normal anatomy   Non-rotation   Malrotation

Figure 18.3 • Schematic illustrations depicting normal intestinal rotation, non-rotation and malrotation. Bold dotted lines illustrate the width of the mesenteric base in each situation.

non-diagnostic but may show a dilated stomach, a 'double bubble' with distal gas, or a relatively gasless abdomen. Upper gastrointestinal contrast study is the preferred examination. A nasogastric tube placed prior to the exam can not only aid in decompression of the stomach, but also the administration of the water-soluble contrast. The chief radiographic signs of malrotation are:

- abnormal position of the duodenojejunal junction;
- spiral, 'corkscrew' or Z-shaped course of the distal duodenum and proximal jejunum; and
- location of the proximal jejunum in the right abdomen.[8]

Abdominal ultrasound may show abnormal orientation of the superior mesenteric artery and vein, or a 'whirlpool sign'.[9]

The operation to correct malrotation involves a laparotomy (although a laparoscopic approach may be undertaken for children without clinical or radiological evidence of midgut volvulus).[10] If there is volvulus, the bowel is untwisted and checked for viability. If there is ischaemia, the bowel is wrapped with warm towels and re-inspected. Grossly necrotic bowel is resected, and the rest is left in, with a second-look laparotomy planned for 24–48 hours later. In children who have necrosis of the entire midgut, a palliative approach without resection should be considered.

If the intestine is viable, a Ladd procedure should be performed. This operation consists of five stages:

1. Division of Ladd's bands.
2. Mobilisation of the colon to the left side of the abdomen.
3. Mobilisation and straightening of the duodenum.
4. Dissection and widening of the small bowel mesentery.
5. Appendicectomy.

Inflammatory conditions

Assessment
The diagnosis of peritonitis in the neonate is complicated by a number of factors, including the patient's inability to communicate with the surgeon, as well as several anatomical and physiological differences between neonates and older children/adults. The very thin abdominal wall may develop oedema and erythema as a result of underlying inflammation. Neonates breathe primarily with their diaphragms, so peritonitis results in rapid, shallow respiration, and ultimately will cause elevation in P_{CO_2} and respiratory

failure. Localised peritoneal signs can be elicited by palpation, but the examiner must be gentle, since the signs of involuntary guarding may be very subtle. In addition, the neonate does not have a well-developed omentum, so ability to localise inflammation may be impaired.

Neonates with peritonitis will often develop systemic sepsis, which may differ in its presentation to older children and adults. Signs of sepsis in neonates may include lethargy, temperature instability (either fever or hypothermia), increased ventilation requirements, thrombocytopenia, a high or low white blood cell count, and acidosis.

Specific forms of abdominal inflammation
Meconium peritonitis
This condition occurs when there has been prenatal intestinal perforation, resulting in chemical peritonitis. Prenatally there may be evidence of free fluid or calcification within the abdomen. In some cases, the fetus is able to localise and wall off the perforation, which may result in a meconium cyst. The aetiology of the perforation is often distal obstruction, usually from meconium ileus or intestinal atresia, but in some cases the perforation is idiopathic.

Management of meconium peritonitis involves fluid resuscitation, nasogastric drainage and antibiotics. If there is evidence of associated intestinal obstruction, a contrast enema may be helpful preoperatively. Laparotomy should be carried out with resection of the involved bowel and either stomas or primary anastomosis, depending on the condition of the child and the bowel.

Necrotising enterocolitis
Necrotising enterocolitis (NEC) is most commonly seen in preterm and small-for-gestational-age infants.[11] The aetiology of NEC is unknown, but a combination of bacterial colonisation, intraluminal substrate and intestinal ischaemia/hypoxia all appear to be important.[12]

NEC should be suspected in neonates with sepsis, increased abdominal girth, feeding intolerance, abdominal wall discolouration, or bloody stools. Abdominal radiograph may show pneumatosis intestinalis, portal venous gas, or free intra-abdominal air (**Fig. 18.4**). Ultrasound may show pneumatosis, free fluid, or intestinal hypoperfusion and hypomotility.

Initial management of NEC includes bowel rest, nasogastric decompression, broad-spectrum antibiotics, parenteral nutrition and supportive measures to optimise perfusion and oxygenation of the bowel. Persistent clinical deterioration and signs of necrosis or perforation are generally considered indications for operative intervention. Options include bedside peritoneal drainage, or laparotomy with resection of grossly necrotic bowel and either primary anastomosis or stomas, depending on the

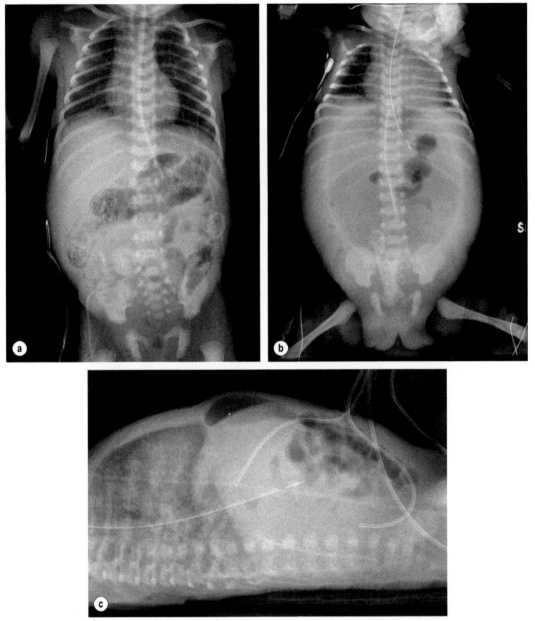

Figure 18.4 • Abdominal radiographs of infants with necrotising enterocolitis. **(a)** Pneumatosis intestinalis. **(b)** 'Football sign' on supine film depicting intra-abdominal free air. **(c)** Free intra-abdominal air on lateral film.

status of the child and the bowel.[11,13] A recent randomised controlled trial in neonates less than 1500 g with perforation found no significant difference in outcomes between peritoneal drainage and laparotomy.[14] Prior to laparotomy, parents should always be informed of the possibility of a long segment of necrosis requiring massive resection that would leave the child with short bowel syndrome. Palliative management should be considered in these infants.

Isolated ileal perforation

This condition resembles NEC, in that it primarily affects preterm and small-for-gestational-age infants. However, infants with isolated ileal perforation do not have any abnormalities of the intestine other than localised perforation, usually in the distal ileum. It is unclear whether this represents a very localised form of NEC, or a distinct entity. Clinically, these infants present with sudden deterioration, sepsis and free air without any evidence of pneumatosis seen on the abdominal radiograph. In general, the same principles of treatment are applied to ileal perforation and NEC.

Other neonatal conditions

Incarcerated inguinal hernia

Inguinal hernias are very common throughout childhood. Hernias in children almost always arise from persistence of the processus vaginalis. If the processus contains only fluid, it is known as a hydrocele; the hydrocele is communicating if the processus remains open, and non-communicating if the processus has become obliterated proximal to the fluid. Communicating hydroceles should be repaired electively if they have not closed by 1 year of age.

In most cases, inguinal hernias are asymptomatic and can be repaired electively. Incarceration of bowel may result in complete bowel obstruction, and represents a surgical emergency since both the bowel and the testis may become ischaemic. The risk of incarceration is greatest in newborns and is approximately 30% in the first 2 years of life. Premature infants are at highest risk.

Neonates and infants presenting with an incarcerated hernia should be resuscitated if necessary, and an immediate attempt should be made to reduce the hernia. In contrast to the adult with an incarcerated hernia, testicular ischaemia is far more common than intestinal ischaemia, and it is appropriate to be aggressive about reducing the hernia. Multiple attempts and the use of sedation may be necessary. Ice should not be applied to the hernia, since it may induce hypothermia. Surgical repair of an incarcerated hernia in an infant is a formidable undertaking. The sac is often thin and oedematous, and the risks of injury to the cord structures and recurrence of the hernia are very high. Therefore, if a general surgeon is unable to reduce the hernia and a paediatric surgeon is accessible, the patient should be referred immediately.

✔ If the hernia is reduced, repair should be undertaken 24–48 hours later, allowing some of the oedema to settle, but hopefully before re-incarceration.[15]

Inguinal hernia repair in infants can be performed using an open or laparoscopic technique.

Abdominal wall defects

Gastroschisis is characterised by an abdominal wall defect to the right of the umbilicus, through which most of the intestinal tract protrudes.[16] Omphalocele (also called exomphalos) is characterised by herniation of bowel with or without solid organs into the umbilical cord. Gastroschisis tends to be an isolated anomaly, whereas omphalocele is often associated with chromosomal, cardiac, renal, limb and facial anomalies.

If the diagnosis is made prenatally, delivery should occur at a centre with paediatric surgical support. Resuscitation and nasogastric decompression should begin in the delivery room. The bowel or sac should be wrapped in warm, saline-soaked, sterile gauze and covered with sterile plastic wrap to minimise heat and evaporative fluid loss.

Repair of both conditions should be done by an experienced paediatric surgeon. Options include primary closure, or staged closure using a preformed Silastic® silo that allows the bowel to be reduced gradually into the abdomen over 1–6 days.[17]

Infancy

Hypertrophic pyloric stenosis

Hypertrophic pyloric stenosis (HPS) is an acquired condition in which the pylorus becomes abnormally thickened, causing gastric outlet obstruction. This occurs in infants during the first 2–12 weeks of life and is characterised by projectile, non-bilious vomiting, usually occurring after feeds. HPS occurs in approximately 1:400 children, with a significant male predominance.[18]

Diagnosis is suspected based on a history of progressive, forceful, non-bilious vomiting in a child of the appropriate age. Physical examination usually reveals some level of dehydration. The presence of a palpable 'olive' in the epigastrium has a 99% positive predictive value for the disease.[19] Vomiting of gastric contents leads to depletion of sodium, potassium and hydrochloric acid, resulting in the typical hypochloraemic, hypokalaemic metabolic alkalosis. The kidneys attempt to conserve sodium at the expense of hydrogen ions, often leading to paradoxical aciduria.[20] The level of dehydration can be estimated by clinical examination, urine output and serum chloride and bicarbonate levels. If the pyloric olive is not palpable, the diagnosis can be confirmed by ultrasound (pyloric length >16 mm and single wall thickness >3 mm). If an experienced sonographer is not available, the diagnosis can be made using a barium swallow (**Fig. 18.5**).

Surgery should be deferred until the infant is fully resuscitated. This is accomplished by using normal saline or Ringer's lactate with potassium. Most children should receive a bolus of 20 mL/kg, and then an infusion consisting of 1.5 times the maintenance requirement (i.e. 6 mL/kg/h for this age group) until the urine output and electrolytes have been normalised.

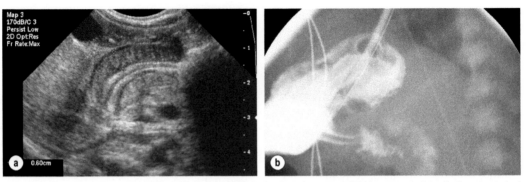

Figure 18.5 • Images of hypertrophic pyloric stenosis. **(a)** Abdominal ultrasound. **(b)** Upper gastrointestinal contrast study.

Surgical management of HPS consists of extramucosal longitudinal splitting of the pyloric muscle. The original procedure described by Ramstedt in 1912 was carried out through a transverse right upper quadrant incision.[21] This technique has been modified in many institutions to utilise circum-umbilical incisions or laparoscopic techniques. Following pyloromyotomy many infants will experience continued vomiting for 24–48 hours, although the majority will eventually tolerate feeds and be discharged. Postoperative complications are rare but include wound infection, duodenal or gastric perforation and incomplete pyloromyotomy.

While intravenous access and fluid resuscitation can occur in most centres some countries have experienced a centralisation of the surgical management of HPS to paediatric surgical centres only. Some evidence exists that there may be shorter postoperative stays and reduced complications in these centres.[22] We recommend that as long as the paediatric, anaesthetic and surgical teams are experienced and competent, and that as long as patient volumes allow for the maintenance of expertise, these patients can be managed in smaller centres. Otherwise, since the surgical procedure can be delayed, transfer to an experienced centre should be considered.

Intussusception

Intussusception, or 'telescoping of the bowel', occurs when one portion of bowel invaginates into a more distant portion. This results in venous congestion, bowel wall oedema, intestinal obstruction and ultimately full-thickness necrosis of the intussusceptum. The peak incidence of intussusception is seen at 6–9 months of age.[23] The majority are ileocolic with hyperplastic lymphoid tissue in Peyer patches acting as a lead point.[24] These are often referred to as 'idiopathic'. Asymptomatic small bowel to small bowel intussusception may be seen incidentally on abdominal ultrasound,

or sometimes may be associated with Henoch–Schonlein purpura or cystic fibrosis. Less than 5% of intussusceptions are due to a pathological lead point such as a Meckel diverticulum, polyp, or small bowel tumour such as lymphoma or leiomyoma. Intussusception occurring outside of the usual age range, or those that recur should raise suspicion for a pathological lead point.

Few children with ileocolic intussusception will demonstrate the classic triad of intermittent severe abdominal pain with drawing up of the legs, palpable abdominal mass and 'red-currant jelly' stool. Physicians must have a high index of suspicion due to the variability of symptoms. Patients may present with irritability, lethargy, abdominal pain, vomiting, diarrhoea or constipation, haematochezia, fever, dehydration or shock. Management should initially focus on diagnosis and resuscitation.

Following fluid resuscitation, imaging should be performed to confirm the diagnosis of intussusception. Abdominal radiograph may show air–fluid levels and distension of the small bowel and there may be a characteristic lack of air in the right lower quadrant. Ultrasonography has a high sensitivity and is currently the test of choice.[24]

> ✔ Traditionally, the treatment of intussusception has been barium enema. More recently, pneumatic reduction using air or CO_2 has been associated with an 80–95% success rate.[24]

If the intussusception is partially, but not completely reduced, it is worth trying again a few hours later, since some of the oedema may have been eliminated by the first attempt and a second attempt may be associated with a 50% chance of success.[25] Pneumatic pressures of 60–100 mmHg are recommended.[26]

Surgical intervention is reserved for those patients who fail hydrostatic or pneumatic reduction, or have signs of infarcted or perforated bowel such as peritonitis, or free air on abdominal radiograph at the time of presentation. At laparotomy, the intussusception is manually reduced if possible. If the intussusception is not reducible, the bowel appears necrotic, or a pathological lead point is identified, a segmental resection should be performed with primary anastomosis. Excellent results using a laparoscopic approach to this condition have been documented.[27]

Children

Appendicitis

Appendicitis is the most frequent abdominal surgical emergency in children.[28] As in adults, the classic presentation is mid-abdominal pain moving to the right lower quadrant, anorexia, vomiting, low-grade fever and localised tenderness with peritoneal signs in the right lower quadrant. Presentation in children may be atypical, particularly in those under 5 years of age. Some authors have attempted to quantify the usefulness of specific findings in children using scoring systems. Clinical scoring systems such as the Alvarado Score and the Paediatric Appendicitis Score have been shown to be both sensitive and specific (Table 18.2).[29–31]

In the otherwise well, stable patient with an equivocal presentation, the diagnostic options include observation with serial examinations, or imaging with ultrasound or computed tomography (CT) (**Fig. 18.6**). There is a great deal of controversy as to which technique is more appropriate. Ultrasound is clearly more operator-dependent, but the overuse of CT scans in childhood should be avoided due to the risk of radiation-induced malignancy later in life.[32] Both have excellent accuracy.

Increasingly, surgeons are using a laparoscopic approach to appendicectomy in children. As in adults,

Table 18.2 • Paediatric Appendicitis Score

Clinical findings	Points
Percussion/hopping tenderness/coughing	2
Anorexia	1
Pyrexia	1
Nausea or vomiting	1
RLQ tenderness	2
Leukocytosis (WBC >10 000/µL)	1
Neutrophilia ('left shift')	1
Migration of pain to RLQ	1

A score of 6 or more has been shown to be associated with a high likelihood of the child having acute appendicitis.[30]
RLQ, right lower quadrant; WBC, white blood cell count.
Reproduced from Samuel M. Pediatric Appendicitis Score.
J Pediatr Surg 2002;37(6):877–81. With permission from Elsevier.

the benefits of the laparoscopic approach include reduced postoperative pain and length of stay, as well as a decrease in wound infection. There is some evidence that the rate of intra-abdominal abscess may be higher after laparoscopic appendicectomy in children with perforated appendicitis.[33] The laparoscopic approach may also be beneficial in children who are muscular or obese, and in adolescent females, where the incidence of ovarian pathology as a cause for the symptoms is higher.

There is some recent evidence in the adult literature that simple, non-perforated appendicitis may be safely managed with antibiotics alone, avoiding appendicectomy.[34] While there are some preliminary studies in children that suggest similar outcomes,[35–37] further evidence will be necessary before this approach can be recommended. This topic is discussed in more detail in Chapter 15.

Approximately 40% of children present with perforation, and the incidence is over 65% in those aged 0–4 years old.[28] In contrast to non-perforated appendicitis, these children usually present with

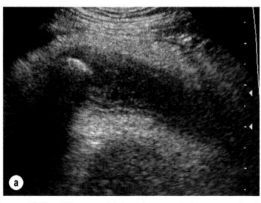
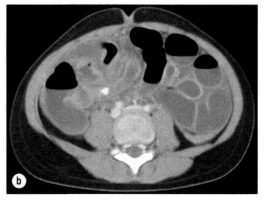

Figure 18.6 • Ultrasound **(a)** and computed tomography **(b)** images of children with acute appendicitis. A faecolith is visible at the base of the inflamed appendix in both images.

prolonged symptoms, higher fever, higher white blood cell count and more diffuse peritoneal signs. Some children present with frank sepsis and diffuse peritoneal contamination; these children benefit from resuscitation, followed by immediate appendicectomy and peritoneal washout. Many children with perforated appendicitis present with a prolonged history and a localised abscess or phlegmon on imaging. This condition can be managed either by early operation, or by non-operative management consisting of broad-spectrum antibiotics and image-guided drainage of any purulent collections. The need for a subsequent interval appendectomy later is controversial. We reserve the use of interval appendicectomy for those with an appendicolith on imaging, since their risk of recurrent appendicitis is over 50%.[38] (See also Chapter 15.)

Evidence-based guidelines have been published to aid surgeons in choosing appropriate antibiotics for appendicitis, whether it is perforated or not.[39] While geographic variations in antimicrobial resistance need to be taken into account, we recommend generally following these guidelines.

Fluid resuscitation of the child with a surgical emergency

Fluid and electrolyte management in children are made challenging by differences in total body water and compensatory mechanisms, as well as changes in physiology throughout childhood. Total body water is as high as 80% of body weight in neonates, and decreases to the adult level of approximately 60% by 1 year. Degree of dehydration can be estimated from the history and physical examination. Children with mild dehydration (1–5% of body fluid volume) show few clinical signs but frequently have a history of 12–24 hours of vomiting or diarrhoea. Those with moderate dehydration (6–10%) are often lethargic, have low urine output (usually evident as fewer wet nappies), weight loss, loss of skin turgor, sunken eyes or fontanelle, dry mucus membranes and crying without tears. If severe dehydration (11–15%) is reached the child may develop cardiovascular or neurological instability. Children have very active peripheral vasoconstriction, so that blood pressure will be maintained until advanced intravascular volume depletion is reached with onset of hypotension, irritability or coma. However, tachycardia is an early sign that should be recognised and treated.[20]

The urgency of fluid replacement depends on the degree of dehydration and the cause of the fluid loss. The goals of treatment are the restoration and preservation of cardiovascular, neurological and renal perfusion. In the event of dehydration resulting from an inflammatory condition that will require urgent surgical intervention, such as appendicitis, isotonic fluid (normal saline or Ringer's lactate solution) should be given in 20 mL/kg boluses until signs of cardiovascular compromise subside. For situations in which there is no urgency to do an operation, such as pyloric stenosis, the fluid deficit can be replaced more slowly. This has the advantage of avoiding sudden fluid shifts, and the possibility of cerebral oedema and seizures, which are particularly likely in neonates and infants. The commonly used protocol is to calculate the fluid deficit and replace half over the first 8 hours, and the other half over the subsequent 16 hours.

Paediatric trauma

The principles of trauma management are the same for children as they are for adults. Securing the airway and ensuring adequate ventilation are paramount before treating bleeding and circulatory collapse. Fluid resuscitation is based on the patient's size, keeping in mind the differences in physiological response to hypovolaemia mentioned in the previous section. As with adults, two boluses of crystalloid (20 mL/kg) should be given through large-bore intravenous lines as quickly as possible. If there is still suspicion for ongoing bleeding, blood products are in a balanced fashion with packed red blood cells, platelets and fresh-frozen plasma. Again, 20 mL/kg boluses should be the goal.

The principles of managing penetrating trauma in children are the same as in adults. However, children sustaining blunt abdominal trauma are more prone to solid organ injury due to the low-lying nature of these organs with respect to the paediatric rib cage and the relative laxity of the abdominal wall. In general, injuries to the spleen, liver and kidney can be managed non-operatively regardless of the grade of injury. Operations are rare for blunt abdominal trauma in children. The indications for laparotomy in a child with blunt abdominal trauma include: evidence of peritonitis on abdominal examination, free intra-abdominal air on imaging, inability to normalise haemodynamic status despite resuscitation efforts, rapidly expanding abdomen associated with persistent hypotension, and need for transfusion of more than one-half of the blood volume over 24 hours.

Key points

- Neonatal and complex surgery in children should ideally take place in specialised paediatric surgical units, with subspecialised paediatric surgical, anaesthetic and intensive care unit support.
- Resuscitation is the first step in the management of all children with surgical problems.
- *Beware the child whose vomit is green!* Bilious vomiting in a neonate or child is usually associated with intestinal obstruction, and every child with bilious vomiting should be assumed to have life-threatening malrotation and midgut volvulus until proven otherwise.
- A high index of suspicion for intussusception should be maintained in children in the high-risk age group (3–12 months of age) presenting with intermittent abdominal pain, vomiting, and/or bloody stools.
- Delayed passage of meconium (>24 hours of life) should arouse suspicion of Hirschsprung disease.
- Incarcerated inguinal hernias should be reduced if possible, and repaired within 48 hours of reduction.
- Tachycardia is an important sign of intravascular fluid depletion in children; hypotension is a late finding.

🌐 References available at **http://expertconsult. inkling.com**

19

Management of trauma for the general surgeon

Valentin Neuhaus
Pradeep H. Navsaria
Andrew John Nicol

Introduction

The global burden of disease related to trauma is immense, with greater than 1.5 million deaths each year due to violence, 1.25 million deaths in road traffic accidents annually, and nearly 1 million children die each year because of injury.[1] These numbers are expected to increase in the next 20 years and trauma is among the top 10 causes of death globally.[2] The numbers of injured survivors have increased, with up to 1 billion patients seeking medical assistance after an injury yearly,[3] and depending on the geographical location every eighth hospital admission now is related to injury. The associated global costs are excessive, approaching 2% of a country's gross national product with respect to road accidents;[4] however, it must be emphasised that there are considerable variations between different countries.

The trimodal death distribution, first described by Trunkey in 1983, may have changed in the past years, but it remains a good model to understand the timing and causes of death following injury.[5] The first peak are patients with non-survivable injuries (e.g. complete aortic rupture). Despite preventive measures (e.g. seat-belts, airbags, helmets, avoiding drunk-driving), which remarkably reduced the first peak and the years of life lost, injuries continue to cause death and morbidity.[3] The majority of patients die within the first 24 hours after an accident,[6] and the second peak comprises patients arriving alive in the emergency department, with head, thoracic and abdominal/pelvic injuries being the predominant lethal injuries. Unrecognised or untreated abdominal injury is one of the most important causes of preventable death.[7] One of the main goals of trauma surgery is to diminish this peak and Advanced Trauma Life Support (ATLS®) with its primary and secondary survey is one way to evaluate and treat severely injured patients in this phase.[8] The third peak comprises patients dying at a later stage due to multi-organ failure and sepsis.

> ✓✓ The Advanced Trauma Life Support (ATLS®) guidelines are a crucial part of the early evaluation and management of all trauma patients.[8]

Trauma surgery has evolved tremendously over the past 50 years. The traditional dogma of mandatory exploration of all penetrating wounds has changed to selective non-operative management in neck and abdominal trauma.[9,10] Damage control surgery and damage control resuscitation have been introduced. Abdominal compartment syndrome and intra-abdominal hypertension have been identified and strategies put in place for prevention. Early institution of blood and lower volumes of crystalloids are seemingly beneficial. There is a far better understanding of coagulopathy in the trauma setting and specific transfusions ratios have been shown to improve survival. Imaging is far more frequently available and the introduction of focused assessment with sonography in trauma (FAST) and eFAST in the resuscitation room is changing surgical algorithms. There is much to be enthusiastic about in our management of the injured patient but we also need to be aware of the fact that clinical signs are vital in our assessment and that there should not be an over-reliance on special investigations.

Evaluation of the injured patient

Primary and secondary survey, damage control surgery, transfer

The goal of the primary survey is to identify and instantaneously treat life-threatening injuries. This early management phase is called the 'golden hour'.[11] Time plays an important role in this resuscitation phase as mortality is highest within the first 24 hours after the incident. Patients are assessed and resuscitated along the ATLS ABCDE algorithm. The following life-threatening injuries must be ruled out:[8]

- Airway: airway obstruction (due to foreign bodies, aspiration, facial or laryngeal injuries)
- Breathing: tension pneumothorax, open pneumothorax with a sucking wound, massive haemothorax, cardiac tamponade, flail chest
- Circulation: shock (mainly caused by haemorrhage)
- Disability: severe traumatic brain injury
- Exposure: hypothermia

The pathophysiological consequences of these injuries are *hypoxia* (caused by airway or breathing problems), *hypotension/hypoperfusion* (caused by circulation problems) and *hypothermia* (exposure problem). Hypoxia and hypoperfusion result in anaerobic metabolism with accumulation of acidic metabolites, a deficiency of adenosine triphosphate (ATP) and failure of the Na/K-ATPase pump. This failure causes cell swelling and damage, and finally organ dysfunction. Serum lactate, pH and base excess are good parameters to assess the adequacy of organ perfusion and oxygenation. Higher lactate level and the duration of hyperlactataemia correlate with mortality after trauma.[12] Hypoperfusion also leads to increased excretion of stress hormones, which consecutively increases the contractility of the heart, the heart rate as an early sign of relevant blood loss and local vasoconstriction with hypoperfusion of the skin, muscles, kidneys and the intestine (centralisation). Blood pressure drops later with ongoing blood loss and exhausted compensatory mechanisms. Heat loss while lying exposed, cold intravenous fluids and opened body cavities during surgery cause hypothermia. Hypothermia itself negatively influences the coagulation system and myocardial function. The three 'hypo'-problems lead to the well-known deadly triad of *hypothermia, acidosis* and *coagulopathy*.[13]

The treatment in this primary phase is priority-oriented and kept as simple as possible.[8]

All patients are given supplemental oxygen. A definitive airway (intubation or surgical cricothyroidotomy) will clear any airway obstruction. Needle decompression and intercostal drains usually resolve any life-threatening tension or open pneumothoraces. A thoracotomy is required for a massive haemothorax (>1500 mL drainage) or for ongoing bleeding (>200 mL per hour for the next 4 hours), patients in profound refractory shock or undergoing cardiopulmonary resuscitation after penetrating trauma. The main goal in circulation problems is to stop the bleeding and restore the volume. Chest (e.g. intercostal arteries), abdomen (mainly spleen, liver, mesentery, or kidneys), pelvis or long bones (fractures) and external wounds (with vascular injuries, extensive scalp or torso injuries) are the main sources. Intercostal drains, direct compression, packing, or (partial) resection of bleeding organs, aortic cross-clamping, Pringle manoeuvre, vessel repair or shunting are some basic techniques to stop the bleeding. Unstable pelvic fractures are temporarily stabilised by a pelvic binder, C-clamp, or external fixator. Long bone fractures are externally or internally stabilised to reduce bleeding, alleviate pain and enable intensive care. A moderate, balanced, volume resuscitation can be carried out, especially in penetrating injuries, until successful bleeding control, but an adequate volume substitution has then to be carried out and adequate urine excretion has to be achieved.[14] Using the Glasgow Coma Scale (GCS) a patient with a score less than 9 must be intubated and evaluated with a computed tomography (CT) scan of the brain. The CT of the brain should be delayed in the case of a patient who is haemodynamically unstable requiring operative intervention. Warm infusions, blankets, or warming devices such as a Bairhugger 3 M© are used to limit and treat hypothermia.

Damage control surgery

Further relevant injuries can now be sought and treated in the next phase, the 'secondary survey', usually carried out from head to toe. Basically, definitive repair of all relevant injuries is the main target. However, the extent of these therapeutic measures as well as the surgical procedures in the primary survey must be considered. Trauma causes a first hit and a consecutive systemic inflammatory response syndrome (SIRS), which can trigger reduced resistance to infection. Early extensive surgical care of all injuries, acting as a second hit, can lead to a further immune response with resultant multi-organ dysfunction, failure, or even death.[15] In addition, if certain criteria are met, only abbreviated operative procedures, so-called *damage control surgery*, should be applied. Damage control surgery is a well-established surgical strategy, mainly in major abdominal trauma, but also in other conditions, and should enable patients not to slip further into an unsalvageable metabolic state of the deadly triad of hypothermia, acidosis and coagulopathy.[16–18] Damage control surgery aims to quickly stop the bleeding and limit contamination without restoration of the anatomy (e.g. to pack or remove solid organs, staple bowel injuries and to temporarily close the abdomen), and to normalise the pathophysiological parameters in the intensive care unit (ICU).[19] No major surgery is carried out during this ICU stage. Oxygen delivery, blood pressure, heart rate, urinary output, body temperature, pH, lactate and coagulation must be normalised in the ICU. Aggressive volume resuscitation, abdominal packing and the accumulation of intra-abdominal blood increase the risk of an abdominal compartment syndrome in some of these patients and the intra-abdominal pressure should therefore be monitored. Reduction in cardiac output, renal failure, impaired ventilation and raised intracranial pressure are several pathophysiological consequences of raised intra-abdominal pressure (see also Chapter 20). After normalisation of these parameters, a re-look is performed with definitive surgical care and abdominal wall closure if possible. The timing here is crucial; the possible consequences are re-bleeding if returned too early, and infection and sepsis if returned too late to the theatre to remove abdominal packing.[20] Patients ideally remain intubated, ventilated, under antibiotic cover and return to theatre 24–48 hours after the first operation.

The following pathophysiological parameters, signs and criteria are indicators to proceed with damage control surgery:[16,21]

- Hypothermia <35°C
- Acidosis pH <7.2
- Lactate >5 mmol/L
- Coagulopathy INR >1.5
- Systolic blood pressure <90 mmHg
- Mass transfusion (10 and more blood units)
- Trauma mechanism (e.g. multiple torso gunshot wounds)
- Injury Severity Score >36 points
- Major vascular (e.g. inferior vena cava) injuries and visceral or pelvic injuries
- Higher age and comorbidities
- Inability to control bleeding by conventional methods
- Inability to close the abdomen
- Abdominal compartment syndrome during attempted abdominal wall closure
- Need to reassess extent of bowel viability.

Referral patterns

Depending on the hospital facilities, some care cannot be provided and the patients must be transferred as soon as possible to a trauma centre or another suitable facility. Typical injuries warranting a transfer are:[8]

- Severe or moderate head injury
- Major pulmonary contusions
- Flail chest
- Cardiac or great vessel injury
- Acute spinal cord injury
- Solid organ injuries
- Unstable pelvic ring injury
- Severe open fractures or amputations
- Several long bone fractures
- Polytraumatised patients
- Severe burns
- Older patients (>55 years) or patients with comorbidities.

Patients with these injuries are ideally treated in a level I trauma centre with a better outcome and survival.[22]

Regional injuries

Injury scoring scales

The American Association for the Surgery of Trauma (AAST) publishes the most widely accepted and used injury classification system for neck, chest and abdominal injuries, which is available online at http://www.aast.org/Library/TraumaTools/InjuryScoringScales.aspx. Organ injuries are graded into five increasing severity categories, grade I being minor haematomas or lacerations and grade V completely shattered or devascularised organ injuries.

✓✓ Injury severity scores are important as they help to guide treatment, have a prognostic value and allow the comparison of results in the literature.[23]

Blunt and penetrating abdominal trauma

Abdominal organs are less protected than those of the chest. General surgeons are consequently often confronted with intra-abdominal trauma. Depending on the country, penetrating (i.e. in South Africa) or blunt (i.e. in Switzerland) mechanisms are predominant. Independent of the mechanism, there are some mainstays.

The timing of assessment and treatment depends on the haemodynamic status of the patient and the clinical evaluation. In the primary survey, a clinical evaluation of the haemodynamic status, the abdomen and a FAST, particularly in blunt trauma or suspected haemopericardium, is required. Haemodynamic stability is defined as systolic blood pressure >90 mmHg, pulse rate <100/min, *and* no more than 1–2 litres of crystalloid infusion.[24] Vital signs must be cautiously interpreted, especially in elderly patients and under the influence of certain medications, and always be correlated with the injuries and metabolic response of the patient.[25] A laparotomy is mandatory in the event of an acute abdomen, or in the haemodynamically unstable patient with a penetrating wound or in the case of blunt trauma where there is a positive FAST and an unstable patient.

A thorough clinical evaluation is required in the secondary survey, with inspection, palpation, percussion and auscultation. Repeated examination is the key as physical signs may be delayed or altered in the case of drunk or drugged patients, patients with traumatic brain injuries, acute spinal cord injuries and with distracting injuries. Adjuncts (nasogastric tube, urinary catheter, FAST, CT of the abdomen, diagnostic laparoscopy) are helpful tools particularly in these patients to rule in or out a relevant intra-abdominal injury.

The most important method in clinically evaluable patients remains serial clinical examination. In penetrating trauma, the authors do not recommend ultrasound of the abdomen or invasive procedures such as local wound exploration or diagnostic peritoneal lavage.

The further priority of assessment and treatment is dictated by the mechanism of injury, the sustained injuries, the haemodynamic status of the patient and the clinical evaluation. Typical indications to proceed with a laparotomy are:[8]

- Haemodynamic instability due to an intra-abdominal injury (positive ultrasound or clinical evidence of intraperitoneal bleeding)
- Peritonitis (tenderness of the abdomen and abdominal guarding)
- Organ evisceration
- Gunshot wounds with a transabdominal trajectory
- Confirmed stomach, rectum, or genitourinary system (bladder, ureter, vagina) injuries after a penetrating trauma
- Free intra-abdominal air
- Hollow viscus rupture or perforation
- Patient develops peritoneal signs or haemodynamic instability after failed non-operative management (NOM).

A few decades ago, all penetrating wounds mandated a laparotomy. More than 30% of the laparotomies were negative (no intra-abdominal injuries) or non-therapeutic (the intra-abdominal injury does not need any intervention).[26] Short-term morbidity of a trauma laparotomy is high (wound infection, intra-abdominal abscess, pneumonia, urinary tract infection, deep venous thrombosis, pulmonary embolus) and long-term complications (small-bowel obstruction and incisional hernia) are encountered in 15% after trauma laparotomy.[27,28] This is independent of whether the laparotomy was therapeutic or unnecessary. To reduce unnecessary laparotomies and their consequences, selective NOM was developed in asymptomatic and haemodynamic normal patients. Lower transfusion requirements, fewer abdominal infections, shorter hospitalisation, lower mortality and lower costs are positive consequences of NOM.[29,30] The decision to proceed with NOM is crucial. The fear of re-bleeding, missing a hollow viscus injury and the consequences of a delayed laparotomy are still constant companions.[31] The fear may be exaggerated since delayed laparotomies do not increase the risk of adverse events if carried out within 12–24 hours.[32] Serial examinations are mandatory to detect failure of NOM and to act appropriately in a timely fashion, with risk factors for failed NOM being age older than 55, haemodynamic instability, higher specific organ and total injury severity grade, size of haemoperitoneum, contrast blush on CT and use of anticoagulants. Angioembolisation may play an important role in patients with these risk factors and solid organ injuries.[33]

Special investigations

Focused assessment with sonography in trauma (FAST)

FAST is a non-invasive, cheap, easily reproducible, focused examination of the chest and abdomen, which can be performed at the bedside by the treating trauma surgeon. The primary goal of FAST is to detect free fluid (presumably blood in a trauma patient) in the abdomen, chest or the pericardium, as an explanation for the haemodynamic instability of a patient. The goal is *not* to detect distinct organ injuries. FAST can be carried out within 5 minutes, with the specificity to detect free fluid in blunt trauma being 90–100% and sensitivity 60–100%.[34,35] FAST, however, is operator-dependent, despite an easy learning curve.[36] False-negative results are misleading and often seen in patients with obesity or surgical emphysema. The ultrasound can be falsely negative if it is performed too early, since it needs more than 500 mL blood in Morrison's pouch to be visible.[37,38] Ideal indications are blunt torso trauma, haemopericardium, children and pregnant patients. The goal of extended FAST (eFAST) is to diagnose a pneumothorax, which can be done with a higher sensitivity than a chest X-ray.[34]

Computed tomography (CT)

Contrast-enhanced CT is the gold standard to detect and grade torso injuries in stable patients. Contrast-blushes can also represent active bleeding spots, which are amenable to angiographic embolisation. It is non-invasive, but it usually requires transport to radiology, time and is expensive.[8] Contrast material can cause allergic reactions and induce nephropathy. The danger of radiation-induced cancer is not clear and where possible radiation exposure should be minimised as much as possible. The overall accuracy and sensitivity is high except for diaphragmatic, bowel and some pancreatic injuries.[39] A special algorithm is needed for diaphragmatic injuries (see later in this chapter). The index of suspicion of bowel injuries is high in the presence of:

- free fluid and no solid-organ injury;
- free extraluminal gas;
- thickened bowel wall;
- mesenteric stranding;
- haematoma surrounding a hollow viscus.

Ideal indications for CT are stable patients with blunt trauma, penetrating back or flank trauma, penetrating trauma with questionable extraperitoneal tract, right upper quadrant/right-sided thoraco-abdominal trajectory (i.e. to exclude liver injury) and haematuria (i.e. to exclude upper urinary tract injury). In transpelvic penetrating wounds with haematuria a CT-cystogram is helpful to guide further treatment.[8,30] It is currently not clear if routine or selective scanning is recommended in polytraumatised patients, where there is a clear trend to a whole-body CT.[31,40]

Diagnostic and therapeutic laparoscopy

Laparoscopy is a minimally invasive procedure; however, it requires special expensive equipment, surgical skills and usually general anaesthesia. There is as yet no role for diagnostic laparoscopy (DL) in the haemodynamically unstable patient, since pneumoperitoneum further compromises the haemodynamic, pulmonary and renal status. In elective trauma situations, it has been successfully used in diagnosis and repair of peritoneal breach, stomach, minor liver, suspected extraperitoneal rectal and, specifically, diaphragmatic injuries. It can help to avoid a laparotomy in a highly selected patient group.[41,42]

Blunt trauma

The spleen (40–55%), liver (35–45%) and small bowel (5–10%) are the most frequently injured organs in blunt abdominal trauma.[8] Major pelvic or chest injuries are commonly associated with relevant intra-abdominal injuries and serial clinical examination usually detects these injuries. A seat-belt sign or a buckle-handle injury raises the suspicion of a mesenteric, duodenal, or pancreatic

injury and such patients need admission and further investigations.[8] NOM has become the standard of care in patients with parenchymatous organs injuries with no indications to proceed with laparotomy (predominantly *haemodynamic instability* due to major haemorrhage). FAST or CT are often used as adjuncts in NOM. *Hollow viscus rupture* and/or *peritonitis* are still clear indications to proceed with operative treatment. Free air or free intra-abdominal fluid without parenchymatous organ injuries must raise the suspicion of a hollow viscus or mesenteric injury and mandates a laparotomy, especially in patients with a severe head injury or complete spinal cord injury due to unreliable physical examinations.[43]

Figure 19.1 presents an algorithm for management of blunt abdominal trauma.

Spleen

The spleen provides important immunological function by clearing intravascular antigens, hence infectious complications are feared after splenectomy. Demetriades et al. analysed 269 patients with blunt splenic trauma,[44] one-third of whom underwent splenectomy. Risk factors for splenectomy were hypotension and a higher degree of splenic injury. Wound infection, intra-abdominal abscess, urinary tract infection, pneumonia and septicaemia were complications encountered in 32% of the splenectomy group versus 5.2% in the splenic

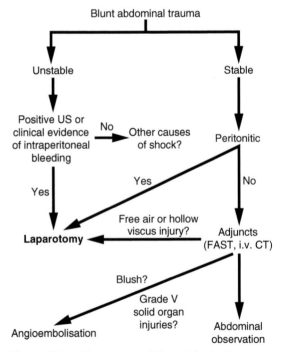

Figure 19.1 • Management of blunt abdominal trauma.

preservation group, with splenectomy raising the infection risk 10 times. Other relevant risk factors for infections were hypotension on admission, an injury severity score (ISS) >16 and hollow viscus injury. The recommendation is therefore to preserve the spleen if possible.

Splenic preservation, however, is not always feasible. *Haemodynamic instability* and a severely blunt-injured spleen remain a clear indication to proceed with laparotomy and probably splenectomy. In a large retrospective case series of the most severe splenic injuries (AAST grade IV and V), 58% of all patients were initially managed non-operatively.[45] NOM failed in 38%, mostly within 48-hours. Risk factors were *grade V splenic injuries*, *concomitant brain injury*, and *contrast extravasation on CT*. Either surgery should be undertaken in these patients, or angioembolisation if patients are stable but have contrast extravasation.[46]

✅✅ Grade V splenic injuries, especially in combination with a head injury, predict failure of non-operative management.[45]

Delayed haemorrhage, splenic artery pseudoaneurysm, splenic abscess or pseudocyst are complications after NOM. However, a 6-hourly serial physical examination and haemoglobin (Hb) estimation in a high-dependency ward (HDU) or intensive care unit (ICU) with bed-rest for 2–3 days seems to be safe to avoid and detect these complications. Deep venous prophylaxis can be started after 48 hours without a higher risk of bleeding in isolated blunt splenic injury.[47] Length of in-hospital observation remains unclear; however, 5–7 days, or even less in isolated minor splenic injuries with unproblematic observation seems acceptable.[48]

All patients after splenectomy should receive active pneumococcal and meningococcal vaccination within 2–3 weeks after the operation.[49]

Liver

Patient selection is crucial for NOM of blunt liver trauma. A recent large study at our institution analysed 134 patients with blunt liver injuries.[29] One in four patients required urgent surgery due to haemodynamic instability (31%), peritonitis (46%), or CT findings mandating surgery other than the liver injury (23%). Haemodynamic instability at admission was present in more patients. However, hypotension on arrival was successfully treated in 70% with a fluid bolus of no more than 1 to 2 litres of crystalloid transfusion. These patients did not need surgery for the liver injury. The remaining patients were non-responders and required surgery. Operative management comprising evacuation of haematoma and drainage only was needed

in 37% of patients. Liver-related complications were encountered in 20% after surgery: necrosis, haemobilia and biliary fistula. NOM was initiated in three-quarters of patients, consisting of serial clinical examinations and Hb estimations in a HDU or ICU, with no routine follow-up CTs. NOM was successful in 95%. Increasing abdominal pain and tenderness, spiking temperature, drop in blood pressure or a fall in Hb level were typical indicators of NOM failure. Liver-related complications were encountered in 7%: bilioma, biliary peritonitis, liver haematoma and abdominal compartment syndrome. Conclusion: NOM is safe, feasible, and successful in selected patients. Patients for NOM must be *stable*, *not peritonitic* and *amenable for clinical evaluation*.

Similar results were presented by Van der Wilden et al., who analysed 393 patients with AAST grade IV and V blunt liver injuries. One-third of the patients had to be operated on because of haemodynamic instability. NOM was started in two-thirds of patients and was successful in 91%. Failure of NOM was due to recurrent liver bleeding or biliary peritonitis. We concluded that even higher-grade liver injuries with haemoperitoneum and contrast extravasation can safely be treated non-operatively, which contrasts with higher-grade splenic injuries.[50] Important to note, nearly 70% of all NOM patients had a diffuse haemoperitoneum, 27% a contrast extravasation on CT and one-quarter of all patients in their NOM group had angioembolisation of the liver.

✅✅ Most blunt liver injuries can be managed non-operatively in the stable patient.[50]

Kidneys

Low-grade blunt kidney injuries, e.g. kidney contusions, are successfully treated non-operatively. The evidence for higher-grade injuries is unclear. Haemodynamic instability and/or urine extravasation are indications to proceed with surgery, which generally means nephrectomy. A study that analysed 206 patients with AAST grade IV and V blunt kidney injuries demonstrated that one in four patients needed an urgent laparotomy due to haemodynamic instability. Nearly 60% of these patients underwent a nephrectomy. In three-quarters of patients, NOM was started and successfully accomplished in 92%. Angioembolisation was undertaken in every sixth patient. Haemodynamic instability, peritonitis, or abdominal compartment syndrome were the reasons for NOM failure. The authors concluded that even higher-grade blunt kidney injuries with urine extravasation in haemodynamic stable patients can safely be treated non-operatively.[51]

Abdominal stab and low-velocity gunshot wounds

Penetrating wounds between the nipple line and the knees can potentially cause intra-abdominal injuries. The difficult questions to answer are: if (1) the peritoneum has been penetrated; and (2) an intra-abdominal injury requiring surgery has occurred. Penetrating wounds with solid organ injuries can still be managed non-operatively in many selected cases.[52]

Stab wounds

Stab wounds do not penetrate the peritoneum in one-third of patients, particularly after being stabbed to the flank or the back, due to the thick muscle layers. If penetration of the peritoneum has occurred, only 50–75% of patients have an injury requiring surgery.[53] Intra-abdominal stab wounds most commonly injure the liver (40%), small bowel (30%), diaphragm (20%) and colon (15%).[8] A study of 186 patients with abdominal stab wounds[54] found that 40% of the patients had a laparotomy. Indications to proceed with surgery were haemodynamic instability, peritonitis, organ evisceration, or a high spinal cord injury in addition to the abdominal stab wound. In 5%, the laparotomy was deemed negative or non-therapeutic and overall mortality rate was only 1%. Sixty per cent of patients were treated non-operatively, which was successful in 90% of cases. The remaining 10% developed positive abdominal signs and underwent laparotomy. In 33% of these patients, the laparotomy was unnecessary. The authors concluded that *unstable* patients, patients with an *acute abdomen* or *organ evisceration* need urgent surgery. Asymptomatic and haemodynamically stable patients can, however, selectively and safely be treated with 4-hourly serial physical abdominal examination, recording of vital signs (blood pressure, heart rate, respiratory rate and temperature) and Hb estimation over a 24-hour period. CT of the abdomen was only recommended in patients with haematuria, since the main indications for operation are reliably detected by serial clinical examination and the tract of the stab wound is hard to visualise on a CT scan.[55]

✅✅ Selective non-operative management for abdominal stab injuries in stable patients is safe and effective.[30,54]

Organ evisceration mandated provisional closure of any apparent perforations and extension of the stab wound under local anaesthesia to reduce entrapped and congested bowel to avoid strangulation in the emergency room. In mildly symptomatic, haemodynamically stable patients, *omentum eviscerating* through the wound was successfully ligated, resected, pushed back into the abdomen, and the fascia closed in the emergency room without laparotomy, as confirmed in another study.[56] *Haematuria* in unstable, peritonitic, or patients with organ evisceration was an indication for a single-shot intravenous pyelogram (IVP) with an iodinated contrast medium (e.g. 100 mL of Ultravist 300 [Bayer, Germany]) to demonstrate both kidneys are functioning in case a nephrectomy is required. In the NOM group, haematuria was further investigated with an abdominal CT scan with intravenous contrast to assess the severity of the kidney injury. Only AAST grade V kidney injuries (completely shattered kidney or avulsion of renal hilum that devascularises the kidney) were an indication for surgery.[54]

Penetrating *retroperitoneal injuries* of the colon, duodenum, or urinary tract are difficult to detect clinically. However, according to a large prospective study stab wounds to the flank or back should be managed the same way as anterior stab wounds.[57] Because of these clinical difficulties, some trauma surgeons ask for a triple-contrast CT to rule out retroperitoneal injures in stable asymptomatic patients with penetrating back or flank trauma. CT findings mandating a laparotomy are:[53]

- Contrast extravasation from colon
- Major urine extravasation from kidney
- Haematoma adjacent to major retroperitoneal vessel
- Free air in retroperitoneum, not attributed to wounding object
- Evidence of injury above and below diaphragm
- Free fluid in peritoneal cavity.

Figure 19.2 presents an algorithm for management of abdominal stab wounds.

Gunshot wounds (GSW)

GSWs transmit a higher energy and are more destructive than stab injuries. If the peritoneum is breached, the likelihood of having an intra-abdominal injury is nearly 100%. Small bowel (50%), colon (40%), liver (30%) and abdominal vessels (25%) are most commonly injured.[8] Some algorithms require prompt laparotomy for abdominal gunshot wounds regardless of the clinical situation. This approach, however, results in 5–30% of unnecessary laparotomies, especially in GSW to the flank or the back, with complication rates up to 40%. On the other hand, the major concern of NOM is missing a hollow viscus injury. The decision to proceed with NOM is critical.

A large prospective study of 1106 patients with an abdominal GSW from our hospital[30] showed that three out of four patients needed an urgent laparotomy. *Peritonitis, haemodynamic instability* or

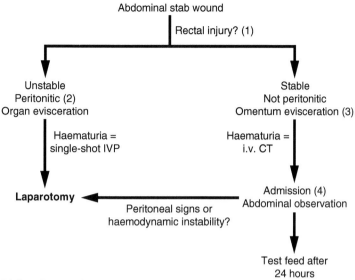

Abdominal stab wound

Rectal injury? (1)

Unstable
Peritonitic (2)
Organ evisceration

Stable
Not peritonitic
Omentum evisceration (3)

Haematuria =
single-shot IVP

Haematuria =
i.v. CT

Laparotomy ◄————— Admission (4)
Peritoneal signs or   Abdominal observation
haemodynamic instability?

Test feed after
24 hours

(1) See 'Rectal injury algorithm'

(2) Low threshold to proceed with laparotomy in patients with a high spinal
cord injury or severe head injury in addition to the abdominal stab wound,
or intoxicated patients

(3) Diagnostic laparoscopy in left thoraco-abdominal omental evisceration
or persistent left upper quadrant tenderness – after 24 hours' observation

(4) No local wound exploration or diagnostic peritoneal lavage recommended

Figure 19.2 • Management of abdominal stab wounds.

ongoing blood loss (more than 4 units of packed red blood cells within 24 hours) were clear indications to proceed with an operation. Only 3.5% were unnecessary laparotomies and the mortality was nearly 7%. On the other hand, one in four patients were treated non-operatively, with a success rate of 95% and no death related to the GSW. The indication for NOM was a haemodynamically normal patient without signs of peritonitis and an intact level of consciousness. Most patients with NOM had a CT and to continue with NOM the CT must show no active extravasation, the tract of the bullet must be away from the stomach, duodenum, small and large bowel. NOM consisted of 4-hourly serial physical abdominal examinations, recording of vital signs (blood pressure, heart rate, respiratory rate and temperature) and Hb estimation over a 24-hour period in a HDU with continuous haemodynamic monitoring. We concluded that NOM is safe and feasible in selected patients with abdominal GSW and serial clinical examination and selective use of CT scanning is essential. Unstable patients and patients with peritonitis remain clear indications for operative management. Furthermore patients with disabilities (severe head injury or acute spinal cord injuries) or intoxicated patients must undergo an urgent operation due to the unreliable physical examinations.

Figure 19.3 presents an algorithm for management of abdominal gunshot wounds.

Small bowel, colon and rectum

Such injuries can usually be primarily repaired if less than 50% of the bowel wall is involved. If more than 50% of the bowel wall is involved or devascularisation of the bowel segment has occurred, resection and primary anastomosis is still possible in haemodynamic stable patients, with an ISS <25, without peritonitis and no significant underlying diseases.[58]

Rectal surgery is technically more demanding and repair not always feasible. Penetrating rectum injuries have a still higher morbidity and mortality and therefore need special considerations. Debridement, distal wash-out, diverting colostomy and presacral drainage were the mainstays of rectal injuries in the past. This has, however, changed to a simpler approach as reported in an analysis of 118 rectal injuries from our institution.[59] Digital rectal and proctosigmoidoscopic examinations were standard assessments in patients with a missile trajectory near the pelvis and a possible rectal injury. The examinations were positive in 73%, and respectively 89% for intraluminal blood. The goal of these examinations was not to visualise the injury but to verify intraluminal blood. All intraperitoneal rectal

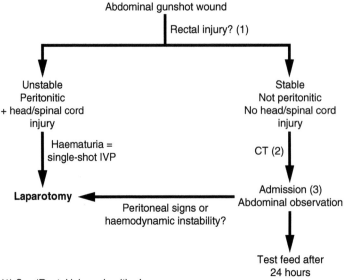

Abdominal gunshot wound

Rectal injury? (1)

Unstable
Peritonitic
+ head/spinal cord
injury

Haematuria =
single-shot IVP

Laparotomy

Peritoneal signs or
haemodynamic instability?

Stable
Not peritonitic
No head/spinal cord
injury

CT (2)

Admission (3)
Abdominal observation

Test feed after
24 hours

(1) See 'Rectal injury algorithm'

(2) Absolute CT indications: trajectory concerns; right upper quadrant/right-sided
thoraco-abdominal trajectory; transpelvic trajectory (inclusive CT-cystogram);
haematuria (if vascular pedicle, renal pelvis or ureteral injuries are present
proceed with laparotomy)

(3) Failure usually implicates a repeat CT-scan +/- percutaneous intervention
in solid organ injuries

Figure 19.3 • Management of abdominal gunshot wounds.

injuries were successfully primarily repaired with or without diversion. Extraperitoneal injuries remained untouched and only a sigmoid loop colostomy protected the rectum for 3 months. All patients received triple antibiotic treatment for 24 hours (penicillin, gentamicin and metronidazole) or until they were afebrile for a period of 24 hours. One-third of patients also had a concomitant penetrating bladder injury. Due to the high risk of rectovesical fistula, all intra- as well as extraperitoneal bladder injuries were repaired in this series, with any extraperitoneal rectal injury unrepaired. Only one rectovesical fistula developed, but healed spontaneously with prolonged urinary catheterisation. Rectal injuries with a purely extraperitoneal trajectory were verified with diagnostic laparoscopy (no peritoneal violation and no intraperitoneal blood) and a loop colostomy was performed.[42,60]

Figure 19.4 presents an algorithm for management of rectal injury.

Kidneys

Haematuria in penetrating abdominal trauma is associated with a renal injury in 80% and requires further investigations,[61] with a single-shot IVP being mandatory in unstable patients to demonstrate both kidneys are functioning. In stable patients, an abdominal CT with intravenous contrast is required to assess the severity grade of the kidney injury. We analysed 95 patients with a kidney GSW,[24] and the following indicators were used to proceed with operative management:

• Haemodynamic instability due to the kidney trauma

• Vascular pedicle, renal pelvis or ureteral injuries (AAST grade V kidney injuries)

• Renal exploration for all suspected kidney injuries without complete preoperative imaging.

Sixty-five per cent of these 95 patients underwent urgent laparotomy. Operative management consisted of nephrectomy in 66% due to hilar injuries or severe irreparable parenchymal disruption. NOM entailed serial physical examination for 48 hours and bed-rest until macroscopic haematuria had resolved. Haematuria for more than 72 hours mandated renal angiography to diagnose and treat false aneurysms or arteriovenous fistulas.[61] The success rate of NOM was 91%, with the remainder (9%, three patients) undergoing laparotomy, in two cases without exploration of the kidneys. There were no kidney-related complications. Ideal candidates for NOM were stable patients amenable to reliable clinical examination with a right-sided thoraco-abdominal or extraperitoneal GSW.

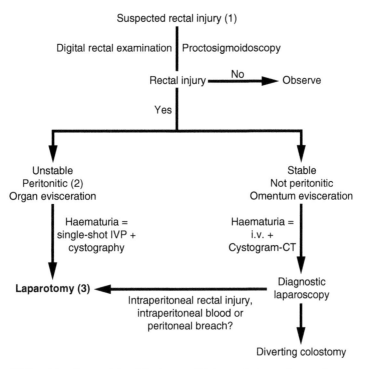

Suspected rectal injury (1)

Digital rectal examination | Proctosigmoidoscopy

Rectal injury —— No ——▶ Observe

Yes

Unstable
Peritonitic (2)
Organ evisceration

Haematuria =
single-shot IVP +
cystography

Laparotomy (3) ◀——

Stable
Not peritonitic
Omentum evisceration

Haematuria =
i.v. +
Cystogram-CT

Diagnostic
laparoscopy

Intraperitoneal rectal injury,
intraperitoneal blood or
peritoneal breach?

Diverting colostomy

(1) Suspicion: transpelvic, gluteal, upper thigh gunshot or stab wound;
   blood per rectum

(2) Low threshold to proceed with laparotomy in patients with a high spinal
   cord injury or severe head injury in addition to the penetrating trauma

(3) • *Intraperitoneal rectal injury:* repair
   • *Extraperitoneal rectal injury:* no touch, but diverting colostomy
   • Intra- or extraperitoneal *bladder injury in combination*
   with a rectal injury: *bladder* repair and prolonged catheter drainage

Figure 19.4 • Management of rectal injury.

Some authors have suggested that there is a higher nephrectomy rate after routine surgical exploration; however, no higher risk of nephrectomy despite routine exploration was found in a previous prospective study.[62]

Duodenum and pancreas

The location and proximity of these organs to other vital structures make injuries complex, difficult to detect and challenging to treat. In addition, they nearly always have concomitant intra-abdominal injuries. Simple surgical management algorithms should be applied to such complex injuries. In a retrospective review of 75 patients with a GSW to the duodenum, the authors showed that most duodenal injuries can be primarily repaired if less than half of the circumference is involved. The injured area may need to be debrided or even resected with a primary end-to-end anastomosis performed. In such circumstances a feeding jejunostomy (14G Foley catheter used in Witzel-type technique) is useful to support enteral nutrition if more than half of the circumference is involved.[63] All repairs were drained with a Penrose-type drain and no pyloric exclusion procedures were required. Pancreatico-duodenectomy was only performed for a devascularised duodenum or head of pancreas, ampullary injury, and/or distal bile duct injuries. In another large review of 219 patients with a GSW to the pancreas from our Trauma Centre, treatment was kept as simple as possible.[64] All patients had a laparotomy, 77% had minor pancreatic injuries without major ductal injury and treatment consisted of control of haemostasis and drainage of the pancreas; 27% had a major ductal injury left of the superior mesenteric vein and underwent distal pancreatectomy; and only 5% had a pancreatico-duodenectomy. On average, there was one emergency pancreatico-duodenectomy per year, usually after a damage control procedure.[65] There is no need for complex enteric diversions or pancreatico-enteric anastomoses. The overall complication and mortality rates were high (up to 69%), especially in patients with higher-grade pancreatic and additional vascular injuries. Haemorrhagic shock and blood loss were the main factors predicting mortality, and they were mostly unrelated to the pancreatic injury.[66] Nearly 18% developed a pancreatic fistula, which resolved with NOM (65%) or with endoscopic sphincterotomy and pancreatic stenting (33%).

Abdominal vena cava

Occasionally the general surgeon may encounter an inferior vena cava injury. Its prevalence is reported as 2.3% of all trauma laparotomies, nearly always after a GSW.[67] Mortality is high (31%) and no complex venous reconstructions were performed in this study. The authors recommend the following procedure: Right-sided medial visceral rotation; temporary control by digital compression of the vena cava against the spine; a Foley catheter may be inserted into the lumen and inflated.

Assessment of the injury:

- if simple and accessible, repair should be performed;
- if difficult, the vena cava can be ligated in infrarenal injuries.

Complications

In general, trauma patients have a considerable risk for ongoing bleeding or rebleeding, disseminated intravascular coagulopathy, deep venous thrombosis, pulmonary embolism, atelectasis, pneumonia, pleural effusion, urinary tract or wound infection and sepsis. The best and cheapest way to avoid many of these complications is mobilisation. In abdominal trauma, intra-abdominal collections, anastomotic leak, enterocutaneus fistula, bowel obstruction, incisional hernia and abdominal compartment syndrome are feared complications. There are also some organ-specific complications and treatment modalities:[24,30,31,54,68]

Liver

- Abscess
- Bilioma
- Bile ascites/haemoperitoneum
- Bleeding
- Haemobilia
- Necrosis

Kidney

- Increased perinephric haematoma
- Persistent haematuria due to a false aneurysm or arteriovenous fistula
- Persistent urinary leak
- Infected perinephric fluid collection

Pancreas

- Bleeding
- Peripancreatic fluid collections (pseudocysts and abscesses)
- Pancreatic fistula

Typical warning signs for complications are:

- Airway/Breathing: Increased respiratory rate, low oxygen saturation
- Circulation: Drop in blood pressure or significant fall in haemoglobin level ($>3\,g/dL$)
- Disability: Diminished consciousness, increasing abdominal pain
- Environment: Fever, elevated white blood cell counts, jaundice

These signs warrant a thorough clinical examination and potentially a repeat CT-scan.

Fortunately, most complications can be successfully treated non-operatively or with interventional procedures:

- CT- or ultrasound-guided percutaneous drainage of biliary or purulent collections
- Angioembolisation in case of bleeding, haemobilia, haematuria, false aneurysm, or an arteriovenous fistula
- Endoscopic sphincterotomy and stenting in case of biliary leaks
- Endoscopic placement of double J ureteric stents in case of urinary leak.

In a large review of 412 patients with liver injuries, 12% developed a biliary fistula with the risk factors being operative management, higher-grade liver injuries and liver packing.[69] A minor biliary leak (less than 400 mL/day) was present in 65% of this group and successfully treated without surgery. All drains were removed within 2 weeks. A major leak (more than 400 mL/day) was apparent in 35% of patients and successfully treated with endoscopic sphincterotomy and stenting, with the stent removed after 6 weeks. Major biliary collections should be drained either percutaneously under ultrasound guidance or laparoscopically.

Pelvic fractures

The severity of pelvic fracture ranges from insignificant to major and frequently fatal. With increasing trauma force the likelihood of having an unstable pelvic fracture, i.e. open book or vertical shear fracture, is increased. In addition, an unstable pelvic fracture is often associated with intra-abdominal (16.5%), chest (i.e. aortic rupture in 1.4%), and diaphragmatic injuries (2.1%).[70] Intra- and/or extra-pelvic bleeding sources can cause haemodynamic instability, with typical extra-pelvic bleeding causes being solid organ injuries. Intra-pelvic sources are either the fractured bone itself, venous plexus, or arterial vessels, but an arterial source is only present in around 10% of pelvic fractures. Unstable patients with a severe pelvic fracture must be assessed clinically, with a chest and pelvic X-ray and with ultrasound (FAST) in blunt trauma. If FAST is positive, patients need urgent laparotomy, some sort of pelvic stabilisation (most easily with a pelvic binder) to tamponade the pelvic haematoma, and extraperitoneal pelvic packing if bleeding persists after any intra-abdominal bleeding has been controlled.[71] Packing will most likely not stop arterial bleeding and in such patients with persistent haemodynamic instability, postoperative angiography with embolisation of arterial bleeding points must be carried out. Stable patients are usually assessed with a contrast CT to identify an active bleeding site. In case of such a blush, angioembolisation can be performed and the patients observed.

A step-by-step guide to trauma laparotomy

In a trauma laparotomy, some steps are mandatory and some procedures depend on the injuries:

- Inform the anaesthetist and the scrub nurse.
- Prepare the theatre: warm theatre and fluids.
- Prepare the patient: supine, low lithotomy position if an extraperitoneal rectal injury is suspected or in the case of a transpelvic gunshot wound with bleeding as this will allow access into the pelvis if required.
- Give preoperative broad-spectrum antibiotics to cover gut bacteria.
- Drape from nipple to the pubic symphysis
  - from chin to groin if sternotomy/thoracotomy/ saphenous vein graft harvesting needed.
- Preoperative WHO checklist.
- Full midline incision.
- **First step** = control the bleeding, evaluate the use of intraoperative blood salvage devices.
  - Remove blood with dry packs and pack all quadrants of the abdomen, try to restore the anatomy of the solid organs with packs.
  - Remove packs systematically.
  - Source of major bleeding: spleen, small bowel mesentery, liver, retroperitoneum:
    - Spleen: mobilise and bring the spleen into the operation field, open the lesser sac and occlude manually the splenic artery, decide on splenectomy.

- Small-bowel mesentery: apply digital pressure, clamping and suturing.
- Liver:
  - Manual compression and packing (ideally six packs), restore the anatomy; most injuries will have stopped bleeding. Do not pack into the liver wound.
  - Get better access to the liver by mobilisation of the liver by taking down the ligamentous attachments.
  - Minor lacerations: use diathermy, argon beam coagulation, fibrin glue.
  - Moderate lacerations: apply Pringle manoeuvre for 20 minutes and suture selectively bleeding vessels and large bile leaks. Remember that packing will not stop arterial bleeding and this needs to be controlled with a polypropylene figure-of-eight suture.
  - Major lacerations: rarely resection or total hepatic vascular isolation is needed, better perform damage control surgery (pack and temporary close the abdomen, transfer to ICU).
  - Drain all liver injuries.
- Retroperitoneal haematoma: central and/or expanding haematomas must be explored, consider inflow control by aortic cross-clamping; supra-colic haematoma = medial visceral rotation from the left/infra-colic haematoma = medial visceral rotation from the right.
- Pelvic haematoma: if haemodynamically stable and not expanding = only external control of the pelvic fracture; If haemodynamic instability or expanding haematoma in penetrating wounds or in open book or vertical shear fractures = extraperitoneal packing. This will not stop arterial bleeding; rather pack and proceed with angioembolisation if haemodynamic status does not improve.
- Stomach: can bleed considerably – close the injury with a running all-layers suture.
- **Second step** = control the contamination.
  - Systemic approach: inspect all hollow viscera; a single-layer interrupted suture with 3/0 polypropylene (Prolene®) is a good repair technique.
  - Duodenum: Kocher's manoeuvre if a duodenal injury is suspected, duodenal repair, drainage.

- Pancreas: haemostasis and drainage is adequate most of the time.
- Small bowel: debride wound edges, suture any bowel perforations, resection and anastomosis in destructive injuries (>50% of the bowel wall).
- Colon: mobilisation along the white line of Toldt, primary repair or resection and anastomosis (>50% of the bowel wall).
- Rectum: sigmoidoscopy to look for fresh blood as an indicator for a rectal injury; if intraperitoneal = primary repair; if extraperitoneal = diverting colostomy and no direct repair.
- Inspect the peritoneum.
  - Diaphragm: all injuries should be repaired. If there is a stomach or bowel injury then the defect in the diaphragm should be opened and the pleural cavity washed out with 4–5 litres of irrigation so as to prevent the development of an empyema. Repair with a 1 non-absorbable, monofilament, continuous, full-thickness suture.
  - Bladder: intraperitoneal bladder rupture must be repaired in a double-layer technique.
  - Closure of penetrating peritoneal wounds.
- Irrigation of the abdomen with warmed isotonic saline.
- No drains routinely.[72]
- Abdominal closure with a continuous 0 nylon or selective temporary abdominal closure for 48 hours if:[20,73]
  - in shock
  - under tension due to visceral oedema or tissue loss
  - abdominal compartment
  - abdominal packing
  - need for second look.

Blunt and penetrating chest injuries

General surgeons often encounter patients with chest trauma and it is therefore worthwhile understanding some of the main injuries and their immediate management. Serial clinical examination and selective non-operative management is the mainstay in chest trauma.[74] Most of these conditions can easily be managed with simple procedures such as intubation and ventilation, needle decompression, intercostal drainage and volume restoration. Surgical repair is seldom needed.

The first goal is to detect and immediately treat life-threatening injuries in the primary survey:[8]

- Tension pneumothorax
- Open pneumothorax
- Massive haemothorax
- Cardiac tamponade
- Flail chest and pulmonary contusion

Potentially life-threatening injuries must be identified in the secondary survey:[8]

- Simple pneumothorax
- Haemothorax
- Pulmonary contusion
- Tracheobronchial tree injury
- Cardiac injury
- Traumatic aortic disruption
- Oesophageal rupture
- Traumatic diaphragmatic injury

Rib fractures, pneumothorax, haemothorax and pulmonary contusions

Rib fracture

Rib fracture is a clinical diagnosis. It can be diagnosed on chest X-ray; however, the main goal of the chest X-ray is to look for relevant concomitant injuries, such as a haemothorax or pneumothorax. Rib fractures may be associated with potentially life-threatening injuries and fractures of the 1st to 3rd ribs are sometimes a marker for major vascular injuries – as seen in blunt aortic injuries, or an indicator of a liver or splenic injury in lower rib fractures. In elderly patients and in patients with multiple injuries, rib fractures are related to a higher risk of morbidity, particularly pneumonia, and mortality.[75] The main treatment consists of adequate *analgesia* (including morphine) to enable the patient to cough. Intercostal nerve blocks or thoracic epidurals are very effective ways to ameliorate the pain level in selected patients. All patients should get chest physiotherapy and supplemental oxygen if needed. In some circumstances, particularly flail chest (three and more ribs are fractured in two places causing a mobile thoracic wall segment) or severely displaced rib fractures, osteosynthesis of ribs can significantly improve thoracic cage stability and hasten recovery.[76]

Pneumothorax and haemothorax

These are both frequently seen after blunt or penetrating trauma. Definitive treatment of pneumo- or haemothoraces usually consists of chest tube insertion and subsequently a chest X-ray to document chest drain position, lung expansion and persistent opacities. In haemodynamic instability, need for positive-pressure ventilation, in tension or open pneumothorax, obvious haemothorax, or flail chest, the indication to insert a chest drain is clear and urgent. In one study of 635 patients with a haemothorax,[77] two-thirds of the haemothoraces were drained and one-third were treated conservatively. The study went on to say that an *ipsilateral flail chest, pneumothorax* and the *size of the haemothorax* were independent predictors for chest tube insertion. A *massive haemothorax* (>1500 mL of bloody pleural effusion or >200 mL per hour for the next 4 hours) is an indication for a thoracotomy. Different chest tube sizes have been compared in patients with traumatic haemothoraces and it would appear that size does not change the efficacy of drainage and does not affect the rate of complications: 28–32 French chest tubes are therefore probably sufficient.[78]

Some pneumo- or haemothoraces, however, can safely be treated without drainage with a shorter length of stay, fewer infectious complications and no increase in mortality.[77] An *asymptomatic pneumothorax* less than 1.5–2 cm in size, measured on a chest X-ray, can be treated without chest tube.[79] An *occult pneumothorax*, found on CT but not visible on a supine chest X-ray, needs careful monitoring but no chest tube insertion, except for patients requiring positive-pressure ventilation, in respiratory distress, proved progression of the pneumothorax, or development of a haemothorax.[80] *Asymptomatic or also retained haemothoraces* with less than *300 mL* or 1.5 cm on a CT scan and no other indication for tube insertion can safely be managed with observation.[81] In the case of conservative treatment a radiological follow-up is recommended after 6–12 hours.

Pulmonary contusions

Pulmonary contusions represent bleeding into lung parenchyma and result in abnormal gas exchange in the affected segment and an arterial blood–gas analysis should be carried out to evaluate the pulmonary dysfunction. The chest X-ray changes are often delayed and initially underestimated, whereas CT of the chest can clearly visualise the affected segments and predict the need for mechanical ventilation.[82] Treatment usually consists of analgesia, chest physiotherapy and supplemental oxygen. Not surprisingly, pulmonary contusions are risk factors for pneumonia and acute respiratory distress syndrome.

Intrathoracic complications

Persistent opacities mandate a chest CT to differentiate atelectasis, consolidation, pulmonary contusion, retained haemothorax, other pleural effusions and their exact location. Empyema (4.4%), pneumonia (4.7%) and retained haemothorax (11.3%) are typical complications in patients with drained haemo- or pneumothorax.[78]

The incidence of *empyema* among patients with a retained haemothorax was 27% in a prospective, multicentre study in the USA.[83] Risk factors were ISS >24, the presence of rib fractures and the number of interventions to evacuate the retained blood. Chest tube insertion significantly increased the length of stay and the risk of empyema.[77] Presumptive antibiotics do not appear to decrease the incidence of empyema, but once present the treatment consists of antibiotics and (CT-guided) drainage. An empyema not responding to non-operative treatment may be approached using video-assisted thoracoscopic surgery with a conversion to a thoracotomy if required.

Pneumonia significantly increases length of stay and mortality. Blunt trauma and ISS >24, but not a retained haemothorax, were significant predictors for pneumonia. Use of periprocedural antibiotics on chest tube insertion does significantly decrease the pneumonia rate.[84]

Fibrothorax and empyema are feared complications after a *retained haemothorax*. Small (<300 mL) retained haemothoraces eventually resolve over time. Some liquefied retained haemothoraces can safely be treated with a second chest tube. However, some retained haemothoraces are clotted and loculated and need more aggressive treatment. Some surgeons advocate the use of local thrombolysis via the chest drain. Video-assisted thoracoscopic surgery is a safe method to successfully treat a retained haemothorax in up to 80%.[85] The earlier the treatment the better is the outcome, with less mortality and less need to convert to a thoracotomy.

Cardiac injuries

Up to 90% of all penetrating heart injuries are already fatal in the prehospital phase. The remainder are those patients arriving alive in the hospital. They may present as:

- lifeless, with signs of life present in the last 5–10 minutes – these patients need an emergency department thoracotomy to relieve a tension haemo- or pneumopericardium, stop any exsanguinating haemorrhage, repair of the cardiac injury and massage the heart;
- in persistent haemorrhagic shock despite resuscitation – these patients need urgent exploration either via sternotomy or thoracotomy, depending on the clinical situation, in the operating theatre;
- symptomatic with cardiac tamponade, three-quarters of them showing the Beck's triad (hypotension, muffled heart sounds and elevated jugular venous pressure) – these patients need a sternotomy in the operating theatre;

- or stable and relatively asymptomatic – there is a high likelihood of a cardiac injury with stab or gunshot wound in penetrating chest trauma or trajectories crossing the heart area – and it must aggressively be ruled out.[86]

While the first three situations are clear clinical situations and clear indications to proceed with surgery, the last situation poses some difficulties for the trauma surgeon. The clinical examination reveals little except for the penetrating skin wound. A penetrating wound in the 'cardiac zone' (**Fig. 19.5**) as well as gunshot wounds to the neck, chest, abdomen and back, depict a high risk of a cardiac injury.[87] A history of prehospital hypotension alerts the general surgeon. A pericardial rub or a cardiac murmur (i.e. traumatic septal defects or valve injuries) can be a guide. Cardiac ultrasound, chest X-ray, ECG and central venous pressure of greater than 15 cm H_2O can also help in diagnosing cardiac injuries.

Ultrasound identifies a haemopericardium; however, the sensitivity is 87% and limited by the presence of a pneumopericardium or a haemothorax.[87] Ultrasound can be falsely negative if the haemopericardium is draining into the pleural cavity (presenting as a haemothorax) through the penetration in the pericardial sac. These false-negative results can have a catastrophic outcome and must be avoided. False-positive results are encountered in patients and may be related to differing amounts of pericardial fluid in normal individuals and a haemothorax. Pericardiocentesis has no role in the diagnosis of penetrating cardiac injuries and is more likely to cause an injury to the heart.

Chest X-ray can raise the suspicion of an occult heart injury. A pneumopericardium or an enlarged heart shadow are possible signs. Up to 10% of patients with a pneumopericardium become unstable and need urgent decompression. Since the pericardium is poorly distensible, a little amount of blood in the pericardium can cause straightening out of the sac at the pulmonary artery concavity. The straight left

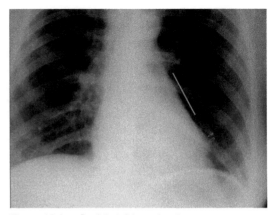

Figure 19.6 • Straight left heart border.

heart border was examined on erect chest X-ray in 162 patients with a cardiac injury[88] (**Fig. 19.6**). While there are some differential diagnoses (status post left lower lobectomy, mitral valve diseases, pectus excavatum), the sensitivity of this radiological sign correlating with an operatively confirmed haemopericardium was 40%, with a specificity of 84% and a positive predictive value of 89%. Hence, the straight left heart border sign was a useful sign in predicting the presence of a haemopericardium.

A J-wave, a small positive reflection on the R-ST junction on a standard ECG, can also be a sign of a possible cardiac injury (**Fig. 19.7**). An analysis of the ECGs of 174 patients with a cardiac injury,[89] demonstrated the sensitivity of the J-wave was 44%, the specificity 85% and the positive predictive value 91%. The authors concluded that a J-wave is a significant sign of an occult cardiac injury if present.

If a haemopericardium is diagnosed, the question remains whether a stable patient needs a sternotomy to treat the cardiac injury or has the cardiac wound already sealed? Many of these cardiac injuries were already found to have sealed or needed no special intervention in view of partial-thickness or tangential wounds if a sternotomy is performed in stable patients

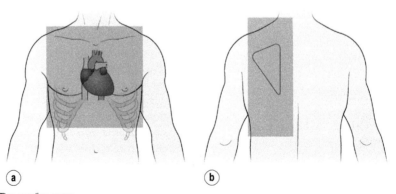

Figure 19.5 • The cardiac zone.

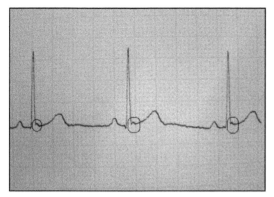

Figure 19.7 • J-wave.

with a haemopericardium.[86] A randomised controlled trial in 111 patients comparing sternotomy versus subxyphoidal window with drainage, determined a stable patient with a haemopericardium can be managed with a subxyphoid pericardial window. If there is no active bleeding the patient can then be

managed without a sternotomy, with lower morbidity and mortality.[90] In summary, stable patients with a haemo- or pneumopericardium need a subxyphoid pericardial window to rule out active bleeding, with a sternotomy only mandatory in the case of active bleeding.[91] Electrocardiogram and echographic follow-up is recommended.

> ✅✅ Subxyphoidal window and drainage is effective and safe in stable patients with a haemopericardium after penetrating trauma. No sternotomy is mandatory.[90]

Figure 19.8 summarises management of penetrating cardiac injury.

Aortic injuries

Aortic injuries rather cause death than haemodynamic instability. Typical trauma mechanisms are fall from a height or excessive deceleration causing a rupture usually just distal to the left subclavian artery at the isthmus. Penetrating aortic injuries

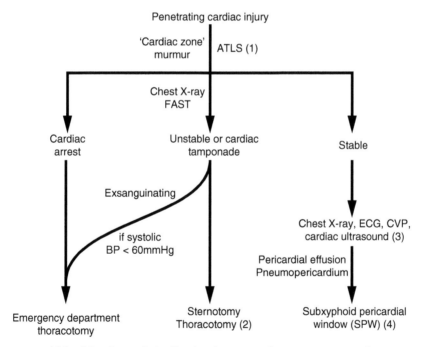

(1) Look for airway obstruction, tension pneumothorax, open pneumothorax, massive haemothorax, cardiac tamponade

(2) Penetrating wound medial to the midclavicular line mandates a sternotomy/lateral thoracotomy on the side of the penetrating wound

(3) A haemothorax or a high index of suspicion despite a negative ultrasound mandates a second ultrasound 24 hours later or a CT scan

(4) Blood (clots) in the pericardial sac is a positive SPW, active bleeding mandates a sternotomy

Figure 19.8 • Management of penetrating cardiac injury.

are usually fatal. A widened mediastinum (>8 cm) on a supine chest X-ray can be a sign of an aortic injury. However, the chest X-ray has a high false-positive and false-negative rate and further work-up is needed. Over a period of 10 years there was a major shift in the diagnosis of blunt aortic injuries. The American Association for the Surgery of Trauma compared the results of two observational studies from 1997 and 2007. They concluded that aorto- and echography are no longer regularly used, and contrast CT represents the current gold standard. Treatment also changed tremendously from open repair to endovascular procedures. Consequently mortality rate as well as procedure-related paraplegia decreased significantly to 13% and 1.6%, respectively. However, early graft-related complications significantly increased to 13.5%. Timing of repair remains controversial and there is a shift to delayed (>12–16 hours) repair – when it can be performed under better or even normalised pathophysiological conditions. This is the current standard in patients with major concomitant injuries if maintaining a low systolic blood pressure to prevent free rupture is possible.[92]

Oesophageal injuries

Oesophageal injuries, either in the neck or in the chest, are rare. The frequency is less than 10 patients per year even in large trauma centres. In a study of 52 patients with penetrating oesophageal injuries over an 8-year period,[93] unstable patients with massive bleeding or an expanding haematoma underwent surgery and had endoscopy during the operation to diagnose the oesophageal injury. Stable patients were further assessed. Subcutaneous emphysema and/or pre-vertebral air were each present in nearly 50% of patients and are the most frequent radiological findings in oesophageal injuries. These patients as well as symptomatic patients (dysphagia, odynophagia, haematemesis or blood in the nasogastric tube, leakage of saliva or gastrointestinal contents from the wound or the intercostal drain) require a water-soluble contrast swallow study to detect an oesophageal injury. Seventy-three per cent of oesophageal injuries can be primary-repaired and widely drained even if the delay to surgery is more than 12-hours. The authors found a delay to diagnose and treat an oesophageal injury as the most important risk factor for oesophageal-related complications. Therefore an expeditious assessment is of paramount importance. For patients presenting late in septic shock, a damage control approach is more suitable, with stapling of the injury with drainage and the later formation of an oesophagostomy, gastrostomy and feeding jejunostomy. At a later stage a total oesophagectomy will be required with a gastric pull-up.

Transmediastinal gunshot wounds

Transmediastinal gunshot wounds are associated with a high pre- and early in-hospital mortality due to cardiac and major vascular injuries. Of 133 such patients reported, 87% were unstable or had no vital signs at arrival and 11% arrived dead at the hospital.[94] The reported injuries were: 71% cardiac, 24% thoracic aorta, 35% liver, 29% splenic injuries. Seventy-three per cent of all patients in this study underwent emergency department thoracotomy – because of loss or imminent loss of vital signs – and only 8% of them were discharged alive. In comparison, all patients arriving stable in the emergency department were discharged home. Stable patients may yet have occult cardiovascular or aerodigestive tract injuries and therefore an intravenous contrast-enhanced CT of the chest in stable patients delineates the suspicious tract and predicts injuries. Mediastinal haematoma or air warrants further testing such as bronchoscopy, oesophagography or endoscopy in theatre in the intubated patient. CT has reduced the need for potentially harmful investigations.[95]

Emergency department thoracotomy

An emergency department thoracotomy (EDT) is rarely indicated, but can be life-saving. Accepted indications are *life-threatening pericardial tamponade* or *exsanguinating haemorrhage with profound shock* (systolic blood pressure <60–70 mmHg not responding to resuscitation) or already *hypovolaemic cardiac arrest after penetrating thoracic trauma*. The success rate depends on the trauma mechanism, the sustained injuries and the presence of signs of life. The survival rate is 1% in blunt trauma and 35% in penetrating cardiac injuries. The main goals of EDT are:[96]

- to release a pericardial tamponade, repair a penetrating cardiac wound, and open heart massage;
- to control major intrathoracic bleeding (either thoracic wall, lung, or great vessel injury);
- cross-clamping of the lung hilum in cases of massive exsanguination from the lung;
- cross-clamping of the descending aorta to improve blood flow to the brain and the heart and limit possible intra-abdominal haemorrhage.

EDT must therefore provide fast access to the pericardium, the pleura, the lung hilum, and the descending aorta. Standard access is via a left anterior thoracotomy.

The limits for EDT are:[97]

- prehospital CPR 10 min after blunt trauma without response;

- prehospital CPR 15 min after penetrating injury without response;
- asystole is the presenting rhythm, and there is no pericardial tamponade.

The Western Trauma Association multicentre group had no survivor after EDT in all these situations. The EDT can further be continued to a clamshell incision providing fast and excellent access to nearly all thoracic structures.[98]

Emergency department thoracotomy technique[99]

- Patient is intubated and ventilated in supine position.
- A thoracotomy set should be available in the emergency department.
- Morphine 10 mg and midazolam 10 mg i.v.
- Rapidly clean and drape the chest.
- Long incision from the edge of the costal cartilage to the left midaxillary line in the 5th intercostal space with the line of incision passing just below the nipple line.
  - Consider a right thoracotomy if the penetrating wound is on the right side.
- Incise the pleura and divide all layers towards the sternum using a Mayo scissors while avoiding injury to the lung and the internal mammary artery.
- Insert a rib spreader to its full extent.
- Evacuate any blood.
1. *Incise the inferior pulmonary ligament* if possible to mobilise the lung.
2. *Heart:* Apply an Allis clamp to the pericardial sac and make a long midline incision of the pericardium; avoid injuring the phrenic nerve running anterior to the hilum of the lung. Remove blood clots if applicable and inspect the heart. Unoxygenated blood is dark and indicates a right-sided heart injury. Apply digital pressure to the wound. Close the wound with an interrupted monofilament 2/0 polypropylene (Prolene®), if necessary with pledgets (Teflon®) (**Fig. 19.9**). A Foley catheter (ventricle) or a Satinsky clamp (atria) can be of some help. An injury near a coronary artery is best sutured with a mattress stitch to avoid narrowing of the coronary artery.

    Consider internal heart massage and defibrillation with an initial energy level of 10–50 joules in cardiac arrest

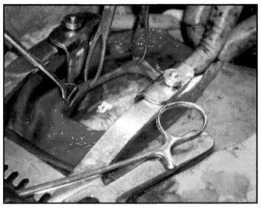

Figure 19.9 • Suture of a cardiac injury with pledgets.

3. *Major bleeding chest, lung or thoracic wall:* Inspect the chest wall (light red blood indicating intercostal artery injury), lung (air-mixed blood for lung and dark blood for hilar injuries) and mediastinum for active bleeding. Stop the bleeding with local compression, swab-on-a-stick, suture or hilar cross-clamping (from cranial).
4. In case of *air embolism* consider hilar cross-clamping.
5. In case of *extrathoracic haemorrhage* consider aortic cross-clamping a few centimetres above the diaphragm to improve blood flow to brain and heart and decrease haemorrhage into the abdomen or pelvis.
6. Consider division of the sternum and a contralateral thoracotomy (clamshell) to get better exposure.

- Temporary closure of the chest and transfer to the theatre for definitive repair and wash-out.

Retained knife blade

This is a very dramatic injury (**Fig. 19.10**). Resist removing the blade as it may be tamponading a major vessel. We reviewed our experience with this injury.[100] In 40% of the patients the entry site was the chest, in 21% each it was the neck and back, but rarely the abdomen. All patients were clinically and radiologically evaluated and all but one patient was haemodynamically stable. X-rays (AP and lateral) were helpful to define the tract and CT angiography was very useful to determine the proximity of the blade to vital structures. After excluding solid organ, hollow viscus or neurovascular injuries, the blade could be extracted in the operating room in nearly 60%. In 5% post-extraction bleeding needed to be addressed. Forty per cent of patients needed either wound exploration or an open operation

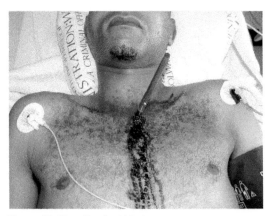

Figure 19.10 • Retained blade.

(thoracotomy, thoracoscopy or laparotomy) and extraction of the knife under direct vision after gaining proximal and distal control of major vessels. All operations were performed under general (94%) or local anaesthesia (6%) in the theatre. Postoperative sepsis was a significant complication after retained thoracic blades.

Thoraco-abdominal trauma

Thoraco-abdominal injuries may cause diagnostic and therapeutic problems and they are often associated with multiple injuries that require surgery. Depending on the trajectory, cardiac injuries are quite often seen in thoraco-abdominal injuries,[101] with diaphragmatic injuries present in up to 60%.[102] Furthermore there is a high rate of negative thoracotomies (22%) or laparotomies (11%) and inappropriate sequencing was found in 44% undergoing thoracotomy and laparotomy.[103]

Cardiac injuries with arrest, hypovolaemic shock, or cardiac tamponade, chest drain output (massive haemothorax: >1500 mL or >200 mL per hour), peritonitis, or haemodynamic instability due to an intra-abdominal haemorrhage are clear indications to proceed with surgery. Which injury is bleeding more and needs to be addressed first is not always clear: the chest drain output may be from an abdominal bleed through the diaphragmatic injury.[103] Ultrasound can be of some benefit, especially to search for a haemopericardium. However, as already mentioned, ultrasound of the heart can be false-negative with a haemothorax. The burden of both, a thoracotomy and laparotomy, is furthermore immense for the patient, and unnecessary surgery must be avoided as mortality is doubled in these patients.

In a cohort of patients with *thoraco-abdominal stab injuries*,[104] half of all patients (53%) needed only a laparotomy, the indications being either a hollow viscus perforation, a diaphragm injury or a bleeding solid organ injury. No surgery was needed in 40%. The remainder had a thoracotomy/ sternotomy, nearly always because of a cardiac injury. The authors in this study concluded that in an unstable patient with a thoraco-abdominal stab wound, a relevant cardiac injury must be ruled out first, followed by abdominal exploration. If clear signs of cardiac injuries are absent, the best approach is to start with a laparotomy and if there remains concern regarding a cardiac injury then a diagnostic transdiaphragmatic pericardial window can be made. If this window is positive (results in blood) then the chest should be opened in the acute phase.

Gunshot wounds producing *thoraco-abdominal gunshot injuries* are more complex and most of these patients (66%) need a laparotomy, with 14% requiring a laparotomy and thoracotomy/ sternotomy.[105] In this series 14% had no surgery. In total one-third needed a thoracotomy; however, most of these patients were in cardiac arrest or agonal and had an EDT with a very poor outcome. The authors summarised that patients either have clear signs of cardiac or major thoracic vascular injuries requiring EDT or have haemodynamic instability requiring a laparotomy. If patients have a clear indication to proceed with a laparotomy but no clear indication to proceed with a thoracotomy, these patients ideally have a transdiaphragmatic pericardial window first to rule out a cardiac injury if the trajectory is close to the heart. Some authors recommend a subxyphoidal approach instead. A subxyphoid pericardial window has a lower risk of pericardial contamination with gastrointestinal contents and can diminish the rate of negative sternotomies and mortality.[101]

Blunt thoraco-abdominal trauma is quite often seen, but rarely needs surgery of one or both cavities. Most of the chest trauma can be managed with supplemental oxygen, chest physiotherapy, analgesia and occasionally with an intercostal drain. Some of the intra-abdominal injuries will require a laparotomy.

In thoraco-abdominal injuries there is a general increased risk of pleural empyema due to the spillage of gastrointestinal contents through the diaphragmatic injury into the chest. One safe way to lower the risk of intrathoracic septic complications is to enlarge the diaphragmatic injury, to wash out and drain the thorax and consequently to close the injury[106] (**Fig. 19.11**).

Diaphragmatic injuries

Up to two-thirds of patients with a penetrating thoraco-abdominal trajectory have a diaphragmatic injury, which usually does not heal spontaneously.[102]

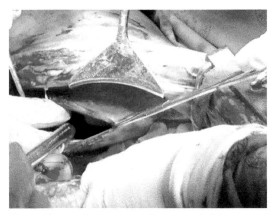

Figure 19.11 • Enlarging the diaphragmatic injury to wash out the chest.

Complications include herniation, incarceration and strangulation of bowel into the chest due to the intrathoracic negative pressure, with a high morbidity of 30% and a mortality of 10%.[107] Delayed or missed diagnosis must be avoided and left-sided diaphragmatic injuries particularly should be addressed as these have a much higher rate of subsequent hernia formation. Some patients present with a clear indication, other than the diaphragmatic injury, to proceed with a laparotomy, at which a thorough examination of the diaphragm must be carried out and an injury repaired. In stable and asymptomatic patients, the algorithm is more ambiguous. Clinical examination cannot clearly establish the diagnosis. Haemo- and/or pneumothorax are most often seen on a chest X-ray; however, one-third have a normal chest X-ray.[108] The overall CT accuracy and sensitivity is low. Although thoracoscopy or laparoscopy have a high accuracy; they are, however, invasive. In a report of 24 highly selected patients with possible diaphragmatic injuries,[108] the patients underwent diagnostic and therapeutic laparoscopy *after* 24–36 hours of uneventful clinical observation (hence no hollow viscus injury). Prevailing indications were:

- omentum herniation through the chest wall;
- persistent left upper quadrant tenderness following abdominal observation;
- free air under the diaphragm despite benign abdominal signs.

The idea of the asymptomatic patient with initially stable abdominal observations being observed is logical but performing laparoscopy on all patients with lower left thoraco-abdominal stab wounds. An early laparoscopy tends to be associated with a high conversion rate to a laparotomy.

Blunt diaphragmatic injuries are usually located on the left side and concomitant with major thoraco-abdominal or pelvic trauma. They are often missed,

since sensitivity of chest X-ray and CT is low. Acute diaphragmatic injuries are best approached via a laparotomy since most patients have relevant abdominal injuries. Chronic diaphragmatic injuries can be repaired via a laparotomy, laparoscopically or by thoracotomy depending on the expertise available.

Neck trauma

Penetrating neck injuries

Penetrating neck injuries are common in urban trauma centres, can be life-threatening and difficult to treat due to complex anatomy and concentration of vital structures.[109,110] As with penetrating abdominal trauma, there is a clear shift from categorical exploration to selective non-operative management. Nowadays, nearly 80% of all patients with penetrating neck injuries can be safely and successfully treated without surgery.[110] Only about 10% of patients with hard signs (explained below) need immediate surgery.[111]

Penetrating neck injuries are generally anatomically divided into anterior and posterior triangle injuries. The anterior triangle is further divided into three zones (**Fig. 19.12**), which helps to appraise possibly injured structures, and guide further diagnostic and therapeutic approaches.

Penetrating neck injuries can be life-threatening. An ABC-approach according to ATLS guidelines is recommended.[8,110]

> ✓✓ The algorithm for penetrating neck injuries is a very useful method of assessing and managing penetrating neck injuries.[110]

All penetrating neck injuries can cause airway compromise due to a local haematoma, secretions, direct laryngeal, or tracheal injuries, surgical emphysema, or decreased level of consciousness with a Glasgow Coma Scale of less than 9. Air bubbling through the wound is also a hard sign.[111] In all these cases, the airway must be secured either via intubation or cricothyroidotomy. Occasionally, a tracheal tube can be inserted via the open tracheal wound. A cervical (C-) spine injury must be assumed, the C-spine accordingly immobilised and a lateral C-spine X-ray ordered. A thoracic injury must be ruled out clinically and by means of a chest X-ray in every patient with a penetrating neck injury. Next, any fatal bleeding must be assessed and stopped. An unstable patient or a patient with a severely bleeding neck wound, an expanding, or a pulsatile neck haematoma (hard signs) must be treated immediately either with surgery or (easier) with a 20-FG Foley catheter balloon tamponade.[112] Balloon tamponade significantly reduces the need for immediate and

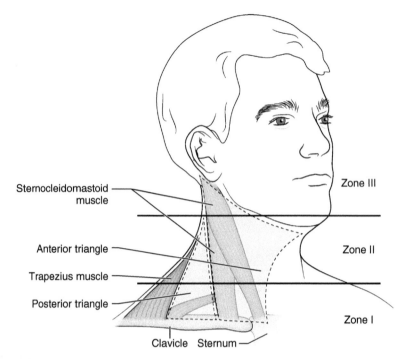

Sternocleidomastoid muscle

Anterior triangle

Trapezius muscle

Posterior triangle

Zone III

Zone II

Zone I

Clavicle   Sternum

Figure 19.12 • Neck zones.

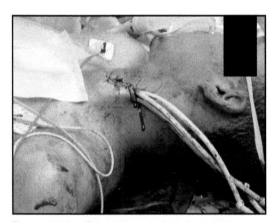

Figure 19.13 • Foley catheter balloon tamponade.

late operative exploration (**Fig. 19.13**). Stable patients must be thoroughly examined (i.e. hard and soft signs for neck injuries, including neurological signs), are admitted to a high-care trauma ward, and regularly, every 4 hours, observed with haemodynamic monitoring, airway and neck examination. Certain symptoms warrant further work-up in a timely fashion:[93,109,110]

- CT-angiography for possible *vascular injuries* in case of a moderate to large neck haematoma, pulsatile but stable haematoma, pulse deficit, bruit, Foley catheter balloon tamponade, any

mediastinal widening on chest X-ray, and a retained knife blade.

- Laryngoscopy and bronchoscopy for *laryngeal or tracheobronchial injuries* if dysphonia, hoarseness, tension pneumothorax, severe surgical emphysema, or persistent air leak from chest drain are present.

- Contrast oesophagography and endoscopy in patients with odynophagia, dysphagia, haemoptysis and haematemesis, or signs of subcutaneous emphysema, blood in the nasogastric tube, leakage of saliva or gastrointestinal content from the wound, prevertebral air on lateral neck radiography or a pneumomediastinum to rule out *pharyngeal or oesophageal injuries*.

- *Transmidline gunshot wounds* need routine CT-angiography

Figure 19.14 presents an algorithm for the management of penetrating neck injury.

Vascular injuries

An arterial injury found on CT-angiography needs to be addressed, either surgically (i.e. common carotid artery) or endovascularly. A common or internal carotid injury needs to be repaired as soon as possible. Primary repair, end-to-end anastomosis,

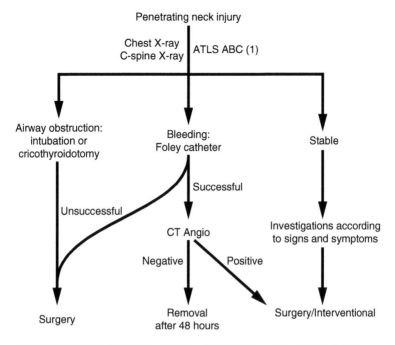

Penetrating neck injury

Chest X-ray
C-spine X-ray | ATLS ABC (1)

Airway obstruction:
intubation or
cricothyroidotomy

Bleeding:
Foley catheter

Stable

Unsuccessful

Successful

CT Angio

Investigations according
to signs and symptoms

Negative

Positive

Surgery

Removal
after 48 hours

Surgery/Interventional

(1) Look for airway obstruction, tension pneumothorax, open pneumothorax,
massive haemothorax, cardiac tamponade

Figure 19.14 • Penetrating neck injury.

saphenous vein or PTFE patching/grafting are possible repair techniques. Carotid ligation is reserved for comatose patients, patients with CT-proved cerebral infarction, or no backflow at surgery. Occluded or dissected vertebral arteries can be treated conservatively. A normal CT-angiography after Foley catheter tamponade suggests venous injury. The catheter can be removed in the operating room after 48-hours and the patient observed for another 24 hours in the hospital. In the rare case of re-bleeding the patient needs to undergo surgical exploration.[109,113]

Oesophageal injuries

Morbidity and mortality are high in oesophageal injuries, especially in delayed diagnosis or presentation. Therefore, the presence of an oesophageal injury must be eliminated in a timely fashion and with a high suspicion. Any air, either cervical or mediastinal, can be a hint for an oesophageal injury and warrants further work-up. Oesophageal injuries must be repaired with a single-layer suture and widely drained.[93,114]

Pharyngeal injuries

Pharyngeal injuries usually heal without surgery. They are treated with antibiotics and nasogastric tube feed. A neck wound must not be sutured for drainage purposes. After a period of 7 days a contrast swallow is repeated to demonstrate healing.

Future developments

Resuscitative endovascular balloon occlusion of the aorta (REBOA)

REBOA is a new technique currently under assessment. This technique can provisionally stop a life-threatening haemorrhage, mainly into the abdomen or pelvis, to gain some time to transfer a patient to theatre or to an angiography suite. A catheter is placed into the aorta and a balloon temporarily inflated to interrupt any blood flow distal to it. Some indications are currently being evaluated.

Enhanced recovery after surgery (ERAS)

ERAS aims at faster recovery after surgery. It is a well-established perioperative multidisciplinary approach in minimally invasive colorectal surgery and increasingly in other areas. Main elements are early mobilisation, no drains or catheters (or early removal), as little intravenous and opioids as possible and early oral nutrition. It is now being applied to trauma patients with current randomised studies about to start.

Key points

- Head, chest and abdominal injuries are the main lethal ones.
- Abdominal injury is one of the most important causes of preventable death.
- Advanced Trauma Life Support (ATLS) is one way to evaluate and treat severely injured patients in the acute phase.
- The traditional dogma of mandatory exploration of all penetrating wounds has changed to selective non-operative management.
- A laparotomy is mandatory in the event of an acute abdomen, or in the haemodynamically unstable patient with a penetrating wound or in the case of blunt trauma where there is a positive FAST and an unstable patient.
- Life-threatening chest injuries are tension pneumothorax, open pneumothorax, massive haemothorax, cardiac tamponade and flail chest.
- A haemopericardium on ultrasound, a straight left heart border on a chest X-ray, a J-wave in the ECG or an elevated central venous pressure raise the suspicion of an occult cardiac injury and require further investigation.
- An emergency department thoracotomy (EDT) is indicated in life-threatening pericardial tamponade, exsanguinating haemorrhage with profound shock (systolic blood pressure <60–70 mmHg not responding to resuscitation) or already hypovolaemic cardiac arrest after penetrating thoracic trauma.
- Hypoxia, hypoperfusion and hypothermia lead to the well-known deadly triad of hypothermia, acidosis and coagulopathy, which mandates damage control surgery.

✔ Full references available at **http://expertconsult. inkling.com**

Key references

8. American College of Surgeons Committee on Trauma. Advanced Trauma Life Support ATLS student course manual. 9th ed. Chicago, IL: American College of Surgeons; 2012 . p. 366S.

23. Moore EE, Moore FA. American Association for the Surgery of Trauma Organ Injury Scaling: 50th anniversary review article of the Journal of Trauma. J Trauma 2010;69(6):1600–1. PMID: 21150537.
This is the most widely accepted and used injury classification system for neck, chest and abdominal injuries.

30. Navsaria PH, Nicol AJ, Edu S, et al. Selective nonoperative management in 1106 patients with abdominal gunshot wounds: conclusions on safety, efficacy, and the role of selective CT imaging in a prospective single-center study. Ann Surg 2015;261(4):760–4. PMID: 25185470.
This large study showed that non-operative management of selected patients with abdominal gunshot wounds is safe and effective.

45. Velmahos GC, Zacharias N, Emhoff TA, et al. Management of the most severely injured spleen: a multicenter study of the Research Consortium of New England Centers for Trauma (ReCONECT). Arch Surg 2010;145(5):456–60. PMID: 20479344.
This multicentre study revealed that grade V splenic injuries, especially in combination with a head injury, predict failure of non-operative management.

50. van der Wilden GM, Velmahos GC, Emhoff T, et al. Successful nonoperative management of the most severe blunt liver injuries: a multicenter study of the research consortium of New England Centers for Trauma. Arch Surg 2012;147(5):423–8. PMID: 22785635.
Even higher-grade liver injuries can be treated non-operatively, as shown by this multicentre study.

54. Navsaria PH, Berli JU, Edu S, et al. Non-operative management of abdominal stab wounds – an analysis of 186 patients. S Afr J Surg 2007;45(4):128–30 . 132. PMID: 18069579.
Non-operative management in selected patients is safe. Serial examination in these patients significantly reduced unnecessary laparotomies.

90. Nicol AJ, Navsaria PH, Hommes M, et al. Sternotomy or drainage for a hemopericardium after penetrating trauma: a randomized controlled trial. Ann Surg 2014;259(3):438–42. PMID: 23604058.
This randomised study showed that subxyphoidal window and drainage is effective and safe in stable patients with a haemopericardium after penetrating trauma. No sternotomy is mandatory.

110. Thoma M, Navsaria PH, Edu S, et al. Analysis of 203 patients with penetrating neck injuries. World J Surg 2008;32(12):2716–23. PMID: 18931870.
This prospective observational study presents an algorithm for penetrating neck injuries.

20

Abdominal sepsis and abdominal compartment syndrome

Jonathan C. Epstein
Iain D. Anderson

Introduction

The diagnosis and management of abdominal sepsis is one of the greatest challenges the general surgeon faces. Optimal patient outcome requires considered decision-making and prompt surgical input. Application of basic principles allied to experience allows even complex cases of abdominal sepsis to be managed confidently and competently. Up to 90% of general surgical mortality follows emergency admission with sepsis[1] yet there are few units where 90% of resource is targeted at non-elective work. Delay to definitive treatment is the single most common reason for adverse outcomes and anastomotic leak the single commonest complication in fatal cases. Given its frequency and severity, a sound understanding of abdominal sepsis must be integral to every general surgeon's professional armamentarium.

This chapter will address the diagnosis and management of abdominal sepsis, including the challenges of looking after patients treated on the ICU (Intensive Care Unit), where management of abdominal compartment syndrome, the open abdomen and enterocutaneous fistulas can create particular difficulties. We also discuss the linked topic of intra-abdominal compartment syndrome. This is a relatively recently understood phenomenon often associated with sepsis where intra-abdominal hypertension (IAH) leads to a spectrum of life-threatening pathophysiological changes. The reader is referred to Chapter 5 for a description of the intensive care management of the surgical patient, and to Chapter 6 for a discussion of surgical nutrition.

Definition of sepsis

Sepsis has been recently re-defined as life-threatening organ dysfunction caused by dysregulated host response to infection.[2] This definition moves away from previous focus on the systemic inflammatory response syndrome (SIRS), which emphasised inflammation but is widely found in hospitalised patients who never develop infection. In the new definition, organ dysfunction is defined by the Sequential (Sepsis-specific) Organ Failure Assessment (SOFA) score: an increase by 2 points or more is associated with in-hospital mortality greater than 10% (see Box 20.1). An abbreviated score (quickSOFA) identifies patients with suspected infection at risk of poor outcomes typical of sepsis based on the presence of any two out of three of:

- respiratory rate $\geq$22/minute;
- altered mentation;
- systolic blood pressure $\leq$100 mmHg.

Septic shock is now defined as a subset of sepsis in which underlying circulatory and cellular metabolism abnormalities are profound enough to substantially increase mortality. Septic shock can be identified by the requirement of vasopressors to maintain mean arterial pressure (MAP) above 65 mmHg and a serum lactate greater than 2 mmol/L (18 mg/dL) in the absence of hypovolaemia. Septic shock is associated with hospital mortality of over 40%.

Box 20.1 • Sequential (Sepsis-related) Organ Failure Assessment (SOFA) score and definitions[2]

- Sepsis is defined as life-threatening organ dysfunction caused by a dysregulated host response to infection.
- Organ dysfunction can be identified as an acute change in total SOFA score >2 points consequent to the infection.
- The baseline SOFA score can be assumed to be zero in patients not known to have pre-existing organ dysfunction.
- A SOFA score of 2 reflects an overall mortality risk of approximately 10% in a general hospital population with suspected infection. Even patients presenting with modest dysfunction can deteriorate further, emphasising the seriousness of this condition and the need for prompt and appropriate intervention, if not already instituted.
- In lay terms, sepsis is a life-threatening condition that arises when the body's response to an infection injures its own tissues and organs.
- Patients with suspected infection who are likely to have a prolonged ICU stay or to die in the hospital can be promptly identified at the bedside with qSOFA, i.e. alteration in mental status, systolic blood pressure 100 mmHg, or respiratory rate 22/min.
- Septic shock is a subset of sepsis in which underlying circulatory and cellular/metabolic abnormalities are profound enough to substantially increase mortality.
- Patients with septic shock can be identified with a clinical construct of sepsis with persisting hypotension requiring vasopressors to maintain MAP 65 mmHg and having a serum lactate level >2 mmol/L (18 mg/dL) despite adequate volume resuscitation. With these criteria, hospital mortality is in excess of 40%.

	0	1	2	3	4
PaO_2/FiO_2 (kPa)	≥53.3	<53.3	<40	<26.7 with respiratory support	<13.3 with respiratory support
Platelets (×1000/µL)	≥150	<150	<100	<50	<20
Bilirubin (µmoL/L)	<20	20–32	33–101	102–204	>204
Cardiovascular system (All inotrope doses in µg/kg/min)	MAP ≥70 mmHg	MAP ≤70 mmHg	Dopamine <5 or dobutamine (any dose)	Dopamine 5.1–15 or epinephrine ≤0.1 or norepinephrine ≤0.1	Dopamine >15 or epinephrine >0.1 or norepinephrine >0.1
Glasgow Coma Score	15	13–14	10–12	6–9	<6
Creatinine (µmoL/L)	<110	110–170	171–299	300–440	>440
Urine output (mL/24 h)				<500	<200

PaO_2, partial pressure of oxygen; FiO_2, fraction of inspired oxygen; MAP, mean arterial pressure.

Pathophysiology of sepsis

The healthy host response to bacterial invasion includes neutrophil- and macrophage-mediated release of proinflammatory mediators including cytokines, chemokines and nitric oxide at the site of infection (documented in standard texts). If this inflammatory response becomes generalised, systemic vasodilatation, increased vascular permeability and microcirculatory dysfunction with decreased capillary flow lead to hypotension, fluid transudation and ultimately tissue hypoxia. The resulting multi-organ dysfunction syndrome (MODS) is associated with high mortality. Once established, this downward spiral is believed to be independent of the precipitating infective insult and is similar in conditions without initiating infection, such as major trauma, burns and pancreatitis.

The hypothesis that septic shock and MODS may be ameliorated by seeking to control the exaggerated, uncontrolled inflammatory response has not been supported by much clinical success to date. Probably due to the complexity and redundancy of the many pathways involved, targeting a single mediator or even single pathway has had limited clinical success. The predominant current theories can be summarised as follows:

1. **Uncontrolled systemic cytokine release.**
   Uncontrolled or exaggerated release of cytokines from macrophages in response to cellular injury is proposed to initiate further mediator cascades resulting in neutrophil and platelet activation. There has been particular focus on the role of mediators believed to play a central role, including tumour necrosis factor alpha (TNF-α) and

interleukins 1 and 6 (IL-1 and IL-6).[3] However, the measured circulating levels of cytokines vary widely between studies and indeed within study populations.[4] Clinical trials of drugs that inhibit the inflammatory cascade (corticosteroids, TNF-α antagonists and specific monoclonal antibodies) have failed to demonstrate a survival advantage.[3] Individual randomised trials examining the clinical effectiveness of activated protein C in severe sepsis showed promising initial results, but a recent Cochrane review concluded no survival advantage[4] and this intervention has now been withdrawn.

2. **Disturbances to coagulation.** Activation of vascular endothelial cells by inflammatory mediators leads to a pro-thrombotic state, by alteration of both the coagulation and fibrinolytic systems. This can result in haematological failure with a consumptive coagulopathy resulting in disseminated intravascular coagulation (DIC).[4,5]

3. **Immunosuppression.** Septic patients display features of immunosuppression including reduced capacity to clear primary infection and predisposition towards secondary infection with nosocomial pathogens.[4] A number of proposed mechanisms have been mooted – for example, reduced secretion of proinflammatory cytokines such as TNF-α, IL-1 and IL-6 in exchange for increased release of the anti-inflammatory cytokines IL-4 and IL-10 by T helper cells may play a central role.[6] This pattern of cytokine release has been observed in septic patients in the intensive care setting.[7,8] However, the possibility of immunotherapy to modify this host response has not yielded a therapeutic target to date.

The slippery slope of sepsis

Some degree of physiological derangement is common amongst surgical patients on the ward, although this is usually resolved by appropriate treatment of the underlying problem. When significant physiological derangement persists beyond 48 hours, outcome is worsened as progression to organ dysfunction is much more likely, an event associated with a mortality rate of up to 40%.[9] Mortality, in general, increases with the number of organ systems affected and with the severity of physiological disturbance at onset.[8] Early recognition of deterioration at a time when prompt intervention may yet avert catastrophe is essential.[10] By the time the patient with abdominal sepsis has developed shock, mortality increases from less than 10% to greater than 50%.[11,12]

It is critical that the surgeon appreciates that deterioration can often start insidiously on the ward, hence early detection is vital as intervention is most successful at this stage. While there are objective criteria that define organ dysfunction as above, clinical findings are helpful pointers. Hypoxia, oliguria, hypotension, deranged liver function tests or clotting, thrombocytopenia, acidosis and confusion are some of the features that indicate that a potentially severe systemic derangement is beginning.

The benefits of managing such high-risk surgical patients with early critical care input are well recognised.[13,14]

> ✓✓ The importance of detecting the subtle signs of abdominal sepsis at the earliest stage cannot be overemphasised and while the rate with which organ dysfunction develops in individual patients will vary, the requirement for rapid identification and treatment is key.

The Surviving Sepsis Campaign (SSC)

In 2008, informed by the results of a number of clinical trials, an international campaign was launched with the intention of improving outcomes in sepsis by standardising care.[15] The emphasis of the campaign was timely identification and treatment of patients with severe sepsis, using goal-directed strategies. Evidence-based guidelines were published in 2004, split into 'bundles' of care to be accomplished within certain time frames (Box 20.2). A total of 165 sites participated in the campaign, submitting bundle compliance and outcome data on 15 022 patients with severe sepsis. Despite incomplete compliance, a significant reduction in unadjusted hospital mortality (37% to 31% over the 2-year study period) was identified in those centres participating in the campaign.[16] The SSC has continued to reissue guidelines and remains active.

> ✓✓ The goal-directed treatment bundles developed by the Surviving Sepsis Campaign are a recommended standard of care. Their use in the timely identification and management of patients with severe sepsis has been shown to reduce mortality.[16]

Systematic assessment

Although effective management of patients with severe sepsis may entail complex investigations and procedures, the results of these manoeuvres are often suboptimal or even lethal without adequate prior resuscitation. A systematic approach such as that described in the Care of the Critically Ill Surgical Patient (CCrISP) course[17] is recommended as it provides a common management structure for problems of any type or severity (**Fig. 20.1**). Having a

Box 20.2 • Surviving Sepsis Campaign bundles[15]

Sepsis resuscitation bundle
To be accomplished within the first 6 hours of identification of severe sepsis:
1. Measure serum lactate
2. Obtain blood cultures prior to antibiotic administration
3. Administer broad-spectrum antibiotic, within 3 hours of A&E admission and within 1 hour for current inpatients
4. In the event of hypotension and/or a serum lactate >4 mmol/L:
    a. Deliver an initial minimum of 20 mL/kg of crystalloid or an equivalent
    b. Apply vasopressors for hypotension not responding to initial fluid resuscitation to maintain mean arterial pressure (MAP) >65 mmHg
5. In the event of persistent hypotension despite fluid resuscitation (septic shock) and/or lactate >4 mmol/L:
    a. Achieve a central venous pressure (CVP) of >8 mmHg
    b. Achieve a central venous oxygen saturation (Scv_{O_2}) >70% or mixed venous oxygen saturation (Sv_{O_2}) > 65%

Sepsis management bundle
To be accomplished within the first 24 hours of identification of severe sepsis:
1. Administer low-dose steroids for septic shock in accordance with a standardised ICU policy
2. Maintain glucose control >70 but <150 mg/dL
3. Maintain a median inspiratory plateau pressure (IPP) <30 cmH$_2$O for mechanically ventilated patients

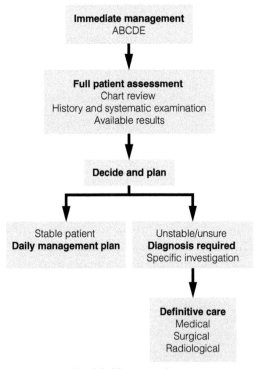

Figure 20.1 • The CCrISP system of assessment. Reproduced from Anderson ID. Assessing the critically ill surgical patient. In: Anderson ID, editor. Care of the critically ill surgical patient. London: Arnold; 1999. p. 7–15. © Hodder Arnold. Reproduced by permission of Hodder Education.

structured approach in times of crisis facilitates speed and is also important in reducing the likelihood of management errors. It certainly provides a common language and transparency that lets other health professionals understand the role of interventions. An integrated team approach involving diagnostic and interventional radiology, anaesthesia and intensive care is often required.

Patients with abdominal sepsis will inevitably have some degree of physiological instability. The CCrISP course advocates rapid immediate resuscitation following ABC principles of assessment with simultaneous correction of life-threatening conditions and initiation of high-flow oxygen therapy, intravenous fluids and monitoring as required. Some patients will deteriorate catastrophically and require intensive care support, but relatively simple interventions will commonly buy sufficient time for a comprehensive assessment. This will aim to determine the cause and severity of any problem and to exclude or optimise other conditions. A thorough appraisal of the patient's notes and charts is essential.

Complications can often be anticipated from the surgical condition in question, knowledge of any recent operative intervention and understanding of comorbidities (Box 20.3). The range of possible diagnoses is often large (Box 20.4) and the initial diagnostic net must be cast wide before drawing it in rapidly with the assistance of selective investigations. Reaching a provisional diagnosis and management plan rapidly is important as outcome worsens with delay and deterioration.

Patients should improve after clinical interventions. Failure to improve or signs of deterioration suggest a new problem or an incompletely treated initial one. The same systematic CCrISP approach forms the basis of ongoing assessment of the critically ill or at-risk patient on the critical care unit or ward. As repeated complications and setbacks are sadly common in complex cases, the surgeon must anticipate a long campaign rather than a single skirmish and be prepared to take a leading role in ongoing management.

- Pyrexia or hypothermia
- Tachycardia
- Tachypnoea
- Confusion
- Oedema
- Metabolic acidosis
- Hypoalbuminaemia
- Thrombocytopenia
- Ileus
- Poor peripheral perfusion
- Hypotension
- Hypoxia
- Lethargy
- Oliguria
- Raised lactate
- Hyponatraemia
- Leucocytosis or neutropenia

Sepsis of other origin (urine, line, chest, etc.)
Cardiac (ischaemia, infarction, dysrhythmias, failure)
Cerebral (toxic confusion, ischaemia)
Pulmonary (atelectasis, collapse, infection, pulmonary embolism)
Fluid imbalance
Other non-septic abdominal complications (e.g. ileus, bleeding)

Lactate measurement

The role of lactate measurement has become less clear-cut in recent years. The SSC has emphasised the importance of a raised lactate in diagnosing sepsis and it can undoubtedly provide an extremely useful guide to diagnosis in patients not making an obvious physiological response. The SSC guidelines emphasise the role of aggressive goal-directed therapy, which should aim to normalise lactate levels rapidly.[18] However, as the pathophysiology of sepsis has become better understood the benefit of targeting lactate correction as a surrogate marker for successful resuscitation has become less certain. The elevated lactate level in sepsis may not be a consequence of global tissue hypoperfusion and anaerobic metabolism as had been assumed but rather a consequence of beta-adrenergic stimulation in aerobic conditions.[19] There is a school of thought that raised lactate may even be a beneficial compensatory mechanism, although refractory high lactate levels tend to be an ominous sign.[20] While it is useful to be aware of this debate, it should not distract from the importance of considering lactate levels as a marker of sepsis and responding to raised levels promptly.

Antimicrobial therapy in abdominal sepsis

Definitive management of abdominal sepsis requires eradication of the source of infection. However, antimicrobial therapy is also vital.[21] Where sepsis is suspected, blood, vascular access sites, urine, wound and sputum should be sampled for urgent Gram staining and culture. Cultures from the main source of sepsis are several times more likely to be positive (75% vs 18%)[22] than blood cultures, but both are important in the critically ill patient. Once samples for culture have been taken, broad-spectrum antibiotic therapy should begin immediately as delay may deleteriously influence outcome.[16] The role of cultures is to enable the antibiotics to be changed selectively if the patient fails to respond to initial therapy. The choice of antibiotic will be influenced by the clinical circumstances and the expected range of infecting organisms. Early combination antibiotic therapy yields significantly improved survival compared to single-agent use in septic shock.[23] The route of administration must ensure adequate plasma levels and the drugs should penetrate adequately into the tissues. Intravenous infusion is usually necessary. Whenever there is doubt concerning the optimal choice of antibiotics, the advice of a medical microbiologist should be sought. For most abdominal sepsis, coverage of Gram-negative and anaerobic bacteria will be necessary. With biliary sepsis, approximately 15% of cases will involve streptococci species that are resistant to cephalosporins, so the addition of a penicillin is a common approach. With hospital-acquired infection, cover against a broader and more resistant spectrum of organisms will be needed.[21] Fungal infection (usually *Candida* species) is not uncommon in complex abdominal sepsis requiring ICU care and additional antifungal therapy will often be required.

✅✅ When severe sepsis is identified, blood cultures should be taken, and broad-spectrum antibiotics administered within 1 hour. This has been shown to reduce mortality as part of a management strategy in sepsis.[16]

✅✅ Combination antibiotic therapy should be used in preference to monotherapy in septic shock as it is associated with a reduction in mortality.[23]

Imaging in abdominal sepsis

A range of imaging techniques may be employed to localise an infective focus (see also Chapter 11) but computed tomography (CT) with intravenous contrast enhancement provides excellent information in thoracic, abdominal and pelvic sepsis. There will be occasions when intravenous contrast is avoided (particularly renal impairment) and/or gastrointestinal contrast utilised via mouth, nasogastric tube, drain, stoma or rectum. The vast majority of surgical patients can be stabilised sufficiently for scanning to take place safely and the guidance that CT provides in diagnosis and therapeutic intervention should not be underestimated. CT is excellent at primary diagnosis and in the complex or postoperative patient where clinical examination is more difficult.[24] Comparison with previous scans is important and the input of a senior, specialist radiologist is priceless. In emergency cases, the surgeon should ideally be present so that decisions about interventional radiological procedures may be made jointly.

It should be remembered that CT (or indeed any diagnostic test) is not perfect. Artefact from drains and metallic prostheses may reduce image quality. Intravenous contrast use is relatively contraindicated in acute kidney injury, although gastrointestinal contrast can still be used to advantage. Even in expert hands, there is a small rate of missed diagnoses and this is inevitably amplified when out-of-hours scans in complex postoperative patients are interpreted by trainees.

The chest radiograph still plays a role in patient assessment and ultrasound has the advantage of being portable, harmless and repeatable. The greatest utility of ultrasound probably lies in assessment of biliary and renal pathology and monitoring identified collections. However, it is operator-dependent, and a negative scan will offer little reassurance when the clinical picture is concerning. When a focus of persistent sepsis cannot be identified on primary imaging, investigations such as magnetic resonance imaging (MRI) particularly for biliary or pelvic pathologies or nuclear medicine modalities such as labelled white cell scanning may help identify occult sources of sepsis.

Early source control in abdominal sepsis

Source control describes the physical measures taken to eradicate an infective focus. This includes the drainage of collections, debridement of necrotic tissue and definitive surgical procedures to correct an anatomical abnormality. It is intuitive that early source control should improve outcomes in abdominal sepsis and there is evidence for this from studies of perforated peptic ulcer.[25] Delay to source control has been shown to significantly increase mortality in septic shock[26] and expedient source control before progression to septic shock is clearly beneficial.[16,27]

In a complex system such as a hospital it is easy for multiple small individual delays to add up. Managing the multidisciplinary team to achieve prompt and timely intervention is a considerable skill, which requires active and continued leadership from the surgeon. The Royal College of Surgeons of England and the Department of Health have issued timelines regarding the urgency of source control in sepsis (Box 20.5), which are commended as a standard of care.

✔ Expedient control of the septic focus is of utmost importance in the management of severe sepsis. Neither overly prolonged resuscitation nor observation should delay this.[13]

Aims of treatment in abdominal sepsis

The management of abdominal sepsis in the emergency surgical admission is relevant to a range of pathology, as covered elsewhere in this volume. Pus should be drained, necrotic tissue excised and specimens submitted for urgent microbiology. While localised collections can be drained percutaneously, generalised peritonitis remains an indication for laparotomy. Spontaneous primary bacterial peritonitis and acute pancreatitis may be considered as exceptions to this rule. Laparoscopy is increasingly used in the management of specific surgical conditions causing abdominal sepsis. It is important to remember that the laparoscopic approach may not allow adequate debridement and drainage and that the physiological sequelae of a pneumoperitoneum may be poorly tolerated in patients with septic shock.

Whether treatment is radiological or surgical, adequate patient preparation is essential (see also Chapters 2 and 5). Coagulopathy must be identified and corrected and blood should be available if required. Although drainage may be essential to resolve sepsis, not infrequently bacteraemia precipitated by the intervention may cause a temporary deterioration in the patient's condition. Indeed, a bacteraemia may represent the 'second hit' that precipitates MODS. Such circumstances should be anticipated and an appropriate level of post-procedure care arranged.

In complex cases in older and sicker patients a compromise treatment pathway may need to be devised, striking a balance between optimum source control and magnitude of intervention. The opinion of senior colleagues and specialist centres can be invaluable as inadequate treatment will condemn the patient to ongoing sepsis and higher risk of a poor outcome.

Image-guided percutaneous drainage of both spontaneous and postoperative intra-abdominal collections has reported success rates of 70–90%.[28,29] Percutaneous procedures will only be effective if good drainage is achieved. Many percutaneous drains are narrow and inadequate when infected fluid is viscous or contains necrotic tissue. Larger or multiple drains may be more effective and daily flushing can be useful. When radiological drains are placed for abdominal sepsis, the responsibility lies with the surgical team to ensure that the patient's condition improves as expected. Failure to respond to radiological intervention is an indication for laparotomy.

When surgery is performed for sepsis, the procedure will vary according to the underlying pathology. In general, the most straightforward adequate procedure is preferable to a complex and time-consuming operation. There is a current trend towards primary bowel resection and anastomosis in the acute setting, but this should be avoided in unstable patients, in the presence of significant comorbidity or when there is extensive contamination. Generous saline lavage is recommended on completion of the procedure but there is nothing to be gained either by removing fibrinous debris piecemeal or by postoperative lavage systems.[21] Delayed skin wound closure may be preferable to primary suture, or wounds may be left to close by secondary intention if sepsis is substantial.

Obtaining informed consent for treatment may involve both patient and relatives. The potential severity of the situation should not be understated and the possibility of death, stoma creation, the need for intensive care treatment and the potential for further surgery should be discussed explicitly. The average mortality for an emergency laparotomy is around 15%, and increases with age and physiological disturbance.[13] Complementing clinical assessment with an objective determinant of risk from a scoring system (such as P-POSSUM) is valuable in helping to focus efforts appropriately.[13,30]

Postoperative care will almost always be delivered on the surgical high-dependency unit (HDU) or ICU. The surgeon is a key member of the multidisciplinary team, and close cooperation between surgeon and intensivist is essential (Box 20.6).

✔ Intraperitoneal abscesses with safe access routes should be drained percutaneously under radiological guidance. This intervention carries high success and low recurrence rates.[29]

Box 20.6 • The surgeon's role on the ICU

Daily surgical input to:
- Wound and stoma care
- Tubes and drains
- Nutrition
- Ongoing management of sepsis
- Further operations
- Compartment syndrome
- Postoperative bleeding
- Preparation for HDU/ward
- Treatment/advice regarding the underlying surgical disease

Abdominal sepsis on the ICU

The surgeon will be consulted in the assessment and management of patients already on the ICU who develop primary or recurrent abdominal sepsis. The outcome of patients with abdominal sepsis who require ICU treatment depends on age, comorbidities, source of sepsis and degree of organ dysfunction. Control of the source of sepsis is critical for survival of patients with MODS. Survival is greater than 60% when sepsis is eradicated successfully whereas survival is close to zero if significant abdominal sepsis continues.[31]

The principal causes of recurrent abdominal sepsis in the ICU are shown in Box 20.7. Anastomotic leak remains the commonest single cause and should be actively suspected in all 'at-risk patients' who are critically ill or deteriorating. Inadvertent enterotomy during difficult surgery may occur in up to 20% of patients[32] and the repair is a potential weakness that can leak. Gastrostomy and feeding jejunostomy tubes inserted into the gut occasionally leak and this is more likely when tissue healing is poor.

Postoperative small-bowel ileus usually resolves within days, regardless of the extent of bowel handling.[33] Opiate analgesia and electrolyte abnormalities (hypokalaemia, uraemia) may delay resolution, but failure to progress may also indicate ongoing retroperitoneal or abdominal pathology.

Box 20.7 • The principal causes of recurrent abdominal sepsis in the ICU

Leaked anastomosis or enterotomy
Leaking gastrostomies and other tubes
Abscesses or collections
Dead or ischaemic gut
Acalculous cholecystitis
Clostridium difficile-associated pseudomembranous colitis
Acute massive gastric dilatation
Neutropenic enterocolits
Continuing sepsis from 'common' peritonitis (perforation of peptic stress ulcer or diverticulum)

Ileus may be difficult to distinguish from adhesive obstruction, and contrast studies help to clarify the situation. Adhesive obstruction frequently resolves but refractory cases occasionally require laparotomy. However, in a hostile abdomen, such as found in abdominal sepsis, considerable caution should be exercised in subjecting the patient to further surgery.[34] Whereas a 3-day period of non-operative treatment might be acceptable in the presence of straightforward adhesion obstruction, one should be prepared to wait for considerably longer when faced with a hostile abdomen provided nutrition can be delivered safely and the patient is regularly assessed. Most cases will resolve but indications for intervention include evidence of bowel ischaemia, closed loop obstruction and recurrent abdominal sepsis. Recognition of these indications requires regular re-assessment, CT imaging and clinical experience.

Assessment on the ICU

Assessing patients on the ICU is difficult for several reasons. Firstly, the patients are often complex yet unfamiliar if they have been treated previously by other surgeons. Secondly, sedated, postoperative patients in organ failure display abdominal sepsis differently to new emergency admissions with peritonitis. Abdominal signs are unlikely to be evident unless gross (e.g. flank cellulitis, bowel contents in a drain, necrotic stoma), and the diagnosis of recurrent abdominal sepsis is often made from deterioration in vital organ function and suspicion based on previous treatment and imaging. Contrast-enhanced CT is of great value, but some patients will be too unwell to transfer to the scanner. For this group exploratory laparotomy may be required. The interpretation of CT images in the recently operated abdomen is not straightforward. Expert reporting will not only confirm the diagnosis but can also potentially identify areas where there is no evidence of inflammation. In a difficult reoperative procedure with dense adhesions, that roadmap can save time and reduce the risk of surgical damage to other organs. Percutaneous drainage has a similar role here as in primary inflammation and the same caveats apply.

The importance of surgeons making their own thorough assessment cannot be overestimated. The surgeon should be satisfied that the diagnosis is secure and that surgery is the best course of action. Part of that process will be engaging in detailed discussion with the intensivist to weigh up alternative diagnoses and sources of sepsis, and to clarify the risks and benefits of intervention at any given point in time. Often this is not clear-cut as patients may have multiple potential sources (e.g.

simultaneous pneumonia and abdominal sepsis) or other complicating factors in the context of comorbidities and other ICU treatments.

Whilst the risks of surgery in the ICU population are often self-evident, conservative management has complications too – patients can sometimes be described as being 'too sick *not* to have an operation'. Clear indications for life-saving surgery include generalised peritonitis, inaccessible or multiple collections and presence of dead tissue. Patients with deteriorating organ function and a strong suspicion of abdominal pathology remain a significant group in whom laparotomy may be unavoidable. In some patients it will be clear that there is no realistic prospect of survival, either from the required operation or, more commonly, the inevitably prolonged ICU course thereafter. It is important that both intensivist and surgeon counsel the family if care is to be limited.

Re-operating in abdominal sepsis

Re-operating in abdominal sepsis is challenging. From 72 hours after the last operation, dense adhesions make surgery significantly more difficult and the risk of bowel damage increases. Entry to the abdomen can be awkward and an extension of the previous midline incision may help to reach virgin territory. Adhesions are generally most dense around any site of inflammation, as well as around incisions. A preoperative CT scan provides a roadmap to guide the surgeon to the correct location. While a full laparotomy may be desirable, prolonged dissection of adhesions in an area not thought from CT to contain inflammation or a collection may be harmful. The surgeon must deal with the sepsis as thoroughly as possible but balance this with the need for simplicity and speed. Prolonged and complex procedures are likely to lead to systemic deterioration and the prospect of bowel anastomoses healing under such adverse circumstances is not as high as one would like. The ability of the patient to withstand further surgery for further complications is very much lower next time around[31] and the surgeon should see the present operation as the best opportunity for salvaging the patient. Intestinal reconstruction can be attempted when the patient is well and recovered, some months later.

Generally, the simplest and safest procedure will be best. This holds true especially in the patient who already has incipient or established organ failure. The principles of damage control defined in the trauma situation apply: drain sepsis, debride necrotic tissue and exteriorise any leaking bowel or anastomoses. Controversy relates to the management of enteric and colorectal anastomotic leaks. While in a well patient, with a small leak and minimal contamination, preservation of a repaired anastomosis with proximal defunctioning and local drainage may be appropriate, this strategy is unlikely to succeed in the critically ill. A first salvage operation in an ICU patient will successfully eradicate sepsis more than 40% of the time, but a second operation carries a success rate of only 25% and a third operation, only 7%.[31]

In difficult cases, the surgeon must be flexible and have a range of strategies available. In the hostile septic abdomen it may not be possible to take down and exteriorise the primary source of sepsis because of dense adhesions or the anatomical location (oesophagus, duodenum). For inaccessible pelvic sepsis arising from distal small bowel or colon, it may be possible to identify and exteriorise a proximal loop of jejunum without entering and damaging the matted pelvic loops other than to achieve necessary drainage. This will usually relieve the sepsis but at the price of a high-output stoma and prolonged intravenous feeding. For oesophagogastric or duodenal sepsis, all that may be possible is to drain collections and leave large tube or sump drains beside the leaking anastomosis or other septic focus. Placing a T-tube in the defect to create a controlled fistula is also of potential merit. Proximal intestinal contents can sometimes be diverted by way of a surgical gastrostomy. In really difficult situations it may only be possible to gain entry to pockets of pus or enteric content and leave the abdomen open as a laparostomy. Further pus or enteric content will usually find its way to the surface, assisted by subsequent manual lavage on the ICU or in theatre as necessary. In addition to their role in draining proximal gut secretions, gastrostomy and enterostomy tubes can be placed to facilitate future enteral feeding.

As these laparotomies are often bloody, prolonged and take place in contaminated fields many surgeons leave large drains (24Ch tube or sump) in the subphrenic spaces and pelvis at the end of the procedure. This may be particularly useful for certain deep cavities (e.g. psoas abscess) or when further leakage is likely or indeed certain. Large Foley catheters can be used to intubate inaccessible bowel to create a controlled fistula (typically the duodenum) and it is often advisable to place an additional large drain just outside the bowel. There is a particular role for local lavage in pancreatic necrosis (see Chapter 14) but, otherwise, continuing lavage via abdominal drains in the postoperative period is of no proven benefit.

Outcome from surgery for abdominal sepsis in the ICU patient depends on multiple factors. The importance of satisfactory source control has been discussed but numbers of failed organs, comorbid conditions, age and the underlying surgical pathology are also relevant. A further factor associated with survival is the early response to the first operation in the ICU. If there is clinical improvement within 48 hours then survival is as high as 80% but if the patient does not respond in this early phase survival is reduced to approximately 10%.[31] Given the cost of intensive care, attempts have been made to define those patients with negligible chance of survival. However, due to the heterogeneity of the patient group and the nature of scoring systems in general, it is not possible to use them for decision-making in individual patients. Clinical judgement is most important and the scoring systems remain primarily tools for audit and research.

Damage control laparotomy

Damage control laparotomy (DCL) is a concept that has expanded from its initial role in trauma surgery (see Chapter 19). Trauma patients can rapidly develop the unholy triad of hypothermia, acidosis and coagulopathy such that surgery becomes un-survivable. Decisive, immediately life-saving manoeuvres are carried out ('staple, pack and go') and the patient returned to ICU for warming and resuscitation, with more definitive surgery deferred for 24–48 hours once coagulopathy has been corrected and homeostasis returned towards normal. Whilst in abdominal sepsis the first laparotomy carries the best chance for salvage,[35] in unstable patients it can be better to make an active decision to quickly drain pus, remove dead tissue, stop bleeding by packing and close overtly leaking bowel with staples (without resection) before terminating the operation. Physiological instability, massive haemorrhage, coagulopathy, abdominal compartment syndrome and acute mesenteric ischaemia are relative indications for this approach.[35] Packs should generally be removed as early as possible once clotting is restored, and this is usually the next day. The small bowel becomes adherent remarkably quickly and can be damaged as packs are removed. Packs should be removed cautiously under direct vision with saline irrigation and gentle finger separation.

Second-look (planned) re-laparotomy

These terms refer to scheduled re-exploration of the abdomen, planned at the initial procedure. The term distinguishes it from 'laparotomy on demand', in which the abdomen is explored only when a new problem is identified. After a damage control procedure a second look is obviously required to complete the necessary definitive procedures but the term is now more commonly applied to 'looking again' after laparotomy for intestinal ischaemia. The extent of intestinal ischaemia may not be fully evident at the first operation and particularly if the bowel has been re-anastomosed, looking again at 48–72 hours can identify further ischaemia before the patient deteriorates. In cases where there is doubt as to the extent of intestinal ischaemia it may be preferable to resect and staple off the bowel ends and re-assess 48 hours later, rather than gamble on anastomosing bowel that might be subclinically ischaemic and doomed to anastomotic failure.

Repeated planned re-laparotomies have been used aggressively for abdominal sepsis with MODS in both Europe and North America for some years. In this method of treatment, the abdomen is typically re-operated upon every 24–48 hours for several days to wash out the peritoneal cavity and remove any ongoing sepsis. A recent randomised trial has shown that this approach is associated with significantly more laparotomies and prolonged ICU stay compared to a 're-laparotomy on demand' approach.[36] There may be a case for a single planned second-look laparotomy in patients with severe faecal peritonitis but this is debatable. This philosophical approach must not divert the surgeon from maintaining a low threshold for early laparotomy on demand when indicated, as delaying necessary surgery worsens outcome.[31]

✓✓ In patients undergoing surgery for severe secondary peritonitis, re-laparotomy on demand is preferable to 'planned re-laparotomy'.[36]

Leaving the abdomen open (laparostomy)

As outlined above, the hostile abdomen may be left open to allow pus and enteric contents to drain. It may also be left open when the alternative is closure with undue tension. In appropriate circumstances this approach can reduce the rate of recurrent sepsis, minimise wound complications and avoid intra-abdominal hypertension (as discussed further below). It may also allow improved organ function, faster weaning from the ventilator and can facilitate early enteral nutrition. However, this is at the expense of increased fluid loss through evaporation, exposure of the bowel to potential fistulation and considerable psychological distress for the patient. The open abdomen is particularly challenging to nurse as comfortable, secure wound care may be difficult to achieve.[37] Healing is slow and unless the fascia is closed later hernia formation is inevitable. It is undoubtedly a valuable and life-saving technique when needed but it is also a significant future burden to the patient in its own right and is not to be recommended routinely.[21]

In closing the abdomen during laparotomy for abdominal sepsis, the surgeon should close the fascia conventionally but avoid tension. Tension sutures have little to recommend them and their continued use is not supported. If bowel distension, oedema, haemorrhage (or packing to control it) or the potential for intra-abdominal hypertension make closure impossible there are several options open to the surgeon. Each end of the wound may be closed conventionally to the point of reasonable tension and the central defect left open. For short-lived oedema (e.g. after aortic aneurysm repair or traumatic haemorrhage) the defect can be covered with abdominal packing changed daily until such time as the defect can be closed or a longer-term solution implemented (see below). Early dressing changes should be carried out by the surgical team. The small bowel will become adherent to any gauze dressings, and gentle separation will be required to avoid injury.

A double-sandwich dressing of semipermeable adhesive dressing with moist gauze between the layers of dressing protects the bowel with less adhesion formation than with standard gauze packs. There are various commercial plastic sheets that can be used. Alternatively, a version of the Bogota bag can be used. In this technique, a sterile 3-litre intravenous fluid bag is slit open and sutured to the fascia, covering and protecting the bowel and providing it with a clean, moist environment. Again, as the oedema subsides, usually within 72 hours or so, the Bogota bag or double-sandwich dressing can be removed and the abdomen either closed or a longer-term technique instituted.

In recurrent sepsis, where recovery is likely to be slow, prosthetic mesh can be used to restrain the viscera. Absorbable polyglactin meshes are preferred to non-absorbable polypropylene meshes, as there is less likelihood of disastrous chronic mesh infection and fistulation to underlying bowel.[38] Caution is required in the use of biological implants in this scenario as they are extremely expensive and without proven benefit.[38]

Use of commercial negative-pressure dressings has become widespread as they make wound management considerably more straightforward. Early cohort studies suggested that vacuum-assisted closure was well tolerated in the open abdomen, with intestinal fistulation rates of only 5%.[39] The only randomised trial on vacuum-assisted closure in the open abdomen, which compared it to polyglactin absorbable mesh, did not show benefit and the rate of fistulation in the vacuum-assisted closure arm was 21%.[40] Controversy regarding the rate of intestinal fistulation after application of negative pressure dressings continues although it is reasonable to note that the most comprehensive series shows no increased fistula incidence.[41]

However, caution is required before contemplating using vacuum dressings in the presence of suture or staple lines, repaired serosal tears or enterotomies.

Many cases of open abdomen management described in the surgical literature relate to cases of trauma or major haemorrhage. These laparostomies can usually be closed within 7 days by conventional techniques. Laparostomy in abdominal sepsis is a different matter and usually runs a much longer timescale, resulting in retraction of the rectus muscles laterally. The above-described techniques have been combined in expert units to use temporary and protected polypropylene mesh traction with vacuum in the septic open abdomen to prevent muscle retraction and to steadily reduce the size of the abdominal wall defect. However, the techniques are complex and timings are specific and carry very significant risks in non-expert hands.[42] Currently, for the general surgeon forced to create a laparostomy for abdominal sepsis, placement of a polyglactin mesh within the muscular defect remains a good option.

The National Emergency Laparotomy Audit (NELA)

The NELA audit is a joint anaesthetic and surgical national audit of emergency laparotomy in the UK. It measures care in every UK hospital against defined standards including timeliness of assessment and intervention, seniority of decision-makers, facilities, critical care use and seniority of surgical and anaesthetic input. The audit provides high-quality comparative data to drive local and national improvements in the quality of care. Data entry began in January 2014 and reports are published annually.[43] Data on specific diseases and operations should be available in 2017.

Abdominal compartment syndrome

Normally, intra-abdominal pressure is low (<10 mmHg), but it is recognised that it can rise in abdominal sepsis (and other acute abdominal conditions, including trauma and pancreatitis) to the significant detriment of the patient. The condition is probably not as rare as previously thought.[44,45] As abdominal pressure rises, venous return is impaired and cardiac output falls. The tense abdomen can cause pulmonary compromise, oliguria, mesenteric ischaemia and even raised intracranial pressure. These features, similar in some ways to a tension pneumothorax, constitute abdominal compartment syndrome (ACS).[46]

ACS most frequently occurs after laparotomy for peritonitis, abdominal aortic aneurysm repair

and trauma, particularly if surgery is prolonged. Tissue oedema results from the combined effects of tissue injury, intravenous fluid infusion and leaky capillaries, bowel distension and haematomas. ACS can even occur in the abdomen that has been left open and packed, especially if there is ongoing haemorrhage. ACS is not restricted to emergency surgery; prolonged elective surgery with a scarred and rigid abdominal wall may also lead to this condition. The anaesthetist may signal an unacceptable rise in the ventilatory pressure as the abdomen is closed but more commonly ACS develops on the critical care unit 12–36 hours after surgery. Oligo/anuria and raised ventilatory pressures are the usual presenting features.

Intra-abdominal pressure (IAP) is measured via the bladder following instillation of 25 mL of normal saline. The IAP is measured through the aspiration port of the catheter tubing using a transducer. The transducer should be zeroed at the level of the mid-axillary line, and IAP measured in the supine position at end expiration.[47] Standardised definitions for ACS were developed in 2006 by an international consensus group[47] (Box 20.8).

A number of medical treatment options are of benefit in reducing IAP.[48] Abdominal wall compliance can be improved with adequate sedation, analgesia and neuromuscular blockade. Intraluminal contents should be evacuated with nasogastric and rectal decompression and the use of pro-kinetic agents. Abdominal fluid collections should be aspirated. Positive fluid balance can be corrected with fluid restriction, diuretics or dialysis/ultrafiltration. However, if pressures above 20 mmHg persist despite these measures, or organ dysfunction worsens, then the abdomen will need to be decompressed and left open using the laparostomy management techniques discussed above.

Box 20.8 • Definitions of abdominal compartment syndrome[44]

Intra-abdominal pressure (IAP)
- Steady-state pressure in the abdominal cavity
- Between 5 and 7 mmHg in critically unwell adults

Abdominal perfusion pressure (APP)
APP = MAP − IAP

Intra-abdominal hypertension (IAH)
Sustained or repeated pathological elevation in IAP ≥12 mmHg

Abdominal compartment syndrome (ACS)
Sustained IAP >20 mmHg (with or without an APP <60 mmHg) that is associated with new organ dysfunction or failure

Enterocutaneous fistulas (ECF)

Intestinal fistulas pose a particular set of challenges and require complex management. They contribute to sepsis, malnutrition, fluid and electrolyte imbalances, difficulties in wound care, as well as posing an enormous psychological challenge to the patient.

A fistula is defined as an abnormal communication between two epithelial surfaces. The overwhelming majority occurring in the context of abdominal sepsis result from anastomotic leakage or an inadvertent enterotomy, either overlooked or unsuccessfully repaired. Fistulation from somewhere in the intestinal tract to the laparotomy wound will occur occasionally in every gastrointestinal surgeon's practice. Severe early sepsis may result but more typically there is a period of intestinal ileus, wound infection and clinical stagnation. When the laparotomy wound ruptures or is opened to treat apparent wound infection, the enteric or faecal nature of the content becomes apparent. This may not be convincing to begin with as the enteric flow is usually preceded by a volume of pus and blood mimicking simple postoperative wound infections. Postoperative fistulas may also occur through drains or along recent drain sites, to the vaginal vault in those who have undergone previous hysterectomy and occasionally to the rectum or other parts of the gut.

An enterocutaneous fistula (ECF) is most likely to occur after emergency surgery for another postoperative complication, i.e. sepsis, obstruction or bleeding. In these re-laparotomies the inherent difficulty of the procedure, brought about by adhesions, bowel distension and friable tissues, makes further bowel damage a real possibility. If that damage is not, or cannot, be repaired effectively and if there is postoperative obstruction, inflammatory phlegmon or an open abdomen, then the likelihood of fistulation increases considerably. The combination of small-bowel obstruction and an undrained abscess is also likely to result in a fistula as the obstructed bowel eventually softens and gives way at or into the collection. Thus it should be self-evident that repairing a leaking anastomosis when the patient is septic and local tissues oedematous and friable is all too often doomed to failure. Bowel exposed in an open abdomen will also inevitably be subject to some degree of trauma even when the dressings or appliances are handled and changed expertly. In the order of 10–20% of 'laparostomies' will fistulate even with expert care.

A proportion of intestinal fistulas heal spontaneously, although they will cause misery and morbidity while they do so. The factors that contribute to persistence of a fistula are shown in Box 20.9.

Box 20.9 • Factors contributing to the occurrence and persistence of postoperative fistulas

Occurrence
Repaired anastomosis
Inadvertent enterotomy (repaired or missed)
New anastomosis in unfavourable circumstances
Persisting abscess or phlegmon causing obstruction
Fistulating disease
Open abdomen

Persistence
Distal obstruction (including constipation)
Open abdomen
Disconnected bowel ends
Local abscess
High output from fistula
Complex fistula
Mucocutaneous continuity

The best-known approach to fistula care is that described at the Irving Intestinal Failure Unit in Salford (UK), defined by the acronym SNAP (Sepsis, Nutrition, Anatomy, Procedure). The first priority is the expedited treatment of sepsis. Once the necessary resuscitation is in hand, an early CT scan of the abdomen, preferably with both enteric and intravenous contrast, is obtained to identify undrained intra-abdominal sepsis. The frequency of intra-abdominal abscess formation is high, in the region of 66%[49] and this may not be clinically obvious. Without diagnosis and control of the sepsis, the prognosis is bleak. As described earlier, sepsis must be eradicated and the same principles of antibiosis, percutaneous drainage if amenable, surgical drainage if not and diversion if the sepsis is inaccessible apply.

An integral part of early management is wound care and control of the fistula effluent. When there is a small fistula orifice in a drain site or through part of a wound a stoma bag will suffice. When bowel contents are leaking into a laparostomy, management may be very difficult. Large fistula bags are available. Reducing fistula output by avoiding enteral feed, and administering proton-pump inhibitors, codeine and loperamide, can help. Octreotide can reduce intestinal secretions in some patients but in our practice its role is relatively limited as it is expensive, unpleasant for the patient and adds little to the steps already described. It is perhaps most useful in pancreatic fistulas.

Immediate fluid management will have been considered as the patient was resuscitated but attention will have to turn rapidly to the optimal means of nutrition. The potentially negative effect that enteral nutrition often has on output and wound care, particularly in the early stages, has already been described. Enteral feeding may also 'feed' the abdominal sepsis if there is complexity to the fistula or a further unrecognised proximal hole in the bowel. There is often partial obstruction associated with the sepsis and in the vast majority of ECF cases it is more reliable to administer parenteral nutrition (PN) while the patient stabilises and the situation with regard to sepsis, wound care and anatomy is clarified. Indeed PN is the mainstay of nutritional support in intestinal fistulation with abdominal sepsis. In some circumstances, enteral nutrition can take over some, or even all, of the role, but this will usually take time and is only possible in selected patients.

ECF can be categorised as high- or low-output (output above or below 500 mL/24 hours). High-output fistulas are likely to have a significant effect on fluid balance and nutrition. Some proximal fistulas produce several litres of electrolyte-rich fluid per day and maintaining fluid balance can be challenging. Senior surgical staff will need to commit to adequate supervision of the recording of the various inputs and outputs, particularly in the initial phase before steady state is reached. Fistula output will often reduce with time. Many fistulas arising from anastomotic dehiscence will be a side hole anatomically and if there is free distal flow, no sepsis, no bowel disease and no distal obstruction (which may be simple constipation) then spontaneous closure may occur. It is uncertain whether restricted oral intake helps, but it is intuitive to minimise flow to encourage healing. If the fistula has not closed by 6 weeks and there is no apparently reversible factor (e.g. abscess, constipation) spontaneous closure is unlikely and introduction of more liberal oral intake may be reasonable.

In the ICU setting, once sepsis is excluded or controlled and any laparostomy is starting to granulate, oral or enteral feeding can be introduced cautiously, maintaining a careful watch for recurrent sepsis. The nutritional benefit of this will depend on the length and condition of gut available for absorption and it will often take time for enteral feeding to be established. During this phase, combined enteral and parenteral feeding is used.

Early surgery is required for abdominal sepsis not amenable to non-operative intervention where washout, exteriorisation and formation of a laparostomy may be necessary. Attempts at re-operation on an unstable patient to try to correct the fistula are likely to cause more harm than good. Surgery for fistulas is best deferred until the patient is well physically, nutritionally and emotionally, and only after the anatomy has been defined radiologically. This is often some months later and in complex cases is a highly specialist undertaking. The appropriate time to operate is a matter of judgement – prolapse of fistulas/stomas is a useful indication that adhesions have softened as is the ability to pinch to re-epithelialised laparostomy skin. It is axiomatic that 'it is impossible to operate too late – only too early'. Careful planning is required for both the intestinal components of surgery and the abdominal wall reconstruction. In the UK central funding is provided to specialist units where established teams experienced in wound management, skin care, nutrition, central venous catheter care, radiological assessment and definitive surgery are based.

Key points

- Abdominal sepsis is associated with high mortality.
- A systematic approach, based on sound understanding of pathophysiology, is fundamental to successful sepsis management. Adequate resuscitation, early diagnosis, rapid definitive treatment, and accurate and ongoing reassessment are essential if the progression to organ dysfunction and failure is to be avoided.
- Identifying and rapidly treating the underlying cause of sepsis ('source control') is fundamental.
- Radiological intervention for localised sepsis is often key and a logistical challenge for health services to provide on a round-the-clock basis.
- Indications for laparotomy include generalised peritonitis, tissue necrosis, multifocal abscesses and failure of radiological intervention.
- Re-laparotomy is often difficult and advanced techniques may be required.
- Intra-abdominal hypertension and abdominal compartment syndrome are probably under-recognised. Medical management has a role, but in refractory cases surgical abdominal decompression will be required.
- Intestinal fistulas can occur following any abdominal intervention, but are more common after emergency surgery. Prompt eradication of sepsis and attention to nutrition is key. Definitive surgery to correct the fistula should be deferred until the patient is well and the anatomy has been clearly defined.
- Abdominal sepsis often runs a prolonged course and the surgeon must play a central role in coordinating management.

⊕ Full references available at **http://expertconsult. inkling.com**

Key references

1. Scottish Audit of Surgical Mortality 2010. http:// www.sasm.org.uk/Publications/SASM_Annual_ Report_2010.pdf.

   This report reviews all inpatient deaths under the care of surgical teams and highlights the high mortality rate associated with emergency abdominal surgery.

2. Singer M, Deutschman CS, Seymour CW, et al. The Third International Consensus Definitions for Sepsis and Septic Shock (Sepsis-3). JAMA 2016; 315(8):801–10. PMID: 26903338.

   Updated definitions of sepsis and septic shock.

15. Dellinger RP, Levy MM, Carlet JM, et al. Surviving Sepsis Campaign: international guidelines for management of severe sepsis and septic shock: 2008. Crit Care Med 2008;36(1):296–327. PMID: 18158437.

   Evidence-based guidelines for diagnosis and treatment of patients with sepsis.

25. Buck DL, Vester-Andersen M, Møller MH, et al. Surgical delay is a critical determinant of survival in perforated peptic ulcer. Br J Surg 2013;100(8):1045– 9. PMID: 23754645.

   This Danish cohort study reported increased mortality with every extra hour of delay to reaching theatre.

31. Anderson ID, Fearon KC, Grant IS. Laparotomy for abdominal sepsis in the critically ill. Br J Surg 1996;83(4):535–9. PMID: 8665253.

   This study of repeat laparotomies on patients on ICU reported increased complications and diminishing benefits to subsequent surgery.

44. Teubner A, Anderson ID, Scott NA, et al. Intra- abdominal hypertension and the abdominal compartment syndrome. (Br J Surg 2004;91:1102–10). Br J Surg 2004;91(11):1527. PMID: 15499645.

   Describes the problem of abdominal compartment syndrome, how to recognise it and how to treat it.

49. Harris C, Nicholson DA, Anderson ID. Computed tomography: a vital adjunct in the management of complex postoperative sepsis. Br J Surg 1998;85:861–2.

   Radiological diagnosis and treatment of sepsis in patients with an enterocutaneous fistula is key to optimal outcome.

Complications of bariatric surgery presenting to the general surgeon and considerations for the general surgeon when operating on the obese patient

Bruce R. Tulloh
Andrew C. de Beaux

Introduction

Obesity is now a global health problem, placing an enormous health burden on our society because of the medical comorbidities that are associated with it, including type II diabetes, hypertension, dyslipidaemia, steatohepatitis, obstructive sleep apnoea, arthritis of the weight-bearing joints, gastro-oesophageal reflux, depression and infertility. In general, these medical problems improve or even resolve in parallel with weight loss. Surgery specifically aimed at weight loss ('bariatric' surgery, from the Greek word *baros* = weight, *iatrikos* = medical) has been developing since the 1950s and in the last 25 years, in the wake of advances in laparoscopy, bariatric surgery has become increasingly popular. Surgery remains the only way to produce significant, sustainable weight loss and improvement/resolution of comorbidities in the morbidly obese and indeed improve life expectancy in this group.[1-3] Most bariatric surgery is now performed in centres staffed by surgeons with a specific bariatric interest, usually as part of a multidisciplinary team.

✔✔ Bariatric surgery is the only method of producing long-term, reliable and significant weight loss with resolution of the associated morbidities of morbid obesity.[2]

Although the number of hospitals providing a bariatric service in the UK is undoubtedly growing, as in many other countries, many patients still have to travel long distances for their surgery – some even going overseas to other countries. Procedures are generally performed using laparoscopic techniques and lengths of stay are short. In the event of postoperative complications, patients can therefore present back to their local hospital or clinic, perhaps far from the hospital where the surgery was performed, where there may be no specialist knowledge or expertise in the field. The aim of this chapter is to inform general surgeons of the disease processes underlying obesity, the current bariatric procedures which are commonly performed, to outline the common complications that may arise from these operations and to provide management guidance for those patients that present in an emergency setting.[4-6] As the incidence of obesity in most countries is rising and such patients will present for other general surgical procedures, specific considerations that help such operations will also be discussed.

Causes of obesity

While obesity is the result of a chronic energy imbalance when food (calorie) intake exceeds energy expenditure, such an explanation on its own is too simplistic. Obesity should be considered a multifactorial socio-psycho-endocrine disease process.

It is now clear that there is a complex physiological adipostatic system in place that works to maintain a constant body weight in the face of daily fluctuations in energy balance.[7] The hypothalamus is an important control centre for this process, integrating a variety of both short-term and long-term energy flux signals. The gastrointestinal (GI) tract produces a number of hormones including ghrelin, glucagon-like peptides (GLP)-1 and 2, peptide tyrosine-tyrosine, insulin and cholecystokinin, which not only influence gut motility and exocrine secretions but also exert positive and negative feedback on the hypothalamus to regulate appetite. Ghrelin, the 'hunger hormone', is released from the gastric body and promotes appetite, while leptin, a hormone that circulates in proportion to the body's fat mass, has a negative feedback on the hypothalamus to promote negative energy balance. Neural pathways are also involved via vagally innervated stretch receptors in the stomach wall, which induce satiety (and even nausea) in response to gastric distension.

There are also social and psychological drivers to eat. Eating is a pleasurable activity and, for many, meals are the hub of family and social events. Eating may also provide comfort to address fear, loneliness or anxiety. There is now evidence that such negative emotions increase food consumption and that obese people eat in response to emotions more than normal-weight people.[8]

Dieting is known to be difficult and, for many, is not successful in the long term.[9] Modern human beings have evolved from nomadic hunter-gatherers and our physiology defaults to energy storing in periods of food shortage. Thus dieting induces a physiological adaptation to starvation. This stimulates appetite, induces the bowel to absorb a greater proportion of food eaten, reduces energy loss by a subtle lowering of body temperature and promotes fat storage.

Surgery is the most effective treatment for severe and complex obesity because it alters the physiological processes at the heart of weight homeostasis. Different procedures do this in different ways.[10]

Mechanisms of weight loss surgery

Traditionally, weight loss operations have been described as either restrictive or malabsorptive, influencing either the volume of food that can be ingested or the absorption of food at the mucosal level, respectively (or both). However, it is more likely that surgery interacts in a beneficial way with the complex adipostatic system outlined above.[10] Patients with gastric bands, for example, who are restricted in their oral intake by the constricting ring around their upper stomach, do not show the normal hormonal adaptation to starving. Part of the band's action appears to be through feedback to the adipostat, possibly via vagal afferents. Similarly, patients undergoing a so-called malabsorptive operation, such as gastric bypass, do not suffer chronic diarrhoea; their weight loss is mediated by a series of gut hormonal changes that influence appetite, food choices and gut motility, amongst other things.

Even so, iatrogenic manipulations of the adipostat are not the full story. In order to achieve the best outcomes, patients still need to make a series of healthy dietary and lifestyle changes along the lines of eating sensibly and being physically active. Most authorities agree that postoperative weight maintenance is improved by the ongoing encouragement, advice and support obtained from long-term follow-up in a bariatric clinic.[11-13]

While weight control is a complex process, the mechanisms behind the postoperative resolution of obesity-related comorbidities are also complex and, even now, not fully understood. Control of type II diabetes mellitus, for example, is known to improve in parallel with the gradual weight loss that follows gastric band surgery.[14] However, the gastric bypass and duodenal switch operations can normalise glucose tolerance much more quickly, even before there has been any appreciable weight loss.[15,16] Such changes are mediated by gut hormones that are stimulated either by a lack of nutrients in the foregut or by the rapid post-prandial delivery of food to the hindgut, with a resultant improvement in pancreatic function and a reduction in peripheral insulin resistance. These processes are well explained elsewhere[7,15,17] and will not be expanded upon here.

Bariatric operations

The commonest weight loss procedures performed around the world at present are the gastric band, the gastric bypass and the sleeve gastrectomy. In very obese patients, an alternative operation is the duodenal switch procedure. The main endoscopic option at present is insertion of a gastric balloon, with newer procedures such as the endoscopic duodenojejunal barrier and gastric plication on the horizon. Implantable neuroregulatory devices (gastric 'pacemakers') represent a new direction for surgical weight control by harnessing neural feedback signals to help control eating.

The reason that so many options exist is because no procedure is perfect. Each brings its own benefits and risks. There is little evidence to indicate which operation suits which patient, although most series demonstrate greater average weight loss from operations with a 'malabsorptive' component over 'restrictive' operations alone.[13,18] In practice, the final choice of operation emerges from a detailed discussion between the patient and their surgeon about the options available and the potential risks and benefits of each one.

Gastric band

The gastric band is an inflatable silicone ring fixed around the proximal stomach to create a zone of

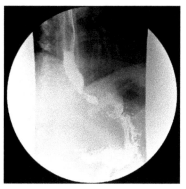

Figure 21.1 • Barium meal showing band sitting at a normal angle of approx 45°, in the 8-to-2 o'clock direction.

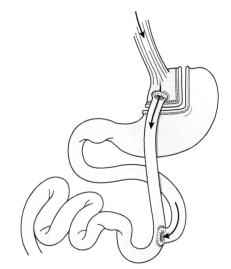

Figure 21.2 • Diagram of a gastric bypass.

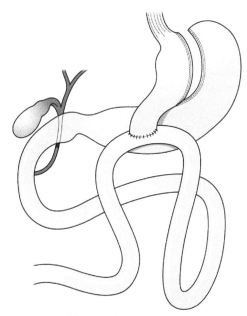

Figure 21.3 • Diagram of a mini-gastric bypass.

constriction with a small proximal gastric pouch of approximately 30 mL. The band sits around the angle of His, runs along the line of the left crus of the diaphragm and typically lies at about 45° to the horizontal in the 8-to-2 o'clock direction (**Fig. 21.1**). Many surgeons secure the band in position with a number of gastro-gastric sutures from the fundus below the band up on to the small gastric pouch. The band connects by tubing to an injection port, which is then secured subcutaneously on the anterior abdominal wall. Instillation or aspiration of saline via the subcutaneous injection port adjusts the degree of constriction produced by the band. The amount of saline required in the band varies from patient to patient and often a number of fine adjustments are needed to achieve just the right level of restriction so that patients can manage small portions of normal food.

Roux-en-Y gastric bypass

This is the most common bariatric operation now performed worldwide. The first step involves using the linear cutting stapler to separate a small proximal gastric pouch, again approximately 30 mL in volume, from the distal stomach, which is left in situ. The small bowel is then divided 50–100 cm beyond the duodenojejunal (DJ) flexure and the distal side anastomosed to the gastric pouch, in an antecolic or retrocolic position. The proximal side, representing the biliopancreatic limb of the Roux-en-Y reconstruction, is anastomosed 100–150 cm distal to the gastrojejunostomy (**Fig. 21.2**). Any mesenteric defects are closed to prevent subsequent internal herniation.

Mini-gastric bypass

A more recent modification of the gastric bypass is the mini-gastric bypass, so called because it

is quicker and easier to perform. The essential differences between this and a conventional bypass are that a longer gastric pouch is created and a Polya-type antecolic loop gastrojejunostomy, rather than a Roux-en-Y configuration, is constructed (**Fig. 21.3**). Early results are satisfactory but long-term outcome data are lacking.

Sleeve gastrectomy

This operation was originally developed as the first stage of a duodenal switch operation but soon

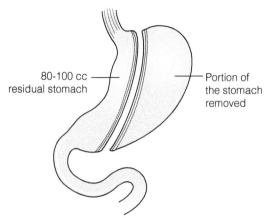

Figure 21.4 • Diagram of sleeve gastrectomy. The omentum (not shown) is preserved on the gastro-epiploic arcade.

became a stand-alone procedure when its weight loss outcomes were, at least initially, similar to what was achievable with a gastric bypass.[19] It is also technically easier to perform than any of the Roux-en-Y procedures, particularly in super-obese patients. The greater curve of the stomach is separated from the omentum from the angle of His to a point 5–6 cm proximal to the pylorus. A bougie, commonly around 34 French in size, is inserted down to the antrum and manipulated up against the lesser curve. Using a linear cutting stapler and with the bougie as a guide, the body and fundus of the stomach are excised and removed (**Fig. 21.4**).

Duodenal switch

The duodenal switch, or biliopancreatic diversion (BPD) operation, can be performed as a two-stage procedure but is more commonly carried out in one sitting.[20] The first stage is a conventional sleeve gastrectomy. The second stage involves dividing the duodenum just distal to the pylorus and then dividing the small bowel halfway between the DJ flexure and the ileo-caecal junction. The distal part of the divided small bowel is then anastomosed to the proximal end of the divided duodenum just beyond the gastric outlet (pylorus). Thus the jejunum is 'switched' for the duodenum. The biliopancreatic (Roux) limb of the divided small bowel is then joined to the ileum 1 metre proximal to the ileocaecal valve. This creates a longer bypassed segment and a much shorter common channel than a standard gastric bypass procedure, resulting in significantly more malabsorption.

Intragastric balloon

This plastic balloon is inserted endoscopically and inflated with saline under vision to between 500

and 700 mL (**Fig. 21.5**). This induces a feeling of fullness and thus reduces oral intake. Because the satiety effect wanes after several months, combined with a small risk of leakage/deflation in situ, with the associated possibility of distal migration of the collapsed balloon, it is recommended that the balloon is removed after 6 months. Removal involves another endoscopic procedure in which the balloon is punctured, aspirated and withdrawn.

> ✔ There is little evidence to indicate which operation suits which patient, although most series demonstrate greater average weight loss from operations with a 'malabsorptive' component over 'restrictive' operations alone.[13]

Older, more obsolete operations

Jejuno-ileal bypass (JIB)

It is rare to see patients with an intact jejuno-ileal bypass today. This operation involved anastomosing the proximal jejunum to the terminal ileum less than 100 cm from the ileocaecal valve. It gained popularity between the 1950s and 1970s before the emergence of the Roux-en-Y gastric bypass operation. The jejuno-ileal bypass resulted in significant protein malabsorption and vitamin/mineral deficiency, with the long blind jejunal limb commonly leading to bacterial overgrowth. Patients were prone to liver failure as a result of both protein malnutrition and toxaemia from bacterial overgrowth in the blind loop.[11] The majority of patients, if still alive, have had their operations reversed.

Vertical banded gastroplasty (VBG)

This operation gained popularity in the 1980s and early 1990s but its high failure rate, and the advent of better procedures, have resulted in it being abandoned. Just above the incisura, a short distance in from the lesser curve, the anterior and posterior walls of the stomach were stapled together with a

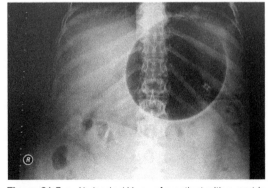

Figure 21.5 • Abdominal X-ray of a patient with a gastric balloon in situ.

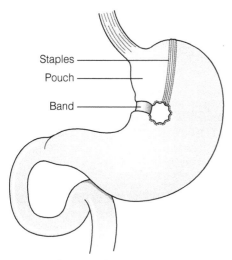

Figure 21.6 • Diagram of the vertical banded gastroplasty (VBG) procedure.

circular stapler. Through the resultant hole made by the stapler, a linear stapler could be applied vertically towards the angle of His. This staple line fixed the anterior and posterior gastric walls together but did not divide the stomach. The outlet of the small gastric pouch thus created was then 'banded' with a 360° ring of tape to prevent dilatation (**Fig. 21.6**). The high failure rate resulted from pouch outlet stenosis and/or pouch dilatation (usually caused by overeating) which was often followed by disruption of the vertical staple line with the consequent loss of restriction to eating.

Newer procedures

Endoscopic duodenojejunal sleeve
This endoscopically inserted tube of thin, impervious plastic material has its proximal end secured to the mucosa of the first part of the duodenum with small barbs and then runs distally, effectively lining the duodenum and upper small bowel, preventing ingested food from making contact with the mucosa until the proximal jejunum is reached. Its effect on the gut hormone milieu mimics that of the gastric bypass and early clinical results have shown a similar improvement in type II diabetes control, along with modest weight loss.[21] At present it is suggested that such barriers be removed at around 1 year. As yet, however, no long-term follow-up information is available regarding the extent of weight regain or the return of glucose intolerance after the barrier is removed.

Gastric plication
Reducing the size of the stomach either endoscopically or laparoscopically has been described where the greater curve of the stomach at the fundus is invaginated to reduce gastric volume.[22] Infolding the gastric wall in this way may also provide stimulation of mural stretch receptors to reduce hunger. Endoscopically this can be performed by firing a series of staples or clips that 'gather' the stomach wall from the inside.[23] Outcomes are not yet known, but the same technology has been described previously for plicating the gastro-oesophageal junction for treating reflux where, despite early successes, long-term results have been disappointing.

Implantable neuroregulators (gastric 'pacemakers')
A number of laparoscopically implantable devices are now undergoing trials. They register the presence of food in the stomach and are designed to mediate satiety by vagal feedback. Lack of outcome data in addition to concerns about battery life and cost are currently a block to their more widespread use.

Complications of bariatric surgery

There are *general* complications such as might follow any abdominal operation, and *specific* complications that relate to the procedure performed.

General complications

It should be within the capability of any abdominal surgeon to manage the general complications of bariatric surgery, which include pulmonary atelectasis/pneumonia, intra-abdominal bleeding, anastomotic or staple-line leak with or without abscess formation, deep vein thrombosis (DVT)/pulmonary embolus and superficial wound infections. Patients may be expected to present with malaise, pallor, features of sepsis or obvious wound problems. However, clinical features may be difficult to recognise owing to body habitus. Abdominal distension, tenderness and guarding may be impossible to determine clinically due to the patient's obesity. Pallor is non-specific and fever and leucocytosis may be absent. Wound collections may also be very deep. These complications in a bariatric patient should be actively sought with appropriate investigations. In particular, it is vital for life-threatening complications such as bleeding, sepsis and bowel obstruction to be recognised promptly and treated appropriately. A persistent tachycardia may be the only sign heralding significant complications and should always be taken seriously.[24]

It is useful to classify complications as 'early', 'medium' and 'late' because, from the receiving clinician's point of view, the differential diagnosis will differ accordingly (Table 21.1). Early complications usually arise within the first few days of surgery but, with ever-advancing laparoscopic surgery and shorter lengths of stay, these may still present to the non-bariatric surgeon after the patient has left the specialist centre.

Specific complications

These relate to the procedure performed. Again, they may be grouped into 'early', 'medium' and 'late', although the 'early' complications overlap with the general complications mentioned above. Medium-term complications are likely to arise while the patient is still overweight and thus may be difficult to diagnose. Late complications may develop many years later. Patients at this stage may be of normal weight, and therefore a link to their previous bariatric surgery may not be obvious (Table 21.2).

Table 21.1 • General complications following bariatric surgery (similar to those that may arise following any GI operation)

Early	Medium or late

Bleeding:
  Intraluminal (staple/
  suture line)
  Intraperitoneal (staple/suture
  line, mesentery, omentum,
  liver/spleen injury)
  Subcutaneous (trocar site)
Staple/suture line leak
Inadvertent GI tract perforation
Port-site haematoma/infection
DVT/pulmonary embolism
Anaesthetic drug reaction, etc.
Chest infection/atelectasis
Port-site hernia with or without
bowel obstruction
	Chest infection
	DVT/pulmonary embolism
	Haematoma or abscess
	Incisional or port-site
	hernia

GI, gastrointestinal; DVT, deep venous thrombosis.

Table 21.2 • Specific complications of bariatric surgery: early, medium and late

Procedure	Early	Medium	Late
Band	Gastric perforation Liver/spleen injury with bleeding	Slippage (with or without gastric necrosis) Injection-port migration or infection	Slippage Erosion Injection-port problems Mega-oesophagus
Sleeve	Reflux oesophagitis Staple-line bleed or leak Splenic infarct Omental necrosis	Intra-abdominal abscess or haematoma	Fistula Stenosis of sleeve
Bypass/duodenal switch/ BPD	Anastomosis/staple-line bleed or leak Small-bowel enterotomy Early small-bowel obstruction	Intra-abdominal abscess or haematoma Roux limb obstruction Biliopancreatic (blind) loop obstruction	SBO (internal hernia, volvulus, adhesions) Anastomotic ulcer Anastomotic stricture Dumping syndrome Micronutrient malnutrition Gastro-gastric fistula Hypoglycaemia
Mini-gastric bypass	As above	As above	As above plus bile reflux
Intragastric balloon	Nausea/vomiting Gastric ulceration Gastric or oesophageal perforation	Dehydration and electrolyte imbalance Reflux oesophagitis	Bowel obstruction from deflated balloon
VBG JIB		Stomal stenosis Bowel obstruction (internal hernia, adhesions)	Staple-line disruption Malnutrition Blind loop syndrome Liver failure

Table 21.2 • Specific complications of bariatric surgery: early, medium and late—Cont'd

Procedure	Early	Medium	Late
Duodenal barrier	Duodenal bleeding Duodenal perforation	Dumping syndrome Food bolus obstruction Migration of the device with mechanical bowel obstruction	Unknown
Gastric plication	Bleeding Splenic or liver injury	–	–
Gastric pacing	Nausea/vomiting Infection of subcutaneous implant	–	–

BPD, biliopancreatic diversion; SBO, small bowel obstruction; VBG, vertical banded gastroplasty; JIB, jejunoileal bypass.

Clinical presentation

Once the receiving clinician understands the operation that has been performed and the specific complications to look out for, the next step is the interpretation of the presenting clinical features and formulation of a management plan.

Gastric band patients

Vomiting and/or dysphagia

These are very common and not surprising symptoms, considering that the band works by causing a constriction ring around the upper stomach. Band patients are accustomed to a degree of dysphagia and occasional vomiting, so for them to present for medical attention implies that it is 'worse than usual'. These symptoms indicate a degree of obstruction at the level of the band and there are three main causes.

Band too tight

Has the patient had an adjustment recently? Perhaps they have a food bolus obstruction. Once the patient begins to vomit, the gastric wall becomes oedematous within the confines of the band and the apparent obstruction becomes worse. The treatment is urgent band decompression using the subcutaneous injection port (see Box 21.1 and **Fig. 21.7**). Once the patient can drink freely they can be discharged, with arrangement for follow-up by their bariatric specialist team.

Acute band 'slippage'

This is the term commonly used to describe what is really a process of gastric prolapse upwards through the band. It typically occurs months or years after the original operation and is possibly more common when no gastro-gastric tunnelling sutures are used to secure the band in place. The patient usually presents with vomiting, often in association

Box 21.1 • Urgent percutaneous band decompression

The subcutaneous injection port should be palpable beneath the skin on the abdominal wall, usually close to one of the longer laparoscopic scars. Some surgeons place it over the lower sternum. The patient usually knows where it is. Using a strict aseptic technique, the port is steadied between the fingers of one hand while the other holds an empty 10-mL syringe with needle attached. Ideally a non-coring 'Huber' or spinal needle is used so as not to damage the port, but in an emergency a conventional 23-gauge hypodermic needle works well (although it may not be long enough). Entering at right-angles to the skin, the rubber diaphragm of the port is punctured. The needle hits the metal base-plate with a 'clunk' and aspiration can begin. The reservoir is aspirated to dryness; it may contain up to 14 mL. The needle is simply withdrawn when finished and a small dressing applied.

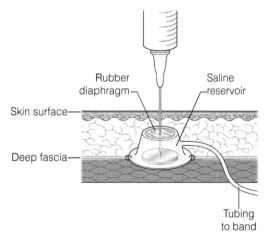

Figure 21.7 • Diagram of needle access to the subcutaneous injection port. Strict aseptic technique is important and a non-coring Huber needle should be used.

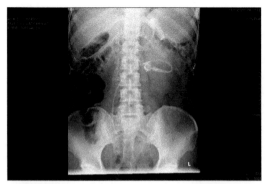

Figure 21.8 • Abdominal X-ray of an acute band slip. The band lies 90° out of alignment (compare with Fig. 21.1).

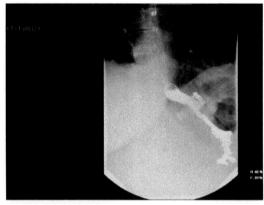

Figure 21.9 • Barium swallow demonstrating band erosion. Note the barium leaking out around the band (compare with Fig. 21.1).

with being able to eat a sizeable meal, as the food accumulates in the large gastric pouch above the band before eventually being regurgitated. Urgent decompression often provides relief but if not, then an urgent contrast swallow should be ordered. Slippage is often evident on a plain abdominal or chest X-rays, with the band lying at an unusual angle (see **Fig. 21.8**), although a contrast swallow provides more conclusive information. The most serious complication of band slippage is ischaemic necrosis of the prolapsed fundus, secondary to distension and/or occlusion of the blood supply to the proximal stomach as it passes through the band. Failure of the symptoms to resolve with percutaneous band decompression is an indication for urgent surgical intervention.

The operation to remove the band is generally by laparoscopy. The tight band must be released. Unclipping it may be difficult, especially laparoscopically, but if possible – and if the stomach is viable – then it may be left in situ for an experienced bariatric surgeon to re-position at a later date. An alternative to unclipping the band is simply to cut it in half, after which it should be removed. Once local adhesions have been divided the band should just slide out. If there is gastric necrosis then laparotomy and some form of gastrectomy will be required along with complete removal of the band, tubing and injection port.

Band erosion

This is not usually an acute problem but presentation may be precipitated by an aggravation of dysphagia with or without pain and sepsis. Symptoms will not improve after percutaneous band decompression. An urgent contrast swallow may also demonstrate band erosion with leakage of contrast around the band (see **Fig. 21.9**) but the most definitive test for erosion is gastroscopy, where a portion of the white silicone band will be visible from within the lumen.

Patients should be referred back to the relevant bariatric team for removal of the band, which is usually possible laparoscopically (see above), leaving a drain to the area. A gastric fistula may result, but this will usually settle with non-operative management.

Abdominal pain

This is uncommon in band patients (as a result of the band) and so should alert the clinician to a serious problem such as visceral distension from acute slippage (see above), inflammation related to band erosion (see above), peritonitis from gastric necrosis with or without perforation or postoperative haematoma. If the symptoms are of recent onset (hours) and pain is a prominent feature, necrosis and/or perforation should be suspected and urgent imaging is required, followed by laparoscopy with or without laparotomy if necessary. Peritonitis is an unlikely consequence of band erosion but may occur with gastric necrosis (acute band slippage) or perhaps foreign body perforation of the gastric pouch.

Chest pain

This is a common reason for anyone to present to the hospital emergency department and cardiac causes need to be excluded. In patients with a gastric band, the possibility of band slippage, erosion and reflux oesophagitis (secondary to a tight band) needs to be considered.

Mega-oesophagus

This is the result of long-standing, excessive restriction and usually follows either a period of excessive band tightness, or chronic malpositioning due to band slippage. It is recognised on a contrast swallow. It usually improves over a period of several weeks following band decompression but may necessitate band removal to prevent recurrence.

Port problems

Migration
The subcutaneous injection port may move about within its subcutaneous pocket, depending on how well it has been fixed in position. This makes it difficult to access for percutaneous needle aspiration and if it has flipped over completely, the band will be impossible to decompress.

Leakage
Repeated attempts to needle the subcutaneous reservoir should be avoided as damage to the rubber diaphragm or perforation/rupture of the tubing can produce a slow leak.

Infection
The injection port may become infected through breach of sterile technique; this may present as abdominal wall cellulitis or an abscess. An infected port will need to be removed but can be replaced at a later date when the sepsis has completely cleared. Sometimes an infected subcutaneous port may be the first manifestation of band erosion (see above), as the tubing effectively acts as a conduit to convey infected material from the eroded band to the skin surface.

Skin erosion
The port may also erode through the skin surface (**Fig. 21.10**). While not an emergency, this situation may present to the general surgeon. Again, plans will need to be made for removal, then later replacement, of the injection port.

Sleeve gastrectomy patients

Early postoperative reflux/vomiting and dysphagia are common as the narrow and oedematous gastric sleeve tends to empty poorly at first. Some degree of reflux oesophagitis is common. Patients are usually discharged from hospital on proton-pump inhibitor (PPI) medication with instructions to adhere to a fluid diet, gradually thickening their intake over several weeks. However, if the problem is severe or associated with early signs of dehydration, then specific complications should be sought.

Staple-line leak or bleed
Any disruption of the staple line along the narrow sleeve of remaining stomach is likely to cause luminal compression, either from oedema or direct pressure such as from a collection or haematoma. A contrast swallow or computed tomography (CT) should demonstrate this, although both imaging modalities may be falsely negative. Furthermore, some obese patients may be too large for the scanner or X-ray table. If there is reasonable clinical concern of a staple-line leak or bleed, perhaps because of grumbling sepsis or worsening anaemia, laparoscopy should be arranged as this is likely to both confirm the diagnosis and allow repair/control/drainage as necessary. A careful gastroscopy could also be considered.

Splenic infarction
As the greater omentum is separated from the fundus of the stomach it is possible to take one or more apical splenic vessels, leading to segmental infarction. This will present as left upper quadrant pain with or without some features of sepsis. A contrast CT should demonstrate this. Non-operative management is usually always successful.

Omental necrosis
The blood supply to the omentum may be compromised if the gastro-epiploic arcade is damaged as it is separated from the stomach. Ischaemic necrosis may be the result, presenting with abdominal pain and features of sepsis. Surgical debridement of the necrotic tissue may be required, depending on the extent of infarction, either laparoscopically or by open surgery.

Sleeve stenosis
This is usually a late complication of a staple-line problem but may be evident within the first week postoperatively if an intense local inflammatory reaction is established, usually following an otherwise undetected leak. After imaging as above, rehydration and possibly nutritional support are all that is initially required. At a later date, once any evidence of active perforation or leak has settled, endoscopic dilatation may help, although this brings its own risk of causing further disruption/perforation. Completion sub-total gastrectomy with conversion to a Roux-en-Y bypass may ultimately be required.

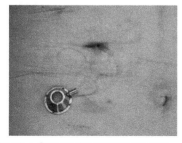

Figure 21.10 • Port erosion through the skin.

Gastric bypass/duodenal switch patients

Staple-line leak

These operations have several staple lines to consider: the gastric pouch, the gastrojejunal anastomosis, the gastric remnant (in a gastric bypass) and the more distal jejuno-jejunostomy. Only the first two of these can be imaged on a contrast swallow. CT may show the others but the receiving surgeon should have a low threshold for returning the patient to theatre for laparoscopy if a leak is suspected. It should be remembered that a tachycardia or elevated C-reactive protein (CRP) may be the only evidence of such a problem in obese patients. If more than 48–72 hours have elapsed since the initial operation, then laparoscopic repair is less likely to be feasible and laparotomy may be required. Surgical treatment should address drainage of sepsis, control of any ongoing leakage and the provision of nutrition (Box 21.2).

Staple-line bleed

Patients may bleed into the GI tract or into the peritoneal cavity. A bleed into the 'blind' gastric remnant after a bypass will only be evident on CT, or by early return to the operating theatre (see Box 21.3). Treatment involves establishing drainage of the collection of the haematoma by gastrotomy and controlling the bleeding point, usually by oversewing the staple line. Placement of a transcutaneous gastrostomy tube is wise, not only to decompress the stomach but also to use for later nutritional support if required. Angiographic embolisation of the bleeding point may be an

alternative but the surgeon must not allow the inherent delays of such intervention to postpone what might be life-saving re-operative surgery.

Small-bowel enterotomy

Full-thickness injury to the small bowel can easily be incurred as a result of handling with instruments and perforations may occur 'off-camera', out of the laparoscopic field of view. Missed enterotomies may take several days to become apparent, usually presenting with increasing abdominal pain, tachycardia and fever. Enteric fluid may leak out from one or more of the laparoscopic port sites. CT may demonstrate free intraperitoneal fluid and even intraperitoneal gas, but these findings are non-specific. Return to theatre for laparoscopy or laparotomy and drainage/repair is required.

Early small-bowel obstruction

Early postoperative small-bowel obstruction is uncommon after laparoscopic surgery and should not immediately be attributed to a paralytic ileus. Port-site bowel herniation, often of the Richter type, is always a possibility but after operations involving Roux-en-Y reconstruction one should always consider internal herniation, small-bowel volvulus and iatrogenic jejuno-jejunal anastomotic stricture or distortion. Vomiting will be absent if the blind gastroduodenal limb is obstructed and abdominal X-rays may be unreliable, especially in a morbidly obese patient. CT is indicated (**Fig. 21.11**). The treating surgeon should not delay operating to correct an established obstruction.

Late small-bowel obstruction

Small-bowel obstruction arising months or years after laparoscopic gastric bypass is a well-recognised problem. A frequent cause is internal herniation, occurring in up to 5% of cases if the mesenteric

---

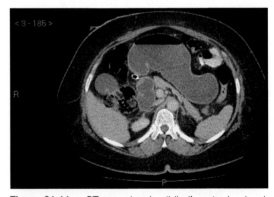

Figure 21.11 • CT scan showing 'blind' gastroduodenal biliopancreatic limb obstruction. Note the dilated, fluid-filled stomach and duodenum and the oral contrast in the non-distended alimentary limb.

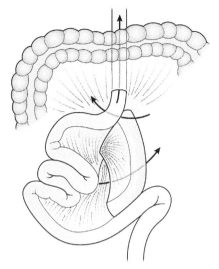

Figure 21.12 • The three common sites for internal hernia after Roux-en-Y reconstruction: the mesocolic defect, Petersen's space and the jejunal mesenteric window.

defects are not closed.[25] Closure of the defects appears to reduce the risk of internal herniation.[26] Hernias typically develop through the mesocolic defect if the retrocolic route is used, the jejunal mesenteric defect at the site of jejuno-jejunostomy, and Petersen's space between the alimentary limb and the transverse colon (see **Fig. 21.12**). For many patients the presentation is insidious, with post-prandial pain and/or bloating. Imaging may not reveal significant small-bowel dilatation. Laparoscopy is the investigation and treatment of choice, where chyle within the abdominal cavity is a clue to the diagnosis. The ileocaecal junction is identified first and then the small bowel is carefully 'walked' back until the point of internal herniation is seen and reduced. The defect is then closed with non-absorbable material to prevent recurrence.

Gastro-gastric fistula

This is a consideration in the medium to long term if a patient develops weight regain. It may also present with dysphagia or pain on eating. It is often associated with stomal ulcers in the gastric pouch, which prove resistant to acid suppression medication, and likely arises following a staple-line leak with abscess formation that discharges into the gastric remnant. The treatment is surgical to divide the fistula and resect some of the distal stomach. This may be achievable laparoscopically.

Dumping syndrome

A recognised complication of gastric resectional surgery, this syndrome comprises post-prandial cramping abdominal pain, nausea, sweating,

light-headedness and sleepiness. It reflects hyperinsulinaemic hypoglycaemia, usually precipitated by a high carbohydrate load in the jejunum from rapid gastric emptying,[27] although it is also described after Nissen fundoplication where vagal injury is the likely cause.[28] Mild forms are common and it is rarely severe enough to present as a surgical emergency, but surgeons should nevertheless be aware of it as a cause of post-bypass malaise. Dietary regulation, medication to slow gut motility and/or somatostatin analogues generally provide relief.

Mini-gastric bypass patients

A similar spectrum of complications can be expected as might follow a Roux-en-Y bypass or duodenal switch. However, because of the loop gastrojejunostomy, bile reflux can be a problem – especially if the efferent limb takes a long time to function.[29] Prolonged nasogastric drainage and nutritional support may be required, with or without the addition of somatostatin analogues or other agents to reduce secretions. If the problem is intractable, conversion to a Roux-en-Y configuration may be necessary.

Gastric balloon patients

Nausea and vomiting are almost universal symptoms after balloon insertion but usually subside by the end of the first week. Patients may need intravenous hydration, PPI medication and parenteral anti-emetics over this time. A small minority of patients cannot tolerate oral intake even after several weeks and, in this group, early balloon removal should be offered and will provide instant relief. Although special equipment is produced for balloon removal, it can easily be performed by using a standard endoscopic injection needle (to puncture and empty the balloon) and some strong grasping forceps, or a snare, to remove the deflated balloon.

Abdominal or chest pain is uncommon and should raise the possibility of reflux oesophagitis, gastric ulceration or even gastric/oesophageal perforation. If relief is not obtained with hydration, PPI and anti-emetic medication, then gastroscopy is warranted – although urgent CT is the preferred investigation if perforation is a serious consideration.

Gastric plication patients

Whether this is done laparoscopically or endoscopically, the procedure-specific risks include gastric trauma (bleeding or perforation), liver/spleen trauma incurred by traction, direct pressure or injury and perforation of the stomach.[22]

Patients with older, now obsolete operations

As patients will have had their operations many years earlier, only late complications will arise. These include exacerbations of long-standing problems such as blind loop syndrome following a JIB and pouch outlet stenosis after a VBG. Nutritional deficiencies, which may manifest in many ways, are also possible complications (see below).

Other postoperative problems

Gallstones

Dramatic weight loss from any cause promotes gallstone formation owing to mobilisation of cholesterol from peripheral fat stores and changes to the enterohepatic cycle. Patients may present with biliary colic, cholecystitis, pancreatitis or obstructive jaundice and should be managed according to established protocols. Laparoscopic cholecystectomy is generally no more difficult after a bariatric surgical operation than otherwise, but the management of common bile duct stones can be problematic because endoscopic retrograde cholangiopancreatography (ERCP) may be impossible if there has been a previous bypass or duodenal switch/BPD. Intraoperative cholangiography is therefore recommended at the time of cholecystectomy, with concurrent surgical common bile duct exploration if required.

Nutritional deficiencies

The common nutritional deficiencies seen in the bariatric surgery population concern thiamine, iron, zinc, vitamin D and vitamin B_{12}. These may have been present preoperatively, in which case replenishment can be difficult, especially if a malabsorptive-type operation has been done. It is common practice for all patients following bariatric surgery to take daily oral vitamin supplements long term. Nevertheless, clinical features of various deficiency syndromes are well documented but, like the neurological manifestations of thiamine deficiency presenting as Wernicke–Korsakoff's syndrome, may not be readily recognised by general surgeons. If one deficiency is diagnosed then others should be sought.[30] These are of particular importance if re-operative surgery is planned because of the possible detrimental effects that nutritional deficiencies might have on wound healing. A good principle is to replenish essential vitamins (especially thiamine) in any patient who

is admitted with complications following bariatric surgery which have resulted in a significant reduction in nutritional intake.

Failure to lose weight

Even the best operations do not work for everyone. While most patients do well in the first few months after surgery, and for many the weight loss is maintained indefinitely as they adopt a new and healthy lifestyle, some degree of late weight regain is very common. This rarely means that the operation has been done incorrectly or failed in some way, although this should be excluded first: bands may become too loose, gastric pouches may stretch, staple lines may disrupt, bypassed bowel may adapt. More usually, however, weight regain reflects a re-emergence of underlying poor eating behaviours – in other words, patients tend to slip back into their old eating habits.[31] Ongoing follow-up with the multidisciplinary bariatric team is important to both prevent and manage postoperative weight regain.[11–13]

Considerations when operating on the obese patient

Obese patients present numerous challenges for surgical as well as anaesthetic and nursing staff, both in the theatre and the wards. For example, obesity has been shown to adversely affect length of operation, hospital stay and postoperative morbidity with gastric cancer resections, without any influence on long-term survival.[32] There are very few open or laparoscopic operations that are not made more difficult, or not associated with more operative morbidity and mortality with increasing BMI. In addition to the comorbidities associated with obesity, obesity itself can influence surgical management at all stages of the perioperative pathway for which a number of extra measures may be helpful and will be outlined here.

Preoperative measures

Specific preoperative counselling as part of the consent process is required to help with the decision-making for the patient to undergo an operation, in view of the increased risk of complications. Areas to consider include the following.

Anaesthesia

Difficult airway access; high airway pressures required (risk of alveolar barotrauma); difficult IV access; tailoring drug doses (especially fat-soluble drugs that may be sequestered in the adipose tissue); positioning and securing on the operating table.[33]

Surgery

Access/visibility, higher risk of conversion of laparoscopic procedures, larger open wounds, higher risk of wound breakdown and infection.

Postoperative care

Pain relief, mobility, chest infection, DVT/PE, wound infection and later incisional hernia.

Patient optimisation

This is an important part of the preparation for any elective operation. Patients should be advised to lose weight in preparation for surgery in order to reduce these risks, although this is easier said than done. Referral to a local Weight Management Service is a good start and an achievable timeline and/or target should be given. For example, it is reasonable to expect someone to be able to lose 5% of their total body weight in 3 months, which for a 150 kg person would be 7.5 kg, or about 1 stone. However, it would be much more difficult for them to lose another stone in another 3 months – that is, the steady weight loss cannot be expected to continue at the same rate. Therefore the urgency of the surgery must be balanced against the feasibility of significant weight loss. In practice this means that the operation is likely to go ahead with the patient still in an obese state, even though they may have achieved the designated weight loss target. Surgeons need to accept this and not delay surgery indefinitely in the vain hope that the patient will, one day, attain a target which is frankly unrealistic.

Consider a very low calorie diet (e.g. 1000 calories per day) for 10–14 days leading up to surgery. Such a regime is widely practised in bariatric surgery and is applicable to other upper abdominal procedures, e.g. cholecystectomy, fundoplication or gastrectomy, laparoscopic or open, *where liver retraction is important.* All obese patients have a very 'fatty' liver, which is usually tense and immobile. In such a state it is difficult to retract and may actually fracture in the attempt. This brief calorie challenge will significantly *reduce liver steatosis* and facilitate its handling during the operation. The diet should be prescribed under the auspices of a dietitian, as a healthy mix of nutrients must be achieved despite the caloric restriction.

Organise appropriate DVT prophylaxis (see also Chapter 2). This involves avoiding unnecessary preoperative immobility and using doses of heparin that are appropriately up-scaled according to body mass. Remember also that compression stockings are designed for normal legs and may not fit the obese patient, perhaps digging in, creating a tourniquet effect and negating any potential benefit.

Intraoperative measures

Care must be taken in positioning the patient on the operating table, not only to provide optimal access for the surgeon but also to prevent movement (e.g. if the table is tilted) and to protect areas from pressure injury. Table side-extensions, extra padding and/or fixation straps may be required (**Fig. 21.13**). For laparoscopic operations a number of special techniques are helpful:

1. Significant table tilt. This requires extra patient safety procedures – see above. Table tilt can create extra working space but be aware that head-up tilt reduces venous return and increases the risk of DVT, while head-down tilt affects diaphragmatic excursion and thus respiratory function.

2. Surgeon stands between the legs (for upper abdominal procedures). With head-up tilt this provides a comfortable and ergonomic position from which to operate. Measures must be taken to prevent the patient sliding down the table, e.g. foot-plates and fixing the knees straight (Fig 21.13).

3. Extra ports to provide extra retraction. These are often more effective than extreme table tilt. Their use may require an extra assistant.

4. Port angulation is critical: passing through the thick abdominal wall, laparoscopic ports are relatively immobile and thus it becomes important to insert ports in the direction of the operative site. If they are angled incorrectly and

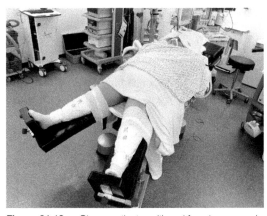

Figure 21.13 • Obese patient positioned for a laparoscopic upper GI operation. The legs-apart position and head-up tilt gives comfortable access for the surgeon standing between the legs. Note the padded foot-plates attached to the table and bandages to keep the knees straight in order to prevent the patient sliding down the table when tilted. Anti-embolism stockings and calf compression are also in use. The arms are securely tucked in by the sides.

cannot 'wiggle' within the abdominal wall, there will be extreme force on the instruments, which is not only uncomfortable for the surgeon but may also lead to instrument malfunction or breakage.

5. Remember that it is where the port emerges on the inside that is important. When correct port angulation is taken into account, the site of skin incision may be some distance from where the surgeon 'usually' places his or her ports. This is especially noticeable in laparoscopic ventral hernia repair, where ports have to be placed more peripherally than usual to maximise working distances inside.

6. Long ports. These are not needed as often as might be expected, especially with correct directional insertion, but sometimes longer ports are needed to traverse a thick abdominal wall, especially with oblique angulation.

For open operations, a longer incision is usually required as well as deeper retractors and/or extra assistance. Closure techniques for open incisions may need to be tailored in obese patients. The lateral tension on the skin owing to the sheer weight of subcutaneous skin flaps indicates the use of slowly absorbable, deep dermal sutures to take the tension off the surface closure, e.g. sutures or skin staples. There is mounting evidence that the use of prophylactic mesh during abdominal wall closure reduces wound dehiscence and later incisional hernia formation in obese patients (see Chapter 7).

Postoperative measures

Good analgesia is critical to allow deep breathing/coughing and early mobilisation and should be planned in discussion with the anaesthetist preoperatively. Preventive chest physiotherapy is worthwhile and DVT prophylaxis should continue at the appropriate dose. Also do not neglect nutrition: obese patients often have a poor dietary range and may be low in the protein, vitamins and minerals that are needed for good postoperative healing. If an obese patient needs to remain fasting for any length of time postoperatively, provision of nutritional support, including enteral or intravenous feeding, should be considered just as for a normal-weight patient.

Key points

- Weight loss operations are becoming more common and complications are increasingly likely to present to the general surgeon on call.
- Knowledge of the operation performed will help the receiving surgeon anticipate any problems that might arise.
- It is wise to contact the original bariatric surgical team as they may provide useful advice but, as for all emergency admissions, the prime clinical responsibility for the patient rests initially with the receiving surgeon.
- Physical examination may be difficult and X-rays may be hard to interpret. Look carefully for clinical and biochemical features of dehydration and sepsis.
- Beware the acute band slippage in a gastric band patient. Percutaneous band decompression may provide short-term relief but definitive operative release/removal/resection may be required.
- Urgent CT to demonstrate a bleed, leak or obstruction in a patient who is unwell following a gastric bypass or duodenal switch procedure can help to make the diagnosis but immediate return to theatre may be a better strategy.
- Incessant vomiting after gastric balloon insertion may respond to inpatient gut rest and anti-emetic medication but instant and permanent relief will be obtained by removal of the balloon.
- Tachycardia should never be disregarded as it may be the only clue to an intra-abdominal catastrophe.
- Consider essential vitamin replacement in all patients admitted with complications from bariatric surgery where there may have been a significant reduction in nutritional intake.
- Because complications may arise some years after bariatric surgery, patients may no longer be overweight and thus the link to the initial procedure may not be obvious.
- Preoperative optimisation is an important area to consider, both in general weight loss but also a 2-week very low calorie diet to reduce liver steatosis.
- Pay close attention to venous thromboembolic prophylaxis.
- Correct and careful positioning on the operating table allows safe movement during surgery, improving access.

🌐 Full references available at **http://expertconsult. inkling.com**

Key references

2. Sjöström L, Narbro K, Sjöström CD, et al. Swedish Obese Subjects Study. Effects of bariatric surgery on mortality in Swedish obese subjects. N Engl J Med 2007;357:741–52. PMID: 17715408

A classic study and the first to show conclusively that bariatric surgery produced lasting health benefits.

7. Tadross JA, le Roux CW. The mechanisms of weight loss after bariatric surgery. Int J Obes (Lond) 2009;33(Suppl. 1):S28–32. PMID: 19363504.

A fascinating account of the effects of bariatric surgery on the incretin-hypothalamic axis and the brain

13. Franco JVA, Ruiz PA, Palermo M, et al. A review of studies comparing three laparoscopic procedures in bariatric surgery: sleeve gastrectomy, Roux-en-Y gastric bypass and adjustable gastric banding. Obes Surg 2011;21:1458–68. PMID: 21455833.

A good review of several series comparing the outcomes of these three popular operations.

24. Abdemur A, Sucandy I, Szomstein S, et al. Understanding the significance, reasons and patterns of abnormal vital signs after gastric bypass for morbid obesity. Obes Surg 2011;21:707–13. PMID: 20582574.

Beware of tachycardia in the early postoperative period.

Index

C